THE BIBLE AND NATURAL PHILOSOPHY IN RENAISSANCE ITALY

The Bible and Natural Philosophy in Renaissance Italy explores the reciprocal relationship between biblical interpretation and natural philosophy in sixteenth-century Italy. The book augments our knowledge of the manifold applications of medical expertise in the Renaissance and of the multiple ways in which the Bible was read by educated people who lacked theological training. Andrew D. Berns demonstrates that many physicians in sixteenth-century Italy, Jewish and Christian alike, took a keen interest in the Bible and postbiblical religious literature. Berns identifies the intellectual tools that Renaissance doctors and natural philosophers brought to bear on their analysis of the Bible and assesses how their education and professional experience helped them acquire, develop, and use those tools. *The Bible and Natural Philosophy in Renaissance Italy* argues that the changing nature of medical culture in the Renaissance inspired physicians to approach the Bible not only as a divine work but also as a historical and scientific text.

Andrew D. Berns is Assistant Professor of History at the University of South Carolina.

The Bible and Natural Philosophy in Renaissance Italy

JEWISH AND CHRISTIAN PHYSICIANS IN SEARCH OF TRUTH

Andrew D. Berns
University of South Carolina

CAMBRIDGE
UNIVERSITY PRESS

CAMBRIDGE
UNIVERSITY PRESS

32 Avenue of the Americas, New York, NY 10013-2473, USA

Cambridge University Press is part of the University of Cambridge.

It furthers the University's mission by disseminating knowledge in the pursuit of education, learning, and research at the highest international levels of excellence.

www.cambridge.org
Information on this title: www.cambridge.org/9781107065543

First published 2015

Printed in Great Britain by Clays Ltd, St Ives plc

A catalog record for this publication is available from the British Library.

Library of Congress Cataloging in Publication data
Berns, Andrew D., 1980–
The Bible and natural philosophy in Renaissance Italy : Jewish and Christian physicians in search of truth / Andrew D. Berns, University of South Carolina.
pages cm
Includes bibliographical references and index.
ISBN 978-1-107-06554-3 (hardback)
1. Bible – Hermeneutics. 2. Bible – Criticism, interpretation, etc. – Italy – History – 16th century. 3. Bible – Criticism, interpretation, etc. – Italy – History – 17th century. 4. Bible and science. 5. Medicine – Italy – History. 6. Physics – Italy – History. I. Title.
BS476.B475 2015
261.5'50945–dc23 2014021774

ISBN 978-1-107-06554-3 Hardback

Contents

Acknowledgments

I would like to thank the following individuals: Nadja Aksamija, Maria Cristina Bacchi, Ann Blair, Robert Bonfil, Francesca Bregoli, Martin Burke, Stephen Burnett, Giancarlo Casale, Roger Chartier, Daniel Cheeley, D'Maris Coffman, Anna Cremaldi, Nicholas de Lange, Theodor Dunkelgrün, Yaacob Dweck, Lynne Farrington, Antonio Feros, Emanuela Ferretti, Paula Findlen, Fabio Finotti, Federica Francesconi, Matthew Gaetano, Anthony Grafton, Allen Grieco, Alessandro Guetta, Josef Gulka, Joseph Hacker, Elliott Horowitz, Moshe Idel, Philippa Jackson, Matt Karp, Arthur Kiron, Judith Leifer, Fabrizio Lelli, Valentina Lepri, Evan MacCarthy, Ian Maclean, Scott Mandelbrote, Bill Marotti, David Myers, Gianfranco Miletto, Mauro Minardi, Benjamin Nathans, Bruce Nielson, Gabriel Piterberg, John Pollack, Maria Portuondo, Eve Troutt Powell, Todd Presner, Renee Raphael, Amnon Raz-Krakotzkin, Laura Refe, Elchanan Reiner, Michael Rocke, David Sacks, Marco Sgarbi, Adam Shear, Pete Stacey, Jonathan Steinberg, Nicholas Terpstra, Piet van Boxel, Giuseppe Veltri, and Beth Wenger.

Thanks are due also to Anna, Giorgio, and Giovanna Bacchelli; Daren Belsby; David Berns; Joan Berns; Sarah Berns; Christopher Boicos; Gregory Borenstein; Deborah Broadnax; Mitchell Charap; Carol Feinberg Cohen; Emanuele Colorni; Antonella Faeda; Jill Feldstein; Flora Filannino; Jeremy Galen; Karen Gilmore; Kieran Hanrahan; Mark Heyman; Jack Higgins; Jim Hinz; Kate Joyce; Nelson Lande; Charles Mayara; Clayton Northouse; Juliana Ochs; Ruth Pearson; Joan Plonski; Andy Rachlin; Jonathan Rosenblatt; Rhonda and Richard Soricelli; Andrew Viterbi; Todd Vladyka; Oriana Walker; Christine Walsh; and Dylan Weller.

I am grateful to these institutions for their support: History Department, University of South Carolina; Villa I Tatti: The Harvard University Center for Italian Renaissance Studies; History Department, Center for Jewish Studies, and Viterbi Family Program in Mediterranean Jewish Studies, UCLA; History Department, Center for Italian Studies, Jewish Studies Program, and Graduate School of Arts and Sciences, University of Pennsylvania; Oxford Centre for Hebrew and Jewish Studies, Oxford; the Philadelphia Area Center for the History of Science; the Foundation for Jewish Culture; Istituto ellenico, Venice; and the Gladys Krieble Delmas Foundation, Venice.

I would like to acknowledge the following libraries and archives: Bibliothèque nationale, Paris; Biblioteca universitaria, Bologna; Biblioteca comunale dell'Archiginnasio, Bologna; Archivio isolani, Bologna; Archivio di Stato, Mantua; Biblioteca Palatina, Parma; Biblioteca Ambrosiana, Milan; Biblioteca nazionale centrale, Florence; Biblioteca marciana, Venice; Archivio di Stato, Venice; Jewish National and University Library, Jerusalem; British Library, London; Cambridge University Library, Cambridge; Peterhouse, Cambridge; Bodleian Library, Oxford; Charles E. Young Library, UCLA; National Library of Medicine, Bethesda, Maryland; Columbia University Library, New York; Jewish Theological Seminar, New York; Fales Library, New York University; Houghton Library, Harvard University; Countway Medical Library, Harvard University; Firestone Library, Princeton University; College of Physicians of Philadelphia; Libraries of the University of Pennsylvania; Chemical Heritage Foundation, Philadelphia.

At Cambridge University Press I would like to thank Brian MacDonald, two anonymous readers, and my editors Beatrice Rehl, Asya Graf, and Isabella Vitti.

My deepest professional debts are to Franco Bacchelli, Sol Cohen, Ann Moyer, David Ruderman, Nancy Siraisi, and Joanna Weinberg. I alone bear responsibility for any errors in this book.

Most of all, Mara Zepeda.

A Note on Translation, Transliteration, and Names

All translations, unless otherwise specified, are my own. Translations of biblical verses are generally those of the Jewish Publication Society. When transcribing Hebrew texts, I have not corrected all grammatical or printing errors. When transliterating Hebrew, I have followed the guidelines laid out in *Encyclopedia Judaica* (Second Edition, 2007). I have preferred vernacular as opposed to Latinate names for the Italian protagonists in this work. Thus David de' Pomi rather than David de Pomis; Ulisse Aldrovandi rather than Ulyssis Aldrovandus; Abraham Portaleone rather than Abraham Portaleonis. One exception: when a Northern European such as Melchior Wieland took on both Italian and Latin names, I have used the Latin appellation Melchior Guilandinus in deference to scholarly precedent.

Abbreviations

BT	Babylonian Talmud
BUB	Biblioteca Universitaria di Bologna
DBI	*Dizionario biografico degli italiani*
EJ	*Encyclopedia Judaica* (Second Edition, 2007)
JQR	*Jewish Quarterly Review*
PL	J. P. Migne, *Patrologiae cursus completus series latina* (Paris: Garnier, 1844–65)
REJ	*Revue des Études Juives*
SG	*Shiltei HaGibborim*

INTRODUCTION

In the dedicatory letter to Pope Leo X that opened his 1521 Polyglot Psalter, Sante Pagnini compared unreliable translations of ancient Greek natural philosophy to unreliable translations of the Bible.[1] Works of natural philosophy, Pagnini stated, were marred by "false interpreters" who were also "blind leaders of the blind" – an expression with clear scriptural allusion.[2] For Pagnini, mistranslations of scientific texts had deleterious effects: they resulted in inaccurate medical prescriptions that poisoned the sick. The damage done from faulty renderings of "sacred literature," however, was worse, since those poor translations lent "evil confirmation to the errors of heretics" and "will be the cause of laughter and contempt."[3]

1 Sante Pagnini, *Psalterium nuper translatum ex hebraeo, chaldaeo, et graeco* (Rome: n.pr., 1521). On this letter, see Anna Morisi Guerra, "Incontri ebraico-cristiani. Il Salterio poliglotto di Santi Pagnini," in her *Itinerari ebraico-cristiani: società, cultura, mito* (Fasano: Schena, 1987), 9–37, esp. 24–27; Morisi Guerra, "Santi Pagnini traducteur de la Bible," in I. Backus and F. Higman, eds., *Théorie et pratique de l'exégèse* (Geneva: Droz, 1990), 191–98, esp. 196; Paul Grendler, "Italian Biblical Humanism and the Papacy," in Erika Rummel, ed., *Biblical Humanism and Scholasticism in the Age of Erasmus* (Leiden: Brill, 2008), 227–76, 242–43. On Pagnini, see T. M. Centi, "L'attività letteraria di Santi Pagnini (1470–1536) nel campo delle scienze bibliche," *Archivum Fratrum Praedicatorum* 15 (1945): 5–51.

2 Pagnini, *Psalterium*, sig. *2r: "utinam vero non etiam falsi interpretes fuerint ac caeci caecorum duces, dum in aequivocis dictionibus alienam a re ipsa significationem accipientes, veram relinquunt et de rebus gravissimis contraria quam oporteat ratione decernunt." Cf. Matthew 15:14.

3 Pagnini, *Psalterium*, sig. *2r–v: "mitto autem quod periculosos humanae vitae errores admiserint, qui nobis graecos medicae facultatis autores male verterunt, dum pro salubri haerba vel pharmaco noxium virus nobis supposuerunt.... Quod autem ad sacrarum literarum pertinet studia, quis non cognoscat tanto periculosius in iis peccatum admitti, quanto sublimiora sunt, quae tractanda suscipiuntur, immortalia scilicet, ac divina? Quae, si quo casu

Pagnini's comparison of scientific and scriptural translation was not merely rhetorical; other scholars of his generation perceived an affiliation between natural philosophy and the study of scripture. Three years before Pagnini published his letter to Leo X, Gianfrancesco Pico della Mirandola wrote to Pagnini in June 1518 to tell him that "aspiring theologians learn natural philosophy." They believe, Pico said, that "many areas of inquiry should be investigated," some of which produce "great anxiety." Nevertheless, according to Pico, these matters "perplexed them not in the least," and they solved them "with relatively little effort."[4] In the century following Pico's observation, a conspicuous number of physicians and naturalists analyzed the Bible from a natural philosophical perspective. They also applied their religious erudition in the service of their scientific pursuits. Many of them lived in central and especially northern Italy. The majority worked in Venice, Bologna, or the Duchy of Mantua. Jews and Christians were equally involved in this endeavor and are equally represented in this book. Whatever their religious faith, they are, for the most part, barely known to modern historians. This project draws from a deep well of writings by Amatus Lusitanus, Melchior Guilandinus, Andrea Bacci, Abraham Yagel, Alessandro Magno, and Giovanni Battista Cavallara. The three primary figures upon whose work it especially relies are only slightly more familiar to modern historians: Ulisse Aldrovandi, David de' Pomi, and Abraham Portaleone. For these sixteenth-century scholars, natural philosophy helped elucidate the Bible. Medical education and natural philosophy provided their recipients and practitioners with the intellectual tools they used to develop a unique approach to the Bible.[5] Scripture, in

male tradita accipiantur, haereticis sinistram erroris occasionem, infidelibus autem risum nostri atque contemptum praebitura sunt."

[4] Santi Pagnini, *Biblia: habes in hoc libro prudens lector utriusque instrumenti novam translationem œditum* (Lyon: Antonius du Ry, 1528), "Ioannis Franciscus Picus Mirandulae Dominus Sancti Pagnino Lucensi Praedicatorii ordinis s.p.d.," sig.*di^v^–dii^r^, sig.*di^v^: "In philosophia vero naturali et in disputatrici, quae nunc plurimum in usu theologia [*sic*: theologiae] candidati praeter illa et condiscent et admonebuntur tractari multas quaestiones apud se (et anxias quidem plurimum), quas eruditissimi viri vix opere longi subsellii dissolvant; quae quidem quam faciles, quam nullo nexu perplexae sint tua ipsa interpretatione manifestum fiet." The letter is dated (Sig. *dii^r^) Calen. Iunii. A partu virginis, MDXVIII, or 1 June 1518. On Gianfrancesco Pico della Mirandola, see Charles B. Schmitt, *Gianfrancesco Pico della Mirandola (1469–1533) and His Critique of Aristotle* (The Hague: Martinus Nijhoff, 1967).

[5] On the close connections between medicine and natural philosophy in Italy at this time, see Giuseppe Olmi, *Inventario del mondo: catalogazione della natura e luoghi del sapere*

turn, helped settle disputes in learned natural philosophy and improve the efficacy of practical medicine.[6]

The Natural Philosophy of the Biblical World explores the reciprocal relationship between biblical interpretation and natural philosophy in sixteenth-century Italy. It investigates people who studied the Bible and pursued natural philosophy with such equal and related ardor that they scarcely perceived a difference between the two. The project describes the fields of study they cultivated, tells the story of how they changed them, and examines the social, educational, and intellectual structures that promoted this extraordinary symbiosis between two ostensibly alien branches of knowledge.

Though the Bible was studied in tandem with natural philosophy in other parts of Europe at this time, Italy presents a unique historical case.[7] In contradistinction to most biblical commentary in early modern Europe, which was colored by confessional polemic, Italian physicians' explorations of the Bible were less dogmatic. Generally, they avoided ideological skirmishes. Natural philosophers, like contemporary theologians, pursued truth.[8] But the truth they sought was of a different kind: they interrogated the precise meaning of natural

nella prima età moderna (Bologna: Il Mulino, 1992), 256, 300; Anthony Grafton and Nancy Siraisi, eds., *Natural Particulars: Nature and the Disciplines in Renaissance Europe* (Cambridge, MA: MIT Press, 1999), 11; Siraisi, "Anatomizing the Past: Physicians and History in Renaissance Culture," *Renaissance Quarterly* 53 (2000): 1–30; Siraisi, "History, Antiquarianism, and Medicine: The Case of Girolamo Mercuriale," *Journal of the History of Ideas* 64 (2003): 231–51; Brian Ogilvie, *The Science of Describing: Natural History in Renaissance Europe* (Chicago: University of Chicago Press, 2006).

6 For mostly Northern European examples of this last point, see Ann Blair, "Mosaic Physics and the Search for a Pious Natural Philosophy in the Late Renaissance," *Isis* 91 (2000): 32–58.

7 For England, see Kevin Killeen, *Biblical Scholarship, Science and Politics in Early Modern England: Thomas Browne and the Thorny Place of Knowledge* (Burlington, VT: Ashgate, 2009); for Spain, see María M. Portuondo, "The Study of Nature, Philosophy, and the Royal Library of San Lorenzo of the Escorial," *Renaissance Quarterly* 63:4 (2010): 1106–50.

8 Claims of arriving at the "truth" or "true meaning" of the biblical texts are commonplace in Italian writings of the sixteenth century. See Abraham Portaleone, *SG*, 86r–v; David de' Pomi, *Tsemaḥ David* (Venice: Giovanni di Gara, 1587), 232; and Andrea Bacci, *L'Alicorno* (Florence: Giorgio Marescotti, 1573) sig. 2Av, all use this language. See also Azariah de' Rossi, *The Light of the Eyes*, trans. and ed. Joanna Weinberg (New Haven: Yale University Press, 2001), 251, 406, and Weinberg, "The Beautiful Soul: Azariah de' Rossi's Search for Truth," in David B. Ruderman and Giuseppe Veltri, eds., *Cultural Intermediaries: Jewish Intellectuals in Early Modern Italy* (Philadelphia: University of Pennsylvania Press, 2004), 109–26.

terminology in the Bible. The quest to find the "true meaning" of biblical language led Italian physicians to compare the Bible's statements about nature to those in pagan texts. They read the Bible in order to solve natural philosophical problems, not theological ones. Historians of early modern history who claim that before the eighteenth century scripture was studied because it revealed "the means to salvation" and that it was only in the Enlightenment that the Bible was to "move beyond theology" miss earlier adumbrations of those eighteenth-century developments.[9] Still, Aldrovandi, Amatus, and their fellow Renaissance naturalists who studied the Bible were more than mere avatars of later periods; they were men of their own time and deserve to be understood as such.

MEDICAL CULTURE IN LATE RENAISSANCE ITALY

Features unique to learned medicine in mid-sixteenth-century Italy facilitated a close scrutiny of passages in the Bible having to do with the natural world. The first was medical education. The education that a young man received at an Italian university in the middle of the sixteenth century retained many traditional features. At the same time it was undergoing significant changes.[10] To begin with, the authority of Galen and Hippocrates was no longer unquestioned.[11] Galenism, which had long dominated the medical curriculum, was becoming increasingly expansive and flexible: by the middle of the sixteenth century doctors added new content to the corpus of Galen's writings.[12] They also

[9] Jonathan Sheehan, *The Enlightenment Bible: Translation, Scholarship, Culture* (Princeton: Princeton University Press, 2005), xiii, 28.

[10] Paul Grendler, *The Universities of the Italian Renaissance* (Baltimore: Johns Hopkins University Press, 2002), 201ff.

[11] I do not mean to conflate these two medical writers or the corpora they left behind. Ian Maclean has introduced a helpful distinction between the two. Whereas students of Hippocratic writings stood for reverence of the past, much as their humanist colleagues did, devotees of Galen believed that knowledge was cumulative. See Ian Maclean, *Logic, Signs, and the Order of Nature in the Renaissance* (Cambridge: Cambridge University Press, 2002), 209. It is perhaps no accident that Abraham Portaleone was critical of the Hippocratic corpus in his medical *consilia*. See herein, Chapter 4.

[12] Between 1490 and 1598, 660 editions of Galen were published. Eighteen of them were *Opera omnia*. See August Buck, "Die Medizin im Verständnis des Renaissancehumanismus," in Rudolf Schmitz and Gundolf Keil, eds., *Humanismus und Medizin* (Weinheim: Acta Humaniora, 1984), 181–98, 187.

criticized him.[13] Medicine's flexible stance toward the authority of tradition, which Ian Maclean has contrasted to the legal profession's tendency to remain faithful to that authority,[14] colored the way Jewish physicians such as David de' Pomi, Abraham Portaleone, and others approached their received Jewish tradition. It similarly altered how Christians such as Ulisse Aldrovandi, Andrea Bacci, and Melchior Guilandinus related to their Christian one.

Another important midcentury shift was that clinical training became more popular and ascended to an unprecedented position in university curricula. At some centers of learning, such as Padua, clinical training – which required bedside visits, pulse measurement, urine sampling, and performance of dissections and autopsies – was so popular that students would matriculate there to receive it after completing the theoretical portion of their studies elsewhere.[15] Anatomy in particular, famously championed by Andreas Vesalius, became after 1525 the defining feature of hands-on, empirical medicine.[16] This emphasis on clinical practice encouraged firsthand observation and attentiveness to natural particulars. When David de' Pomi scrutinized biblical gemstones and Abraham Portaleone studied biblical incense, they applied lessons they had learned as medical students at, respectively, the Universities of Perugia and Pavia to their study of the Bible.[17] One additional aspect of medical education had a strong influence on biblical studies in the late sixteenth century: the emphasis on Greek philology.

In the fifteenth century, scholars learned Greek with private tutors or in small circles.[18] By the beginning of the sixteenth century, Aldus

[13] Nancy Siraisi, "Giovanni Argenterio and Sixteenth-Century Medical Innovation: Between Princely Patronage and Academic Controversy," *Osiris* 6 (1992): 161–80, 178–9. Perhaps the best example of criticism of Galen is Vesalius's *De humani corporis fabrica* (Basel: Johannes Oporinus, 1543). Vesalius criticized some aspects of Galen's work while remaining a committed Galenist.

[14] Maclean, *Logic, Signs, and the Order of Nature*, 231.

[15] Jerome J. Bylebyl, "The School of Padua: Humanistic Medicine in the Sixteenth Century," in Charles Webster, ed., *Health, Medicine and Mortality in the Sixteenth Century* (Cambridge: Cambridge University Press, 1979), 335–70, 351.

[16] Vivian Nutton, "'*Prisci dissectionum professores*': Greek Texts and Renaissance Anatomists," in A. C. Dionisotti, Anthony Graton, and Jill Kraye, eds., *The Uses of Greek and Latin: Historical Essays* (London: Warburg Institute, 1988), 111–26, 115.

[17] For more on Pavia, especially its Greek curriculum, see herein Chapter 3.

[18] N. G. Wilson, *From Byzantium to Italy: Greek Studies in the Italian Renaissance* (Baltimore: Johns Hopkins University Press, 1992), 4.

Manutius had established the Neakademia, a "new academy" devoted to the cultivation of Greek language and literature. Indeed, the members of that group even made a pact not to speak to each other in any language other than classical Greek, and infractions were penalized with a stiff fine. In practice, few members of Aldus's circle truly spoke Greek.[19] The fact that the members of the Neakademia advertised their devotion to that ancient tongue explains their passion more than their skill.[20] Apart from these ephemeral gatherings and ad hoc arrangements dedicated to Greek language and culture, universities played an important role in Greek instruction. In sixteenth-century Europe, medical faculties in Italian universities taught more Greek to a greater number of pupils than any other institution, with the possible exception of the Collège de France.

The sixteenth-century revival of interest in ancient Greek medical texts shaped the study and practice of Renaissance medicine.[21] Even as most medical learning continued to be acquired and disseminated in Latin, sixteenth-century physicians routinely mined ancient Greek texts for nuggets of information about famed cures and rare plants.[22] To the mind of Andrea Mattioli, a famous sixteenth-century naturalist, elite physicians and elite scholars of Greek were indistinguishable from one another.[23] Ulisse Aldrovandi himself invoked an oft-repeated trope when he mused that improved knowledge of Greek was the major reason why medicine had progressed so far in his century.[24]

[19] Ibid., 133.

[20] Martin Lowry, *The World of Aldus Manutius: Business and Scholarship in Renaissance Venice* (Ithaca, NY: Cornell University Press, 1979), 196–99; Martin Davies, *Aldus Manutius: Printer and Publisher of Renaissance Venice* (London: British Library, 1995).

[21] Bylebyl, "The School of Padua," 340. See also Nancy Siraisi, *Avicenna in Renaissance Italy: The Canon and Medical Teaching in Italian Universities after 1500* (Princeton: Princeton University Press, 1987), 65–6, 96–7, and bibliography there.

[22] For a detailed periodization of Greek studies in sixteenth-century medicine, see Vivian Nutton, "Greek Science in the Sixteenth-Century Renaissance," in J. V. Field and Frank A. J. L. James, eds., *Renaissance and Revolution: Humanists, Scholars, Craftsmen, and Natural Philosophers in Early Modern Europe* (Cambridge: Cambridge University Press, 1993), 15–28 and Nutton, "John Caius and the Eton Galen: Medical Philology in the Renaissance," *Medezinhistorisches Journal* 20 (1985): 227–52. On the continued dominance of Latin, particularly until the middle of the sixteenth century, see Nutton, "Hellenism Postponed: Some Aspects of Renaissance Medicine, 1490–1530," *Sudhoffs Archiv* 81:2 (1997): 158–70.

[23] See Pietro Mattioli's letter "agli studiosi lettori," in his *I discorsi di M. Pietro Andrea Matthioli* (Venice: Vincenzo Valgrisi, 1568), sig **5v.

[24] Ulisse Aldrovandi, *Discorso naturale,* BUB Ms. Aldrovandi 91, 530r.

The emphasis on Greek in Renaissance medical education inspired its recipients to deploy their philological skills in different ways. They edited, translated, and commented on classical Greek writers such as Galen, Aristotle, Dioscorides, and Theophrastus. They also sought out Bible translations in Greek that they deemed potentially authoritative, or which, at the very least, could illuminate obscure scriptural passages.[25] Early modern Italian physicians used their knowledge of Greek to investigate alternatives to the Latin text of the Vulgate and the Hebrew text of the Bible.

In sixteenth-century Italian universities conversations about the Bible took place informally. Modern scholars insist that theological studies were marginalized at that time and place.[26] But that argument is based on research that attends to official university records and church pronouncements. The day-to-day realities of life at a university like Bologna or Padua may have been quite different. In midcentury Bologna, for example, Gabriele Paleotti, the future bishop of that city, organized a group of university students united by their interest in spiritual issues.[27] More to the point, at Padua the theology professor Girolamo Vielmi mentioned in his lectures on Genesis a series of "informal conversations" with the botanist Melchior Guilandinus, whom Vielmi credits with helping him understand a difficult verse in that book.[28] Naturalists and theologians helped each other study the Bible. Even if theological study had a limited role in sixteenth-century Italian universities, the scrutiny of sacred texts, most notably the Bible, did not.[29]

The kinds of conversations that Vielmi and Guilandinus were having at Padua intimate a second feature of sixteenth-century medical culture that stimulated a renewed interest in the Bible: the social dynamics of

[25] On interest in Greek Bible texts in the context of diminishing faith in the Vulgate's accuracy, see Hildebrand Höpfl, *Beiträge zur Geschichte der Sixto-Klementinischen Vulgata* (Freiburg im Breisgau: Herder, 1913), 1–43.

[26] Charles B. Schmitt, "Philosophy and Science in Sixteenth-Century Italian Universities," in André Chastel et al., eds., *The Renaissance: Essays in Interpretation* (London: Methuen, 1982), 297–336, 314.

[27] Paolo Prodi, *Il Cardinale Gabriele Paleotti*, 2 vols. (Rome: Edizioni di Storia e Letteratura, 1959–67), 2:217.

[28] Girolamo Vielmi, *De sex diebus conditi orbis liber* (Venice: Giunta, 1575), 335. See herein Chapter 2.

[29] See also Grendler, *The Universities of the Italian Renaissance*, chap. 10.

the medical profession. In the sixteenth century, Italian universities such as Bologna and Padua replaced French and Spanish universities such as Paris, Montpellier, and Salamanca as those that attracted Europe's best and most ambitious students. An international and polyglot group of young men flocked to Italian medical faculties. The University of Padua presented a unique environment in which Jewish students from different ethnic backgrounds forged lifelong friendships.[30] At Padua and other Italian universities, students came into contact with members of different religious communities, too.[31] Relationships manifestly interfaith and not merely intraconfessional flourished. Jews and Catholics alike met students whose unfamiliar perspectives on classical and sacred texts complemented and challenged their own. Dialogues that began at university continued to develop in later years through the international network that Ian Maclean has called the Medical Republic of Letters.[32] Occasionally, conversations between Jews and Christians morphed into epistolary exchanges later in life. For example, Girolamo Mercuriale wrote several letters to Moses Alatino, a Jewish physician from Spoleto, that were published in Mercuriale's printed medical responses and consultations.[33] The letters indicate not only Mercuriale's respect for Alatino's "learning and skill in practicing medicine" but also

[30] David B. Ruderman, *Jewish Thought and Scientific Discovery in Early Modern Europe* (New Haven: Yale University Press, 1995), 100–17; Ruderman, *Early Modern Jewry: A New Cultural History* (Princeton: Princeton University Press, 2010), 127–28.

[31] For examples beyond Padua, see I. Zoller, "I medici ebrei laureati a Siena negli anni 1543–1694," *Rivista Israelitica* 10 (1913): 60–70, 100–10; and A. Franceschini, "Privilegi dottorali concessi ad Ebrei a Ferrara nel secolo XVI," in *Atti e memorie della Deputazione ferrarese di storia patria*, ser. 3, 19 (1975): 173–4. In general, see Vittore Colorni, "Sull'ammissibilità degli ebrei alla laurea anteriormente al secolo XIX," in Colorni, *Judaica minora: saggi sulla storia dell'ebraisimo italiano dall'antichità all'età moderna* (Milan: Giuffrè, 1983), 473–89. Originally published in *Rassegna mensile di Israel* 16 (1950): 202–16.

[32] Ian Maclean, "The Medical Republic of Letters before the Thirty Years War," *Intellectual History Review* 18:1 (2008): 15–30.

[33] *Hieronymi Mercurialis Foroliviensis responsorum, et consultationum medicinalium tomus primus* (Venice: apud Iolitos, 1587), consultatio 16, p. 43: "De uteri tumore, urinae acrimonia, aluique suppressione, Pro nobili iuvene Hebraea, ad Moysem Alatinum Medicum Hebraeum." See also *Hieronymi Mercurialis Foroliviensis responsorum, et consultationum medicinalium tomus tertius* (Venice: apud Franciscum de Franciscis Senensem, 1597), "De vena in pleuritide secanda quaenam ea sit, Moysi Alatino medico," 66v–67v. The responses and consultations are not numbered in this volume. It is not known where Alatino studied medicine. We do know, however, that Alatino visited the University of Padua in 1572, where Mercuriale was teaching at the time. See Cecil Roth, *The Jews in the Renaissance* (Philadelphia: Jewish Publication Society of America, 1977 [1959]), 84.

the affection between the two men.[34] Another of Mercuriale's correspondents was Abraham Portaleone, to whom he wrote, expressing high regard for the Mantuan physician's work and signing off as his "faithful friend."[35] Exchanges between Jews and Christians eventually motivated innovative research in those students' mature writings. Portaleone wrote about the Bible and the Talmud when he corresponded with non-Jewish physicians such as Alessandro Magno and Giovanni Battista Cavallara, whom he may have known from university.

There were several other ways Portaleone may have met and developed relationships with non-Jewish colleagues: colleges of physicians and courts. Those two social, professional, and political settings changed significantly in the sixteenth century, and their occasional admission of Jews tells us much not only about the careers of physicians like David de' Pomi and Abraham Portaleone but also about more general contacts between Jews and Christians in late Renaissance Italy. Mantua is a unique case. While certain academies in that city, such as the Accademia degli Invaghiti, did not admit Jews, the Gonzaga family welcomed them into its court as physicians and entertainers.[36] The city's College of Physicians

[34] Mercuriale, *Responsorum et consultationum medicinalium tomus primus*, 43: "et haec sunt, quae in proposito casu ad te scribenda putavi. Reliquum est, ut me ames ac tuam doctrinam et in medendo peritiam a me plurimum aestimari putes. Bene vale. Patavii." The letter is undated. The phrase "ut me ames" is likely an allusion to Cicero, *Epistulae ad Familiares* 13:47: "tu fac, quod facis, ut me ames, teque amari a me scias."

[35] *Hieronymi Mercurialis Foroliviensis responsorum, et consultationum medicinalium tomus primus* (Venice: apud Iolitos, 1587), Consultatio 8, p. 25, "De mensibus inordinatis atque imminutis ac de sterilitate ad Abrahamum e Portalionis Medicum Hebraeum." "De vivendi ratione, quam in cunctis medicamentis scis esse necessariam, nihil dico, quod mihi persuadeam te nihil quod ad ipsam pertineat esse ullo tempore omissurum. Bene vale, tibique de Mercuriali ea omnia pollicearis, quae a fideli amico expectari possunt" (p. 26). Nancy Siraisi notes this letter in her *Communities of Learned Experience: Epistolary Medicine in the Renaissance* (Baltimore: Johns Hopkins University Press, 2013), 25.

[36] The dramatist Leone de' Sommi was refused membership in the Accademia degli Invaghiti; he was appointed secretary instead. See David Kaufmann, "Leone de' Sommi Portaleone (1527–92): Dramatist and Founder of a Synagogue at Mantua," *JQR* 1 (1898): 445–61. On the Gonzaga family and the Jews, see Shlomo Simonsohn, *History of the Jews in the Duchy of Mantua* (Jerusalem: Kiryath Sepher, 1977); Simonsohn, "The Theater Troupe of the Mantuan Jews" (Hebrew), *Paragod* (1963): 13–17; Don Harrán, "Jewish Dramatists and Musicians in the Renaissance: Separate Activities, Common Aspirations," in Siegried Gmeinwieser et al., eds., *Musicologia Humana: Studies in Honor of Warren and Ursula Kirkendale* (Florence: L. S. Olschki, 1994), 291–304; Daniel Jütte, "Abramo Colorni, jüdischer Hofalchemist Herzog Friedrichs I., und die hebräische Handelskompanie des Maggino Gabrielli in Würtemberg am Ende des 16. Jahrhunderts," *Aschkenaz. Zeitschrift für Geschichte und Kultur der Juden* 15 (2005): 435–98.

had Jewish members.[37] Mantua's court and College of Physicians enabled interconfessional relationships between Catholics and Jews.

The third feature of late Renaissance medical culture that influenced the study of sacred literature was a set of paraprofessional interests that many physicians shared. Of these, two deserve further consideration: collecting and the embrace of alternative sources of knowledge, chiefly empirical. Many early developers of cabinets of curiosity and, later, museums were either pharmacists or physicians.[38] From Francesco Calzolari to Ferrante Imperato, sixteenth-century medical professionals wanted more than to know nature; they wanted to acquire it.[39] The desire to acquire nature led many Renaissance physicians to seek out samples of it. In Mantua, for example, the court physician Marcello Donati owned and operated a museum of curiosities.[40] Some of the

[37] Archivio di stato di Mantova, *Libro dei Decreti* Nr. 46, pp. 24–37. These documents are published in G. Carra and A. Zanca, "Gli statuti del collegio dei medici di Mantova del 1559," in *Atti e memorie dell'accademia virgiliana di Mantova, Classe di scienze fisiche e techniche* 2 (1977). On Jews, see ¶ 21, "De Judeo Phisico," pp. 29–30 and ¶ 28, "De Chirurgo Judeo," 34–35. Italian translations of the Latin text are available in Carra and Zanca, "Gli statuti," 70–1 and 77–8. See also Gianfranco Miletto, *Glauben und Wissen im Zeitalter der Reformation: Der salomonische Tempel bei Abraham Ben David Portaleone (1542–1612)* (Berlin: de Gruyter, 2004), 2–3. Carra and Zanca also published Mantua's "Catalogo o ruolo o matricola del Collegio dei medici (1539–1783)," Part V of which is titled "Magistri Medici Hebrei Admissi per Collegium ad Medendum in Dominio." See Carra and Zanca, "Gli statuti," 114–15. From the list's beginning in 1539 until the sack of Mantua in 1630, six Jewish physicians appear. See also Gianfranco Miletto, "Die Zulassung der jüdischen Ärzte in Italien während der Gegenreform: der Fall Portaleone," *Biblische Notizen* 116 (2003): 48–55. On court physicians more generally, see the contributions of Richard Palmer and Hugh Trevor Roper to Vivian Nutton, ed., *Medicine at the Courts of Europe, 1500–1837* (London: Routledge, 1990).

[38] Paula Findlen, "The Formation of a Scientific Community: Natural History in Sixteenth-Century Italy," in Anthony Grafton and Nancy Siraisi, eds., *Natural Particulars: Nature and the Disciplines in Renaissance Europe* (Cambridge, MA: MIT Press, 1999), 369–400; Findlen, "The Museum: Its Classical Etymology and Renaissance Genealogy," *Journal of the History of Collections* 1 (1989): 59–78; Findlen, *Possessing Nature: Museums, Collecting, and Scientific Culture in Early Modern Italy* (Berkeley: University of California Press, 1994).

[39] Findlen, *Possessing Nature*, 43.

[40] Franco Dotti and Attilio Zanca, "Fatti e figure della medicina mantovana durante il tardo rinascimento," in *Mantova e i Gonzaga nella Civiltà del Rinascimento. Atti del convegno dall'Accademia Nazionale dei Lincei e dall'Accademia Virgiliana con la collaborazione della città di Mantova sotto l'alto patronato del Presidente della Repubblica Italiana Giovanni Leone, Mantova 6–8 ottobre 1974* (Mantua: Accademia Virgiliana, 1977), 393–97, 393. Dotti and Zanca list other museums in Mantua at p. 395. Donati was the author of *De medica historia mirabili libri sex* (Mantua: per Franciscum Osanam, 1586). On Donati, see Attilio Zanca, *Notizie sulla vita e sulle opere di Marcello Donati da Mantova (1538–1602) medico, umanista, uomo di stato* (Pisa: Giardini, 1964).

specimens physicians collected were understood as the equivalents – and not merely the derivatives – of biblical products.[41] The institution that encouraged this pursuit of new plant samples and facilitated the effort to handle biblical *naturalia* was the botanical garden. Botanical gardens proliferated in the 1520s and 1530s, and Padua's enjoyed a particularly prestigious continental reputation.[42] Many of the new drugs that were imported to Venice and its nearby university in the 1530s, 1540s, and 1550s were exotic, and of those exotic drugs a high number came from the Near East.[43] Melchior Guilandinus, for one, believed that he had in his garden the mysterious *kikayon* (gourd) mentioned in the book of Jonah. Similarly, Aldrovandi enthused about Luca Ghini's sending him, from Padua, a branch from the specific kind of cedar tree mentioned in the book of Jeremiah.[44]

In sixteenth-century Italy, especially in the medical community, there was a widespread tendency to study nature with recourse to alternative sources of knowledge. The most prominent of these were vernacular writings (in Italian) and artisanal experience. Recent scholarship on a variety of early modern settings has explained how physicians learned from those bereft of Latinate educations, artisans, and those involved in the mechanical arts.[45] Scholars have not neglected this aspect of Renaissance Italy, either.[46] But we know much less about people who not only let manual trades and vernacular literature inform their medical practice and natural philosophy but also let it transform their study of the Bible. In different ways de' Pomi's and Portaleone's lives and works

41 See herein, Chapters 1, 2, and 5.

42 Findlen, "The Formation of a Scientific Community," 370.

43 Loris Premuda, "La medicina e l'organizzazione sanitaria," in Girolamo Arnaldi and Manlio Pastore Stocchi, eds., *Storia della cultura veneta: Il Seicento,* vol. 4, pt. 2 (Vicenza: N. Pozza, 1984), 115–50, 139.

44 See herein Chapter 2.

45 See, respectively, William Eamon, *Science and the Secrets of Nature: Books of Secrets in Medieval and Early Modern Culture* (Princeton: Princeton University Press, 1994), and Deborah Harkness, *Jewel House: Elizabethan London and the Scientific Revolution* (New Haven: Yale University Press, 2007); Pamela H. Smith, *The Business of Alchemy: Science and Culture in the Holy Roman Empire* (Princeton: Princeton University Press, 1994); Tara Nummedal, *Alchemy and Authority in the Holy Roman Empire* (Chicago: University of Chicago Press, 2007).

46 Matteo Duni, *Tra religione e magia: storia del prete modenese Guglielmo Campana (1460?–1541)* (Florence: L. S. Olschki, 1999); David Gentilcore, *Healers and Healing in Early Modern Italy* (Manchester: Manchester University Press, 1998), 1–28, 156–76.

exemplify this trend, and examining their use of these types of sources expands our understanding of Jewish intellectual life as well as learned medicine in early modern Europe.

The fourth feature of sixteenth-century medicine that drew its practitioners closer to studying the Bible is epidemiological. New diseases and unprecedented problems emerged that required physicians to reach beyond the standard practices they deployed. In an environment of "medical pluralism," some patients – wealthy and poor alike – eschewed the services of university-trained physicians entirely and visited mountebanks, women healers, or other alternative practitioners.[47] But doctors with university degrees still attracted plenty of patients. In fact, there were many more university-educated physicians in Italy than elsewhere in Europe at the time. New World drugs, unknown to ancient writers and medieval pharmacists, could be put to use in fighting new diseases, such as *morbus gallicus* or syphilis. Plagues posed an even bigger challenge than sexually transmitted diseases. Katherine Park has argued that the devastation wrought by plagues in the later Middle Ages provoked a crisis of confidence in traditional medieval medicine.[48] If plagues in thirteenth- and fourteenth-century Florence released a tremor that shook the foundations of scholastic medicine, the plagues of the later sixteenth century, especially that which struck Venice in 1571–2, generated a shock wave that produced equal if not greater damage to the profession of learned medicine.[49] Jewish physicians had a ready-made response to the anxiety and illness produced by plagues: they encouraged the intensified recitation of certain portions of Jewish liturgy, namely those that list the ingredients of ancient incense, or *pitom qetoret*. Recitation of those passages was thought to have salubrious effects, and Jewish doctors such as Abraham Yagel and Abraham Catalano advocated and testified to the diffusion of that practice.[50] Some Jewish physicians did more than

[47] See Gentilcore, *Healers and Healing*; Matteo Duni, *Under the Devil's Spell: Witches, Sorcerers, and the Inquisition in Renaissance Italy* (Syracuse: Syracuse University Press, 2007), 71.

[48] Katherine Park, *Doctors and Medicine in Early Medieval Florence* (Princeton: Princeton University Press, 1995) and herein, Chapter 3.

[49] Paolo Preto, *Peste e società a Venezia nel 1576* (Vicenza: N. Pozza, 1978).

[50] See Abraham Yagel, *Moshia Ḥosim* (Venice: Zuan di Gara, 1587), 17r–18r, for biblical incense curing the plague, and 21v for biblical showbread as a prophylactic against various maladies. Abraham Catalano, who died in 1642, wrote about the plague of 1630–1 in his *Olam Hafukh*, which was published by Cecil Roth in *Kovez̧ al Yad* 4 (1946): 67–101, 74.

read religious literature in times of contagion; a few put it directly to use. David de' Pomi, for example, responded to the challenging circumstances of those years by using biblical cures – in his case the *tarshish* stone mentioned in Exodus 28 – to treat his patients. De' Pomi touted his own unusual methods in a bold letter to Pope Sixtus V, and he was even recognized for his efforts in a 1589 dispatch from the papal nuncio in Venice to the pope in Rome.[51]

Finally, Renaissance doctors were greatly interested in biblical and postbiblical sacred texts. Many Jewish physicians in the fifteenth and sixteenth centuries were rabbis or teachers in Jewish communities, and nearly all had advanced training in Talmudic dialectics and other forms of religious study. That the scrutiny of nature brought one closer to God was a trope in Hebrew writings of the period, many of which approvingly quoted the psalmist's pronouncement that "the heavens declare the glory of God."[52] Christian physicians were no less pious. In 1548 Mattioli wrote of the "spiritual pleasure" he derived from looking at plants.[53] In the same period his Northern European colleague Leonhart Fuchs insisted that by studying "the various forms and natures of plants, the divine presence and benignity is illuminated."[54] But medical men were interested in more conventional spiritual pursuits, too: they studied biblical literature. For example, Françoise Lehoux has shown how, in the libraries of sixteenth- and seventeenth-century Parisian doctors, after medical books the second most common classification was "les sciences religieuses." A few, such as René Chartier and Ponce Privat, who are hardly known to history as religious thinkers, let alone Hebraists, owned and read Hebrew Bibles.[55]

[51] See herein Chapter 3.

[52] Psalm 19:1. See, for example, Judah Sommo, *Ẓaḥut Bediḥuta de-Kiddushin*, ed. J. Schirmann (Jerusalem: Sifre Tarshish, 1965 [orig. written ca. 1550]), 36; Gedaliah ibn Yaḥya, *Shalshelet ha-Kabbalah* (Warsaw, 1877 [1st ed., Venice: Zuan di Gara, 1586]), 146; Leon Modena, *Ari Nohem* (Leipzig: K. Tauchnitz, 1840 [orig. written 1639]), 18–19.

[53] Richard Palmer, "Medical Botany in Northern Italy in the Renaissance," *Journal of the Royal Society of Medicine* 78 (February 1985): 149–57, 150.

[54] Leonhart Fuchs, *De historia stirpium commentarii insignes* (Basel: in officina Isingriniana, 1542), sig. *2v. Quoted in Brian W. Ogilvie, "Natural History, Ethics, and Physico-Theology," in Nancy Siraisi and Gianna Pomata, eds., *Historia: Empiricism and Erudition in Early Modern Europe* (Cambridge, MA: MIT Press, 2005), 75–104, 90.

[55] Françoise Lehoux, *Le cadre de vie des médecines parisienes aux XVIe et XVIIe siècles* (Paris: Éditions A. & J. Picard, 1976), 485–6.

THE BIBLE AND MEDICINE IN LATE RENAISSANCE ITALY

The Bible was central to both Jewish and Christian education in the sixteenth century. In Italian Jewish culture of the Renaissance, the Bible was particularly esteemed. The education that Jewish students received placed a heavy emphasis on biblical literacy.[56] Numerous sources bear witness to the fact that children as young as three or four years of age were able to read and chant portions of scripture.[57] Even if these sources exaggerate the accomplishments of precocious children, they are valuable to the historian as they indicate a cultural aspiration as much as a reality. In late fifteenth-century texts, such as Yoḥannan Alemanno's study program, the Bible is prominently featured.[58] The same is true of sixteenth-century educational documents, such as the Provenzali family's proposal for a Jewish academy.[59] Seventeenth-century sources are even

[56] Shlomo Simonsohn, "Jewish Education in the Renaissance (until the 17th century)" (Hebrew), in *Entsiklopedyah Ḥinukhit*, 4 vols. (Jerusalem: Mosad Bialik, 1959–74), 4:376–81.

[57] A note in a prayer book of the Italian rite, written in 1514 by Daniel ben Shmuel of Rosina, who in that year resided in Ferrara, observed that "at four and a half years of age [a child] recited the *haftorah* in synagogue." Jewish National and University Library, Ms. Roth 3. The note is reproduced in Simḥa Asaf, *Meḳorot le-toldot ha-ḥinukh be-Yiśra'el* (New York: Bet ha-midrash le-rabanim ba-Amerikah, 2001–9 [Tel Aviv: Devir, 1925–29]), 1:255. See also David Reuveni's comment that the physician Moses Abudrahin of Rome had "a young daughter who read the twenty four [books of the Bible.]" ויש לו בת בחורה הקוראה בעשרים וארבע in E. Z. Eshkoli, ed., *Sipur David ha-Re'uveni* (Jerusalem: Bialik, 1993), 39. Finally, see also Leon Modena's comment in his *Istoria de' riti ebraici* (Paris, 1637), Hebrew translation Solomon Ruben (Vienna, 1867), 104: כאשר יבין הנער לדבר אביו מחנכו לקרוא בתורה, ואח"כ הוא מלמדו לתרגם את המקרא ללשון הארץ אשר הוא מתגורר בה "When the boy is able to speak, his father instructs him how to read the Torah, and afterward he teaches him to translate scripture into the language of the land where he lives."

[58] On Alemanno, see Fabrizio Lelli, "L'educazione ebraica nella seconda metà del '400: poetica e scienze naturali nel *Ḥay ha-'Olamim* di Yoḥanan Alemanno," *Rinascimento*, n.s., 36 (1996): 75–136, and Moshe Idel, "The Study Program of R. Yoḥanan Alemanno" (Hebrew), *Tarbiẓ* 48 (1979–80): 303–31.

[59] On Provenzali, see Gianfranco Miletto, "The Teaching Program of David ben Abraham and His Son Abraham Provenzali in Its Historical-Cultural Context," in David Ruderman and Giuseppe Veltri, eds., *Cultural Intermediaries: Jewish Intellectuals in Early Modern Italy* (Philadelphia: University of Pennsylvania Press, 2004), 127–48. To these examples one could add a seventeenth-century curricular text: the Cretan Jewish polymath Joseph Delmedigo's *Mikhtav aḥuz*. However, that document's history and interpretation have been subjects of deep scholarly debate. See Ruderman, *Jewish Thought and Scientific Discovery in Early Modern Europe* (New Haven: Yale University Press, 1995), 146–52. More recently, see Jordan S. Penkower, "S. D. Luzzatto, Vowels, and Accents and the Date of the *Zohar*," in Robert Bonfil, Isaac Gotlieb, and Hannah Kasher, eds., *Samuel David Luzzatto* (Jerusalem: Magnes Press, 2004), 79–130: 128. See also Arthur Lesley, "Il richiamo agli 'antichi' nella

more abundant and detailed: curricula from Jewish primary schools, such as one from midcentury Verona, indicate the dominant role the Bible played in early education.[60]

In late medieval and early modern Jewish culture, one area of knowledge whose acquisition was especially prized, and whose deployment in the service of biblical study was highly praised, was natural philosophy. There were strong practical reasons for this endorsement of scientific literacy. For example, community rabbis were poorly paid: in sixteenth-century Venice, they earned as much in a year as a master builder earned in a month.[61] Practicing medicine was a licit and respected way for rabbis to earn a living wage in Renaissance Italy, and many did so.[62]

But there were strong cultural forces that legitimized and encouraged the study of natural philosophy. In the high and late Middle Ages, Jewish thinkers as diverse as Baḥya ibn Paqudah, Maimonides, Judah Ha-Levi, and Gersonides all proclaimed that studying natural sciences promoted piety.[63] Their works were frequently printed and often read in the sixteenth century.[64] In Renaissance Mantua, for example, Judah Messer

cultura ebraica fra quattro e cinquecento," in Corrado Vivanti, ed., *Storia d'Italia Annali 11/1, Gli ebrei in Italia* (Turin: Einaudi, 1996), 387–409, esp. 394–400.

60 One document dating from 1688, and published by Isaiah Sonne, makes it plain that children between five and seven years of age studied scripture and its cantillation marks in the morning, early afternoon, and early evening. Asaf, *Meḳorot le-toldot ha-ḥinukh be-Yiśra'el*, 1:284–5; for Sonne's introduction to this document, see 1:280–3.

61 Robert Bonfil, *Rabbis and Jewish Communities in Renaissance Italy*, trans. Jonathan Chipman (New York: Littman Library, 1990), 157–68, esp. 160.

62 Ibid., 189–90 and notes there.

63 For Baḥya, see *Ḥovot ha-levavot*, trans. Moses Hymanson, 2 vols. (Jerusalem: Kiryat ne'emanah, 1962), 1:133; G. Vajda, *La theologie ascétique de Bahya ibn Pakuda* (Paris: Imprimerie Nationale, 1947). For Maimonides, see *Mishneh Torah, Hilkhot Yesodei ha-Torah* 2:2. For Ha-Levi, see *Sefer ha-Kuzari* 1:68. On Gersonides, see Charles Touati, *La pensée philosophique et théologique de Gersonide* (Paris: Éditions de minuit, 1973), 33; Gad Freudenthal, ed., *Studies on Gersonides: A Fourteenth-Century Jewish Philosopher-Scientist*, Collection de travaux de l'Académie Internationale d'Histoire des Science 36 (Leiden: Brill, 1992); Freudenthal, "Spiritual Success and Astronomy: Gersonides' War against Ptolemy" (Hebrew), *Da'at* 22 (1989): 55–72; Freudenthal, "Cosmogonie et physique chez Gersonide," *REJ* 145 (1986): 295–314; G. Dahan, ed., *Gersonide en son temps. Science et philosophie médiévales* (Louvain: E. Peeters, 1991). Much of this literature is discussed in Ruderman, *Jewish Thought and Scientific Discovery*, 21–44.

64 For Gersonides in sixteenth-century Jewish libraries, see Shifra Baruchson, *Sefarim ve-ḳor'im: tarbut ha-ḳeri'ah shel Yehude Italyah be-shilhe ha-Renesans* (Ramat-Gan: Bar Ilan University Press, 1993), 125–7, 149, 151, 166–7; J.-P. Rothschild, "Les listes de livres, reflet de la culture des juifs en Italie du nord au XVe et au XVIe siècle?," in G. Tamani and

Leon operated a school for young men whose purpose was to prepare them to study medicine at university.[65] Judah's son David queried one of his generation's leading scholars, Jacob ben David Provenzali, about the permissibility of studying natural sciences in the eyes of Jewish law.[66] Provenzali's response was unambiguous: while works that denied *creatio ex nihilo* were to be avoided, given that they challenged pious conceptions of God's role as creator, medicine was not only unthreatening but even appealing. He lauded "the *artes naturales*, and above all medicine, for there is no science in the world today that sustains its masters with honor as this one does .... accordingly I praise it [medicine] and say that it is good to hold fast to it as many of our rabbis, may peace be upon them, held fast to it."[67] Judah Messer Leon's *Sefer Nofet Ẓufim* (Book of the Honeycomb's Flow) explained how knowledge of secular subjects could enrich one's understanding of Scripture. "After we have come to know all the sciences," Messer Leon explained, "or some part of them, we study the words of the Torah, then the eyes of our understanding open to the fact that the sciences are included in the Torah's words, and we wonder how we could have failed to realize this from the Torah itself to begin with."[68] Those were words that David de' Pomi or

A. Vivian, eds., *Manoscritti, frammenti e libri ebraici nell'Italia dei secoli XV–XVI* (Rome: Carucci, 1991), 163–93, esp. 175–6, 180–1; Bonfil, *Rabbis and Jewish Communities*, 272–80; Bonfil, "Le biblioteche degli ebrei d'Italia nel Rinascimento," in Tamani and Vivian, *Manoscritti, frammenti e libri ebraici*, 137–50.

[65] Messer Leon's school was open from 1473 to 1475. On 21 February 1469, Messer Leon was granted the right to confer degrees on other Jews by Emperor Frederick III. See Isaac Rabinowitz, ed. and trans., *The Book of the Honeycomb's Flow* (Ithaca, NY: Cornell University Press, 1983), xxiv–xxvi. For similar examples from Padua in the sixteenth century, see Ruderman, *Jewish Thought and Scientific Discovery*, 100–15. For Jewish students elsewhere in Europe, see Yosef Kaplan, "Sephardi Students at the University of Leiden," in Kaplan, *An Alternative Path to Modernity* (Leiden: Brill, 2000), 196–210; Israel Bartal, "Jews in Eastern European Higher Education" (Hebrew), in Michael Heyd and Shaul Katz, eds., *Toledot ha-Universita ha-Ivrit bi-Yerushalayim* (Jerusalem: Magnes Press, 1997), 75–89.

[66] See Miletto, "The Teaching Program," 134.

[67] See E. Askenazi, *Divrei ḥakhamim* (Metz: J. Mayer Samuel, 1849), 63–75, 71: והמלאכות הטבעיות וכש"כ הרפואה שהרי אין חכמה היום בעולם שתחיה את בעליה בכבוד כזו. . . ועל זה שבחתי אותה ואמרתי שטוב להחזיק בה כמו שהחזיקו בה הרבה מרבותינו ע"ה The locution "hold fast to it" is an allusion to Proverbs 3:18, where the referent is God's law.

[68] *Sefer Nofet Ẓufim*, book 1, chap. 13, Rabinowitz ed., 145, Hebrew at 144: כי אחרי ידענו כל החכמות או חלק מהם, א"כ נתבונן בדברי התורה, אז תפקחנה עיני שכלנו שהם נכללות בדברי התורה, ונתמה איך לא הבננו זה ממנה מתחלת הענין I have used Rabinowitz's translation. On Messer Leon, see Robert Bonfil, "The Book of the Honeycomb's Flow by Judah Messer Leon: The Rhetorical Dimension

Abraham Portaleone could have uttered with conviction. The belief that expertise in areas of study such as rhetoric, poetics, and natural philosophy was compatible with, and even complementary to, study of the Bible was a tenet of Jewish culture in early modern Italy. Leone Modena freely admitted to drawing from "the best Latin Bibles" in compiling *Galut Yehudah*, his dictionary of difficult biblical words.[69] A quarter century earlier, as Joanna Weinberg has observed, Azariah de' Rossi elucidated rabbinic texts "by means of non-Jewish sources divested of all ideological or religious bias."[70] This interdisciplinary approach to biblical study was one that Christian intellectuals such as Ulisse Aldrovandi, Melchior Guilandinus, and Andrea Bacci advocated and practiced as well.

David de' Pomi and Abraham Portaleone could turn to Jewish writings from the late fifteenth and early sixteenth centuries for expressions of the compatibility of general culture and biblical literacy. Their Christian contemporaries could, too. The clearest example is Erasmus. Though condemned as a heretic in 1559, Erasmus had considerable influence in post-Tridentine Italy.[71] Aldrovandi, for example, was even accused of, and punished for, participating in circles where "Lutheran" texts were read and discussed.[72] Erasmus's *Ratio seu methodus compendio perveniendi ad veram theologiam* urged interpreters of the Bible to study the geography and natural history of the ancient Near East.[73] Knowledge

of Jewish Humanism in Fifteenth-Century Italy," *Jewish History* 6:1–2 (1992): 21–33, 26; Daniel Carpi, "Rabbi Judah Messer Leon and His Activity as a Doctor" (Hebrew), *Michael* 1 (1973): 277–301; reprinted in *Qorot* 6 (1974): 395–415, and also in Carpi, *Be-tarbut ha-Renesans u-ven ḥomot ha-geṭo* (Tel Aviv: University Publishing Project, 1989), 57–84, and in abbreviated form in "Notes on the Life of Rabbi Judah Messer Leon," in Elio Toaff, ed., *Studi sull'ebraismo italiano in memoria di Cecil Roth* (Rome: Barulli, 1974), 37–62.

69 Leone Modena, *Galut Yehudah* (Venice: Giacomo Sarzina, 1612), "L'autore alli benigni lettori," Sig *Av, where he notes that he used "i migliori dittionarii ... il mikhlol, e il חשק שלמה, spagnolo ottimo, e le miglior Bibie latini." Modena's book was dedicated to a Christian physician, "il signor Gioanni Vislingio Cavalliero, lettor primario d'Anatomia, e de Simplici nello Studio di Padoa." Unnumbered folio following title page.

70 Weinberg, *The Light of the Eyes*, xxxi.

71 Gigliola Fragnito, "The Central and Peripheral Organization of Censorship," in Fragnito, ed., *Church, Censorship, and Culture in Early Modern Italy* (Cambridge: Cambridge University Press, 2001), 13–49, 30. For the circulation of Erasmus's works in sixteenth-century Italy, see ibid., n. 57.

72 See herein Chapter 2.

73 Kristine Louise Haugen, "A French Jesuit's Lectures on Vergil, 1582–1583: Jacques Sirmond between Literature, History and Myth," *Sixteenth Century Journal* 30:4 (1999): 967–85, 979.

of natural philosophy was especially praised: "He seems truly learned," Erasmus observed, "and [his learning] is increased if he adds the following things: names of precious stones, kinds of trees, and species of animals."[74] To attain such knowledge, Erasmus did not hesitate to use pagan works of natural philosophy, such as Pliny and Dioscorides in his explication of scripture.[75]

In the Renaissance, studying the Bible was an inclusive undertaking that welcomed many diverse disciplinary perspectives.[76] Throughout the early modern period, from Desiderius Erasmus in the early sixteenth century to Joseph Scaliger in the early seventeenth and beyond, virtually all serious students of the Bible drew on classical texts to supplement their understanding of it, often without questioning the implications of using pagan literature to elucidate sacred literature. Joseph Scaliger exhorted aspiring biblical exegetes to "read good authors, Ovid's *Metamorphoses*, and the Talmud: they are necessary for [an understanding of] the Bible."[77] If Ovid's *Metamorphoses* was relevant to the Bible, Dioscorides' and Theophrastus' works certainly were, since they described plants, minerals, and animals that early modern scholars understood to be the equivalents of those mentioned in scripture.

From the mid-sixteenth century on, a conspicuous number of studies were devoted to identifying and describing the natural particulars in the Bible. Medieval precedents are not entirely lacking. A few Christian commentators such as Nicholas of Lyra (1270–1340) had made an effort to identify and describe the plants, animals, and minerals of scripture.[78] But in the sixteenth century the number of scholars interested in biblical natural

[74] *Erasmi Roterdami Methodus*, originally published with his *Novum Instrumentum*. See *Desiderius Erasmus Roterdamus Ausgewählte Werke*, ed. Hajo Holborn and Annemarie Holborn (Munich: Beck, 1933), 154: "abunde doctum videtur, si tantum adiecerint: est nomen gemmae, aut species est arboris aut genus animantis."

[75] Jacques Chomarat, *Grammaire et rhétorique chez Erasme*, 2 vols. (Paris: Belles Lettres, 1981), 1:553.

[76] Deborah Shuger, *The Renaissance Bible: Scholarship, Sacrifice and Subjectivity* (Berkeley: University of California Press, 1994), 4.

[77] *Scaligerana, ou Bons mots, rencontres agreables, et remarques judicieuses & sçavantes de J. Scaliger* (Amsterdam: n.p., 1695), 453. For discussion, see H. J. de Jonge, "The Study of the New Testament in the Dutch Universities, 1575–1700," in Th. H. Lunsing Scheurleer and G. H. M. Posthumus Meyjes, eds., *Leiden University in the Seventeenth Century*, trans. J. C. Grayson (Leiden: Brill, 1975), 65–110, 84.

[78] For recent scholarship on Nicholas of Lyra, see the essays collected in Phillip D. W. Krey and Lesley Smith, eds., *Nicholas of Lyra: The Senses of Scripture* (Leiden: Brill, 2000). On Lyra

philosophy swelled, and the scope of their investigations expanded. One impetus for the proliferation of these studies was the revival of certain patristic writings. The work of Augustine in particular endorsed the pursuit of natural philosophical knowledge. In the second book of his *De doctrina christiana*, Augustine emphasized that Christians have a duty to study scripture's natural world.[79] Augustine was widely read and enjoyed an enhanced reputation in the fifteenth and sixteenth centuries, as more attention was paid to some of his theological positions.[80] As such, a number of church authorities and devout humanists took his prescriptions for study seriously. For example, Gabriele Paleotti explicitly cited Augustine when he challenged Ulisse Aldrovandi to examine the natural world of the Bible. Aldrovandi willingly took up the charge and mentioned Augustine's support for natural philosophy in several of his writings.[81] And Paleotti was by no means the only theologian to enlist the support of a natural philosopher. Girolamo Vielmi, as we have seen, referred to his helpful conversations with Guilandinus about plants in Genesis. The close attention Vielmi paid to natural topics in his *De sex diebus conditi orbis liber* (Book on the six days of the creation of the world) may well have been motivated by his reading of Augustine.

and Jewish texts, see Deeana Copeland Klepper, *The Insight of Unbelievers: Nicholas of Lyra and Christian Reading of Jewish Text in the Later Middle Ages* (Philadelphia: University of Pennsylvania Press, 2007). On the availability of de Lyra in print, see E. A. Gosselin, "A Listing of the Printed Editions of Nicholas de Lyra," *Traditio* 26 (1970): 399–426. For Nicholas of Lyra's antiquarian and scientific interests, see B. Roussel "Connaissance et interprétation du Judaïsme antique: des biblistes chrétiens de la seconde moitié du XVIe siècle," in Chantal Grell and François Laplanche, eds., *La République des lettres et l'histoire du judaïsme antique XVIe–XVIIIe siècles* (Paris: Presses de l'Université Paris-Sorbonne, 1992), 21–50, 28.

[79] *PL* 34:46–9. See herein Chapters 1 and 2. Augustine also raises similar issues in his *De Genesi ad litteram, PL* 34:219–486. For an English edition, see John Hammond Taylor, *St. Augustine: The Literal Meaning of Genesis*, 2 vols. (New York: Newman Press, 1982).

[80] Charles Trinkaus, *In Our Image and Likeness: Humanity and Divinity in Italian Renaissance Thought*, 2 vols. (Chicago: University of Chicago Press, 1970), 1:18, 2:529; Heiko Augustinus Oberman, *The Harvest of Medieval Theology: Gabriel Biel and Late Medieval Nominalism* (Cambridge, MA: Harvard University Press, 1963), 370; Heiko Augustinus Oberman, ed., *Via Augustini: Augustine in the Later Middle Ages, Renaissance and Reformation. Essays in Honor of Damasus Trapp*, O.S.A. (Leiden: Brill, 1991); Charles Stinger, "Italian Renaissance Learning and the Church Fathers," in Irena Backus, ed., *The Reception of the Church Fathers in the West: From the Carolingians to the Maurists*, 2 vols. (Leiden: Brill, 2001), 2:473–510.

[81] BUB Ms. Aldrovandi 54, *Theatrum biblicum naturale* (2 vols.), 1:5v–6r; BUB Ms. Aldrovandi 91, *Discorso naturale*, 542r; and in a letter of 12 November 1567 to the *protettore* of the Collegio di Spagna, BUB Ms. Aldrovandi 66, 355–67, 362v.

A patristic revival was one reason a diverse group of Italian scholars carefully examined the Bible in the sixteenth century. Another was the influence of interconfessional Christian debates. Historians have analyzed the ways that followers of Luther and Calvin studied the Bible with renewed enthusiasm in the second third of the sixteenth century. Luther's rejection of church authority and proposal of a *sola scriptura* approach to matters of faith understandably drove many of his followers to the Bible. But in the Catholic world there was a contemporary and no less powerful incentive to biblical analysis: the Council of Trent.

The Council of Trent (1545–63) instituted a number of changes, including the refinement of church policies regarding a wide variety of interpretative, juridical, and political matters.[82] But one legacy of the council that was equally important has received considerably less attention. More than a century ago, Charles DeJob argued that, as a direct result of the council, many Italians strengthened their commitment to the study of sacred texts.[83] Scholars such as Pietro Galesini, Latino Latini, and Fulvio Orsini, none of whom was a professional theologian, made conscious decisions to shift the focus of their research from profane to sacred studies.[84] The genre of Bible commentaries expanded after Trent. The antiquarian Orsini, in a letter to Cardinal Guglielmo Sirleto, wrote about his newfound pleasure in reading commentaries on Joshua, Judges, and Ruth.[85] In a more familiar instance, the Spanish theologian Benito Arias Montano mused in 1593 that Christian scholars had long been immersed in the study of classical antiquity; it was now time to study sacred antiquities.[86] But it was not only theologians and antiquaries who shifted their attention from pagan to sacred literature; medical men began to search scripture more diligently, too.

82 Eric Cochrane, *Italy, 1525–1630* (London: Longman, 1988), 106–64.

83 Charles DeJob, *De l'influence du Concile de Trente sur la littérature et les beaux-arts chez les peuples catholiques: essai d'introduction à l'histoire littéraire du siècle de Louis XIV* (Paris: Ernest Thorin, 1884), ii.

84 Ibid., 8.

85 Quoted in ibid., 25–26. For more on Orsini, see William Stenhouse, *Reading Inscriptions and Writing Ancient History: Historical Scholarship in the Late Renaissance* (London: Institute of Classical Studies, 2005).

86 Benito Arias Montano, *Antiquitatum iudaicarum libri IX* (Leiden: Plantin, 1593), sig *A2.

Certain features of sixteenth-century medicine, when applied to the study of sacred texts, altered the way religious works had previously been read. In addition to the several features of late Renaissance medical culture already enumerated, three other epistemological and cognitive assumptions enjoyed wide circulation in that culture and had a strong influence on biblical studies. First, many sixteenth-century physicians believed that truth, to use their expression, was *filia temporis*, the "daughter of time."[87] As such, they embraced two related ideas: that as traditions age they can absorb new findings and jettison old ones, and that alien disciplines should be mastered in order to obtain more perfect knowledge.[88] Second, for physicians experience was more important than authority.[89] Girolamo Cardano, Jean Riolan the Elder, and others all maintained that the practice of medicine made doctors rely on their senses more than on received tradition. Jean Riolan the Elder went so far as to claim that "it is stupid to refute the senses and experience with reason out of reverence for antiquity."[90] Third, at the beginning of the seventeenth century the *converso* physician Rodericus a Castro, reflecting on his profession, pointed out a crucial difference between law and medicine: lawyers, like theologians and classicists, prioritized words; doctors, on the whole, prioritized things.[91] These three features of

[87] See Fritz Saxl, "Veritas Filia Temporis," in R. Klibansky and H. J. Paton, eds., *Philosophy and History: Essays Presented to Ernst Cassirer* (Oxford: Clarendon Press, 1936), 197–222.

[88] See Maclean, *Logic, Signs, and the Order of Nature*, 23, and the literature cited at n. 47. Most studies focus on French-, English-, and German-speaking contexts. A notable exception is Nancy Siraisi's article "Cardano and the History of Medicine," in Marialuisa Baldi and Guido Canziani, eds., *Girolamo Cardano. Le opere, le fonti, la vita* (Milan: F. Angeli, 1999), 342–62, 346.

[89] On early modern medical authors' efforts to balance experience, innovation, and authority, see Richard Toellner, "Zum Begriff der Autorität in der Medizin der Renaissance," in Rudolf Schmitz and Gundolf Keil, eds., *Humanismus und Medizin* (Weinheim: Acta Humaniora, 1984), 159–79.

[90] See Maclean, *Logic, Signs, and the Order of Nature*, 196 and the literature cited at nn. 203 and 204. Cardano wrote "cum igitur medicus sit sciens, et non purus artifex, et habeat operari circa subiectum suum, et subiectum non constet unquam sub uno affectu propter materiam: cogitur medicus solus inter omnes scientes diiudicare ex sensus, non ex rei veritate." Cardano, *Opera Omnia* (1663), 6, 415, quoted by Siraisi, *The Clock and the Mirror: Girolamo Cardano and Renaissance Medicine* (Princeton: Princeton University Press, 1997), 51. For the Riolan quotation, "stultum est ratione pugnare contra sensum et experientiam pro antiquitatis reverentia," see Maclean, *Logic, Signs, and the Order of Nature*, 196.

[91] See Rodericus a Castro, *Medicus-politicus: sive de officiis medico-politicis tractatus* (Hamburg: Froben, 1614), 44–53. See also Maclean, *Logic, Signs, and the Order of Nature*, 231 n. 113. On a Castro, see Ruderman, *Jewish Thought and Scientific Discovery*, 295–6.

medicine encouraged physicians to adopt a critical stance toward received traditions and to relate to textual artifacts much as they did to physical ones. This creative interpretation of ancient texts and tireless pursuit of the physical realia listed within them enabled Aldrovandi to search for *manna* in the Dolomite foothills and Portaleone to reconstruct biblical incense in the *piazze* of Mantua. As such, this book presents a history of material culture as well as of textual analysis. These professional habits and cognitive skills led to and justified a desire not only to control the language of scripture but to handle the physical objects that language described.

BIBLICAL COMMENTARY IN JEWISH AND CATHOLIC LEARNED COMMUNITIES

In scholarship on Jewish culture in early modern Europe, biblical commentary has not received sufficient attention.[92] Given the centrality of the Bible to premodern Jewish life, one might naturally ask why not. One reason that explains this relative dearth of scholarship is that biblical commentary, or *parshanut*, attracts close attention only when early modern Jewish authors wrote in a recognizable genre. Isaac Abravanel, Ovadiah Sforno, and Moses Alshekh – to choose three well-known authors – all either composed line-by-line glosses or expatiated in late medieval forms on key questions.[93] However, explorations of the Bible

[92] An exception is Kalman P. Bland, "Issues in Sixteenth-Century Jewish Exegesis," in David Steinmetz, ed., *The Bible in the Sixteenth Century* (Durham, NC: Duke University Press, 1990), 50–67.

[93] On Abravanel, see Benzion Netanyahu, *Don Isaac Abravanel, Statesman and Philosopher* (Philadelphia: Jewish Publication Society of America, 1953). Also, see Eric Lawee, *Isaac Abravanel's Stance Towards Tradition: Defense, Dissent and Dialogue* (Albany, NY: SUNY Press, 2001); Cedric Cohen Skalli, "The Humanist Rhetoric of Don Isaac Abravanel: Rhetoric, History and Tradition in his Introductions and Letters" (PhD thesis, Tel Aviv University, 2005) (Hebrew); and the essays collected by Menahem Kellner and Abraham Melamed in *Jewish History* 23:3 (2009). On Sforno, the work of Ephraim Finkel, *R. Obadja Sforno als Exeget* (Breslau: Druck von T. Schatzky, 1896) is still reliable. See also the editors' introduction to *Kitvei Rabbi 'Ovadyah Sforno*, 2 vols. (Jerusalem: Mosad Ha-Rav Kuk, 1983). See also Robert Bonfil, "Il Rinascimento: la produzione esegetica di 'O. Servadio Sforno," in Sergio S. Sierra, ed., *La lettura ebraica delle Scritture* (Bologna: EDB, 1995), 261–77; Saverio Campanini, "Un intellettuale ebreo del Rinascimento: 'Ovadyah Sforno a Bologna e i suoi rapporti con i cristiani," in Maria Giuseppina Muzzarelli, ed., *Verso l'epilogo di una convivenza: gli ebrei a Bologna nel XVI secolo* (Florence: Giuntina, 1996), 99–128. On Alshekh,

may be found in other genres as well, such as dictionaries, encyclopedias, personal letters, and medical treatises. In order to understand Jewish Bible exegesis more fully, scholars must widen their lens and look at many different sorts of texts. Much biblical commentary is to be found in works not explicitly advertised as such. Neither David de' Pomi nor Abraham Portaleone wrote in a genre that was immediately – or even eventually – recognized as a channel for biblical analysis.

While these genres have not received much attention, others, especially sixteenth-century printings of the Bible and anthologies of medieval commentaries on it, have. Of these, the most important is the Rabbinic Bible published at Venice by Daniel Bomberg in 1517, and again in expanded format in 1524–5.[94] The Rabbinic Bible was innovative in two ways: it featured a new, complete set of notes on the Masorah, or authoritative text of the Hebrew Bible, and it contained important medieval Hebrew commentaries, chiefly those of Rashi and Abraham Ibn Ezra. Although the publication of a newly edited Masoretic text by Jacob ben Ḥayim ibn Adonijah was a watershed moment in the printing of Hebrew Bibles, and the inclusion of several commentaries changed the way scripture was studied by both Jews and Christians,[95] the Rabbinic Bible was a harvest of medieval learning. While its format was innovative, its content

see Albert van der Heide, "Created at Dusk: Abraham's Ram in Medieval Jewish Bible Exegesis," in Ulf Haxen, Hanne Trautner-Kromann, and Karen Lisa Goldschmidt Salamon, eds., *Jewish Studies in a New Europe: Proceedings of the Fifth Congress of Jewish Studies in Copenhagen, 1994* (Copenhagen: C.A. Reitzel A/S International Publishers, 1998), 365–71; Simon Shalem, *Rabbi Moses Alshekh* (Hebrew) (Jerusalem: Ben Zvi Institute, 1966); Bland, "Issues in Sixteenth-Century Jewish Exegesis," 62 and literature there.

94 Jordan Penkower, "Jacob ben Hayyim and the Rise of the Biblia Rabbinica" (PhD diss., Hebrew University, 1982); Penkower, "The Chapter Divisions of the 1525 Rabbinic Bible," *Vetus Testamentum* 48:3 (1998): 350–74.

95 Elchanan Reiner, "The Ashkenazi Élite at the Beginning of the Modern Era: Manuscript versus Printed Book," in Gershon Hundert, ed., *Polin*, vol. 10: *Jews in Early Modern Poland* (Oxford: Basil Blackwell Institute for Polish-Jewish Studies, 1997), 85–98; Reiner, "The Attitude of Ashkenazi Society to the New Science in the Sixteenth Century," *Science in Context* 10 (1997): 589–603; Reiner, "Transformations in the Polish and Ashkenazic Yeshivot during the Sixteenth and Seventeenth Centuries and the Dispute over Pilpul" (Hebrew), in Israel Bartal, Chava Turnianksy, and Ezra Mendelsohn, eds., *Ke-Minhag Ashkenaz ve-Polin: Sefer Yovel le-Khone Shmeruk* (Jerusalem: Zalman Shazar, 1989), 9–80, 45–6. Stephen Burnett, "The Strange Career of the Biblia Rabbinica among Christian Hebraists, 1517–1620," in Matthew McLean and Bruce Gordon, eds., *Shaping the Bible in the Reformation: Books, Scholars and Readers in the Sixteenth Century* (Leiden: Brill, 2012), 63–84. I would like to thank Stephen Burnett for sharing a draft of his chapter with me before publication.

was not.[96] The medieval commentaries included represent a sampling, and not a summary, of medieval biblical interpretation. Works by Menaḥem Recanati and Moses Naḥmanides, to select two conspicuous examples, were widely read but not to be found between the Rabbinic Bible's covers.[97] Of the Rabbinic Bible's two features, the newly edited Masoretic text was perceived at the time as much more important than the medieval commentaries. Jacob ben Ḥayim ibn Adonijah's own introduction to the 1525 edition of the Rabbinic Bible, for example, says almost nothing about the novelty of the exegesis included therein. At the same time, it expatiates about the quest for, and use of, the far-flung Masoretic manuscripts from which ibn Adonijah carried out his exhaustive research.[98] The impact of the Rabbinic Bible in Eastern Europe was profound, and many rabbis reacted unfavorably to it, as they perceived in its Sephardic content a challenge to Ashkenazi hegemony on biblical interpretation.[99] We know less about how Italian scholars and educators reacted to this text. To intellectual omnivores like David de' Pomi and Abraham Portaleone, the gleanings of the medieval commentaries they read in the Rabbinic Bible could not satiate their hunger to demonstrate that broad culture, derived from diverse disciplines, could explicate scripture.

By and large, sixteenth-century Italian Jews declined to comment on the Bible in traditional forums. One reason for this may have been the effects of what Ann Blair has described as information overload.[100]

[96] David Stern, "The Rabbinic Bible in Its Sixteenth-Century Context," in Joseph R. Hacker and Adam Shear, eds., *The Hebrew Book in Early Modern Italy* (Philadelphia: University of Pennsylvania Press, 2011), 76–108. I would like to thank David Stern for sharing an earlier draft of his essay with me.

[97] On Recanati, see Moshe Idel, *Rabbi Menaḥem Recanati ha-Mekubal* (Jerusalem: Shocken, 1998). A second volume of Idel's work was to have included three chapters (22–24) on Recanati's commentary on the Pentateuch; to date it has not appeared. See 1:77–78, however, for brief remarks on Recanati as a Bible commentator. On Naḥmanides, see Isidore Twersky, *Rabbi Moses Naḥmanides: Explorations in His Religious and Literary Virtuosity* (Cambridge, MA: Harvard University Press, 1983).

[98] For the Hebrew text with an English translation, see Christian D. Ginsburg, ed. and trans., *Jacob ben Chajim ibn Adonijah's Introduction to the Rabbinic Bible, Hebrew and English … and the Massoreth ha-Massoreth of Elias Levita, being an exposition of the Massoretic notes on the Hebrew Bible or the ancient critical apparatus of the Old Testament* (London: Longmans, Green, Reader & Dyer, 1867).

[99] See Reiner's studies listed earlier in note 95.

[100] Ann Blair, "Reading Strategies for Coping with Information Overload, ca. 1550–1700," *Journal of the History of Ideas* 64:1 (2003): 11–29; Blair, *Too Much to Know: Managing Scholarly Information before the Modern Age* (New Haven: Yale University Press, 2010).

A flood of late antique and medieval commentaries on the Bible was printed in the second third of the sixteenth century. For example, from 1543 to 1547, thirteen different homiletical and exegetical works rolled off the press – in Venice alone.[101] Late antique and medieval commentaries were not the only Hebrew works on the Bible to be printed in the sixteenth century; contemporary scholars in the Ottoman Empire such as Isaac Caro and Moses ben Baruch Almosnino published printed works on the Bible as well.[102]

In this book I try to avoid the allures of historical hindsight. I refrain from judging the achievements of Italian Jewish scholars of the Bible according to the standards of later periods. As Donald Kelley observed about sixteenth-century French historians, their work should be assessed in terms not only of their results or the extent of their direct influence but also of the questions they thought of asking and of the means they devised to answer them.[103] This project argues that the questions David de' Pomi and Abraham Portaleone thought of asking and the means they devised to answer them originated in the culture of sixteenth-century learned medicine.

Recently, scholarship on Jews in early modern Europe has moved away from trying to ascertain how Jews contributed to surrounding culture, since such a question presupposes that Jews were outside of, and apart from, those cultures. Current work instead shows how Jews were integrated members of premodern societies and has suggested that social and legal interactions between Jews and Christians should be understood as "a two-way street."[104] Intellectual interactions might

[101] See Julius Fürst, *Bibliotheca Judaica: Bibliographisches Handbuch der gesammten jüdischen Literatur mit Einschluss der Schriften über Juden und Judenthum und einer Geschichte der jüdischen Bibliographie*, 3 vols. (Leipzig: W. Engelmann, 1849–63), 3:452.

[102] Isaac Caro, *Toledot Yitzhak* (Constantinople, 1518; Mantua, 1552; Riva di Trento, 1558; Salonika, 1571). Moses ben Baruch Almosnino, *Yedei Moshe* (1582), a commentary on the Five Scrolls; Almosnino, *Tefilah le-Moshe* (Constantinople, 1563), on the Pentateuch and prayer book. On Almosnino, see N. Ben-Menahem, "Towards a Bibliography of R. Moses Almosnino" (Hebrew), *Sefunot* 11 (1978): 135–85.

[103] Donald R. Kelley, *Foundations of Modern Historical Scholarship: Language, Law and History in the French Renaissance* (New York: Columbia University Press, 1970), 308.

[104] David Biale, ed., *Cultures of the Jews: A New History* (New York: Schocken Books, 2002), part 2; Kenneth Stow, *Theater of Acculturation: The Roman Ghetto in the Sixteenth Century* (Seattle: University of Washington Press, 2001), 69. See also David N. Myers's introduction to Stow et al., *Acculturation and Its Discontents: The Italian Jewish Experience between Exclusion and Integration* (Toronto: University of Toronto Press, 2008), esp. 5.

be profitably understood in this way as well. When Portaleone treated the Gonzaga family and when de' Pomi administered cures to afflicted Venetians during the plague of 1571–2, they may have been perceived as Jews but they acted, respectively, as Mantuan and Venetian subjects. As Jews themselves were part of the fabric of early modern Italian society, their scholarly achievements deserve to be included in narratives of Renaissance intellectual history.

The investigation of how Jewish thought contributed to the Jews' host societies, common in previous generations, has a strong parallel in canonical studies of Renaissance biblical scholarship. Arnold Williams, for example, strived to delineate how Renaissance commentators contributed to the knowledge of their day. His answer was not at all. Instead, he wrote, they "only mirror the dominant concepts of the culture of which they were a part."[105] I submit that Williams's question is the wrong one to ask. If we were to judge the works of early modern Jewish physicians by this standard, they would surely come up short. At the end of the seventeenth century, Tobias Cohen, who held a medical degree from Padua, denounced Copernicus's heliocentric theories and assured his readers that the sixteenth-century Polish astronomer was "in the cauldron of Satan."[106] Rather than probe the historical record for signs of progress, this project analyzes how sixteenth-century students of the Bible used the culture of their own day to elucidate a sacred text. Doing so leads us to reach richer conclusions from our investigations – conclusions not about how Renaissance Jews contributed to the general knowledge of their day but about how they created it, just like their Christian contemporaries.

In Renaissance history and the history of medicine, a similar set of issues persists. Modern scholars of Renaissance medicine have charted the evolution of the medical profession in the sixteenth century and noted the expanding interests of Renaissance physicians.[107] At the same time

[105] Arnold Williams, *The Common Expositor: An Account of the Commentaries on Genesis, 1527–1633* (Chapel Hill: University of North Carolina Press, 1948), 198.

[106] Tobias Cohen, *Ma'aseh Tuviyyah* (Venice: Bragadin, 1705), 52r: כי בכור שטן הוא

[107] See Giuseppe Olmi, *Inventario del mondo: catalogazione della natura e luoghi del sapere nella prima età moderna* (Bologna: Il Mulino, 1992); Paula Findlen, *Possessing Nature: Museums, Collecting, and Scientific Culture in Early Modern Italy* (Berkeley: University of California Press, 1994); and most recently the studies collected in Nancy Siraisi and Gianna

they have largely neglected their acute interest in the Bible, perceiving neither the tendency of doctors to study and write about the Bible nor the strong connections between natural philosophy and biblical analysis. One problem is linguistic: during the Renaissance many Italian scholars with medical degrees worked with a bewildering array of Near Eastern tongues. Ulisse Aldrovandi, whose work is the subject of Chapters 1 and 2, interlards quotations in Hebrew, Aramaic, and Syriac throughout his work. But the general neglect of this topic is more complicated and ideological. After all, linguistic deficiencies may be overcome; deeply rooted ideological biases are harder to loosen.

One of these biases, inculcated by generations of Anglophone scholarship sympathetic to Protestant societies, is an overemphasis on Northern Europe at the expense of Southern Europe. Students of biblical studies in early modern Europe miss key sources because of their preference for Northern European texts. They assume that the main instigation of renewed study of Greek and Hebrew was the Protestant Reformation and associated confessional strife, and that northern writers such as Erasmus, Reuchlin, and Melanchthon led the way.[108] In short, according to this line of thinking, Catholics did not take the Bible seriously and their church was too repressive and regressive to allow them to.[109]

But Europeans south of the Alps also took the Bible seriously. From the fifteenth to the seventeenth century, people who trained, worked, or spent significant time in Italy contributed greatly to the advancement of this field. As Charles Trinkaus observed, Italians of the Renaissance studied the Bible with more ardor than is generally assumed. Trinkaus also

Pomata, eds., *Historia: Empiricism and Erudition in Early Modern Europe* (Cambridge, MA: MIT Press, 2005).

[108] See, for example, Peter Harrison, *The Bible, Protestantism, and the Rise of Natural Science* (Cambridge: Cambridge University Press, 1998); D. C. Allen, *The Legend of Noah: Renaissance Rationalism in Art, Science, and Letters* (Urbana: University of Illinois Press, 1949), 43. For exceptions to this trend, see Michael O'Connor, "A Neglected Facet of Cardinal Cajetan: Biblical Reform in High Renaissance Rome," in Richard Griffiths, ed., *The Bible in the Renaissance: Essays on Biblical Commentary and Translation in the Fifteenth and Sixteenth Centuries* (London: Ashgate, 2001), 71–94; Guy Bedouelle, "Le débat catholique sur la traduction de la Bible en langue vulgaire," in *Théorie et pratique de l'exégèse: actes du troisième Colloque international sur l'histoire de l'exégèse biblique au XVIe siècle (Genève, 31 août–2 septembre 1988)* (Geneva: Droz, 1990), 39–59.

[109] Gigliola Fragnito, *La Bibbia al rogo: la censura ecclesiastica e i volgarizzamenti della Scrittura (1471–1605)* (Bologna: Il Mulino, 1997); Fragnito, *Proibito capire: La Chiesa e il volgare nella prima età moderna* (Bologna: Il Mulino, 2005).

demonstrated how biblical studies were an outgrowth of Renaissance humanism rather than an import from Protestant Northern Europe.[110] Besides the scholars discussed in this book, Gianozzo Manetti, Sante Pagnini, Augustinus Steuchus, Antonio Brucioli, Benito Arias Montano, Angelo Canini, Marco Marini, and Athanasius Kircher – the list could go on – all scrutinized the Old Testament and aided their contemporaries' understanding of it. Some work has begun to examine these figures, but much more remains to be done.[111] The study of Hebrew was a key component of their intellectual lives. Sixteenth-century Italian biblical humanists, as Paul Grendler has shown, integrated Hebrew learning into "mainstream Catholic biblical scholarship."[112] One direction for future research might be to improve our understanding of the motivations for intensified study of Hebrew and Greek in Renaissance Italy. Both, after all, were taught in Rome at La Sapienza from 1480 on, well before Erasmus could have learned either at the Collegium Trilingue in Leuven.

[110] Trinkaus, *In Our Image and Likeness*, 1:559.

[111] On Kircher, see Paula Findlen, ed., *The Last Man Who Knew Everything* (New York: Routledge, 2004); Daniel Stolzenberg, ed., *The Great Art of Knowing: The Baroque Encyclopedia of Athanasius Kircher* (Stanford: Stanford University Libraries, 2001); Stolzenberg, "Egyptian Oedipus: Antiquarianism, Oriental Studies and Occult Philosophy in the Work of Athanasius Kircher" (PhD diss., Stanford University, 2003); on Canini, see Joanna Weinberg, "A Sixteenth-Century Hebraic Approach to the New Testament," in C. R. Ligot and J.-L. Quantin, eds., *History of Scholarship* (Oxford: Oxford University Press, 2006), 231–49; on Arias Montano, see María Asunción Sánchez Manzano, *Prefacios de Benito Arias Montano a la Biblia Regia de Felipe II,* Colección Humanistas Españoles 32 (León: Universidad de León, 2006); Stefania Tuzi, *Le colonne e il Tempio di Salomone: la storia, la leggenda, la fortuna* (Rome: Gangemi, 2002), 128–30; on Marini, see Giovanni Luigi Mingarelli's "Marci Marini Vita," in *Marci Marini Brixiani Canonici Regularis Congregationis Rhenanae Sanctissimi Salvatoris Annotationes Literales In Psalmos* (Bologna: apud Thomam Colli ex Typographia Sancti Thomae Aquinatis, 1748), x–xxii, which has not yet been surpassed. See also Vincenzo Peroni, *Biblioteca bresciana* (Bologna, 1818–23), 2:222–3; Gustave Sacerdote, "Deux index expurgatoires de livres hebreux," *REJ* 30 (1896): 262–71, 264; Fausto Parente, "La Chiesa e il Talmud," in Corrado Vivanti, ed., *Storia d'Italia, Annali II: Gli ebrei in Italia* (Turin: Einaudi, 1996): 521–643, 605; on Manetti, see Trinkaus, *In Our Image and Likeness*, 1:230–70; on Steuchus, see Ronald Keith Delph, "Italian Humanism in the Early Reformation: Agostino Steuco (1497–1548)" (PhD diss., University of Michigan, 1987), and Charles B. Schmitt, "Perennial Philosophy: From Agostino Steuco to Leibniz," *Journal of the History of Ideas* 27:4 (October–December 1966): 505–32; on Brucioli, see Giorgio Spini, *Tra rinascimento e riforma: Antonio Brucioli* (Florence: La Nuova Italia, 1940); on Pagnini, see T. M. Centi, "L'attività letteraria di Santi Pagnini."

[112] Paul Grendler, "Italian Biblical Humanism and the Papacy," in Erika Rummel, ed., *Biblical Humanism and Scholasticism in the Age of Erasmus* (Leiden: Brill, 2008): 227–76, 276.

Similarly, Hebrew studies flourished in Spain, at places like Salamanca and Alcalá, before they took root in the Netherlands or in the Holy Roman Empire. Even more intriguing is the notion, expressed by a variety of Italian thinkers, that Hebrew had merit as a language of science and culture, not merely as a language of scripture.[113]

Another blind spot in this field is the presumed hegemony of religious authorities. A generation ago Williams insisted that only theologians and "church dignitaries" commented on scripture; his assumption was subsequently reified and has yet to be dethroned.[114] This book takes a close look at five figures – both Jewish and Christian – who, though neither rabbis, nor theologians, nor priests, undertook serious projects to study the Bible. Those projects have been ignored, in part because the Bible was not a sanctioned field of investigation for university-trained physicians. But that does not mean that only theologians studied or wrote about it. To a surprising degree, medical men did too. Physicians are rarely, if ever, seen as important scholars of the Bible. Recent trends in Renaissance scholarship, of which Deborah Shuger's work is exemplary, argue that the beginnings of biblical scholarship in the Renaissance may be traced to French legal culture.[115] According to this argument the efforts of jurists like Jacques Cujas to contextualize the late antique law code of the emperor Justinian developed tools that were used to dissect the biblical corpus. To understand the nature of biblical studies in early modern Europe, a history that acknowledges the lasting contributions of physicians as well as lawyers is needed. Physicians were interested in

[113] See Ulisse Aldrovandi, "Quanto essattamente la lingua hebrea esprime la natura delle cose," in BUB Ms. Aldrovandi 83 *Bibliologia*, 444–5. Marco Marini makes a similar point in his "prefatio ad φιλεβράιον lectorem," in *Arca Noë thesaurus linguae sanctae novus* (Venice: Giovanni di Gara, 1593), sig. *3r; De' Pomi expressed a similar attitude in his *Tsemaḥ David*, preface "alli signori lettori," unnumbered pages. For a discussion of the latter two sources, see herein Chapter 3. Fifteenth-century Italians advanced similar arguments, though with less emphasis on natural philosophy. For example, Poggio Bracciolini, in a letter to Niccolò Niccoli from the baths in Baden in May 1416, wrote that Hebrew has utility for *studia humanitatis*: "confert tamen aliquid ad studia humanitatis." See Helene Harth, ed., *Lettere: Poggio Bracciolini*, vol. 1: *Lettere a Niccolò Niccoli* (Florence: L. S. Olschki, 1984–7), 45. See also Eugenio Garin, "L'umanesimo italiano e la cultura ebraica," in Vivanti, *Gli ebrei in Italia*, 361–83. For a similar argument about Hebrew scholarship in the Netherlands, see Theodor Dunkelgrün, "The Hebrew Library of a Renaissance Humanist: Andreas Masius and the Bibliography to his *Iosuae Imperatoris Historia* (1574), with a Latin Edition and an Annotated English Translation," *Studia Rosenthaliana* 42–3 (2010–11): 197–252.

[114] See Williams, *Common Expositor*, 10.

[115] Shuger, *Renaissance Bible*, 52.

a wide range of natural objects not only in their role as *materia medica* but also as collectibles. That passion for collecting drew their attention to descriptions of the natural world in the Bible as in other ancient texts. Although I would like this book to compensate for deficiencies in Jewish and Renaissance history, my primary objective is different. The book attempts to bridge two well-cultivated fields and create dialogue where monologue currently prevails. I would be gratified if Renaissance historians who study natural philosophy and medicine attended more closely to the writings of sixteenth-century Jewish physicians. Conversely, scholarship on the Jews in Renaissance Europe has much to gain from a more rigorous engagement with European culture. This preference for interdisciplinary work is not newfangled; it underlies some classic books of Jewish historiography. Umberto Cassuto, in his magisterial volume on Jews in Renaissance Florence, urged historians of the Jews to "always have regard for events that unfold and phenomena that manifest themselves in contemporary Italian society."[116] I have tried to do just that.

CHAPTER SUMMARY

This is a work of synthetic and interpretive history. Although I focus on the writings of a select group of individuals, some of whom have received limited scholarly attention, I have not written a series of intellectual biographies. Rather, this book aspires to write the biography of an idea – or, more precisely, several ideas. Even though medicine and natural philosophy are essential to my interpretation, they are not, strictly speaking, the only areas of learning studied here. The protagonists of my story cultivated broad interests and lived in a climate where ideas flowed easily between the realms of philology, history, biblical studies, and natural philosophy. In fact, Aldrovandi, de' Pomi, and Portaleone spent their careers in the space that connects those different fields. In a sense, this book does too.

The following chapters are structured around the topics that sixteenth-century Italian natural philosophers wrote about: botany, mineralogy,

[116] Umberto Cassuto, *Gli ebrei a Firenze nell'eta del rinascimento* (Florence: L. S. Olschki, 1965 [1918]), vi.

zoology, and alimentation. However, those topical groupings are merely taxonomic points of entry into conceptual themes that emerge from close readings of Aldrovandi's, Guilandinus's, de' Pomi's, and Portaleone's natural philosophic writings. Those themes include the compatibility of scientific and religious research; the application of the former to the latter, and vice versa; the deprecation of ancient and medieval authorities in favor of more recent writings and more diverse sources of knowledge; and the relevance of biblical medicine in modern times.

Chapters 1 and 2 are case studies in the history of Renaissance textual scholarship. They mine the writings of physicians who occasionally sallied out into the hills and botanical gardens but who spent the lion's share of their time reading books and writing them. Chapter 1 presents commentaries on Dioscorides' *De materia medica*, which attempt to clarify biblical language in contemporary scientific terminology and to evaluate the *hebraica veritas* of scripture. The *converso* physician Amatus Lusitanus and, later, Andrea Bacci and Ulisse Aldrovandi were key contributors to this project. While Chapter 1 tells the story of bringing the Bible to life by using science, Chapter 2 is about reviving science by using the Bible. The chapter shows how Aldrovandi and Melchior Guilandinus, the prefect of Padua's revered botanical garden, used the Bible to adjudicate disputes about the historical veracity and scientific accuracy of Pliny the Elder's *Natural History*. It explores how the two natural philosophers read the Bible as both a historical source and a religious one. In doing so, they elided some of the differences between sacred and profane literature and created an example of scholarship that would irritate church authorities and inspire later biblical critics.

The remaining three chapters shift course. They tell the story of doctors venturing out of their studies and into the world. Chapter 3 introduces a new figure: the Jewish physician David de' Pomi. It presents evidence of early modern physicians entering the marketplace rather than the library in order to understand scripture. And it tells the tale of a doctor who not only used his scientific expertise to explicate the Bible but drew on the Bible and its medical traditions to solve contemporary epidemiological problems. In de' Pomi's lexicographical work *Tsemaḥ David / Dittionario novo* (Venice, 1587), profane science and sacred literature were co-dependent. That co-dependence signals a strong desire to relate to the Bible as a text with contemporary relevance.

For Abraham Portaleone, one of David de' Pomi's coreligionists and fellow physicians, the Bible had multifaceted applications as well. In fact, Portaleone drew on his knowledge of the Hebrew Bible and post-biblical Jewish traditions to aid him in his medical practice and enrich his correspondence with non-Jewish colleagues. On the basis of new evidence – Portaleone's unpublished medical letters – Chapter 4 explores two themes in sixteenth-century natural philosophy: ancient alimentation and embryology. It argues that the medical profession in sixteenth-century northern Italy promoted and facilitated meaningful social and intellectual contact between Jews and Christians. By analyzing several of Portaleone's letters, it considers the nature of Jewish-Christian relations in the Medical Republic of Letters. Religious texts, rather than serving as theological proofs, were valuable to this community of learned physicians as confirmations of early modern scientific developments.

The fifth and final chapter studies Abraham Portaleone's printed Hebrew encyclopedia of biblical antiquities. The chapter explores how Portaleone combined bookish erudition with an empirical bent – nurtured by information gleaned from Mantua's pharmacists – in order to reconstruct a composite ingredient in biblical incense. I argue that transposing habits of thought characteristic of the medical profession and the natural philosophic community to the study of religious texts engendered a highly critical stance toward received tradition, rabbinic and scientific alike.

Of the cases discussed in this book, the majority comes from places famously tolerant of their Jewish populations: the Duchy of Mantua and the Republic of Venice. Jewish-Christian interaction in medical contexts flourished on the Italian Peninsula in other places as well as in different periods. For example, in the fifteenth century many Jewish physicians practiced medicine throughout the Kingdom of Naples: they treated Christian patients, gained citizenship, and were active in literary and scientific circles.[117] Furthermore, Italian settings outside of large cities were propitious for Jewish physicians.[118] For example, a Hebrew manuscript

[117] See Nicola Ferorelli, *Gli ebrei nell'italia meridionale dall'età romana al secolo XVIII* (Bologna: Arnaldo Forni, 1980 [orig. 1915]), 116–23, for examples from Barletta, Lecce, Naples, Salerno, Venosa, and other cities.

[118] For Umbria, see Ariel Toaff, *Love, Work, and Death: Jewish Life in Medieval Umbria*, trans. Judith Landry (Portland, OR: Littman Library of Jewish Civilization, 1996), chap. 10. See

miscellany in Florence's Biblioteca Laurenziana contains the letters of a young Jew, Solomon, who practiced medicine in a variety of towns and hamlets in what is today northern Lazio and southern Tuscany.[119] He was particularly well established in Stimigliano, having been asked by the local cardinal to live in his court and serve as his private physician.[120] Even more detailed evidence survives from midcentury Pitigliano, part of a fiefdom under the control of the Orsini family, where Niccolò IV Orsini had as his personal physician the Jew David de Panis.[121] However, rural life, though conducive to Jewish integration, could not create the extensive professional contacts or provide the institutional support that facilitated the unique intellectual activity of larger northern cities. Conversely, while the Aragonese Kingdom of Naples boasted courts and vibrant urban centers, medical culture in the fifteenth century did not encourage the form of interdisciplinary research into the natural history of the biblical world that it would a century later. Between 1545 and 1612 in urban centers such as Venice, Bologna, and Mantua, conditions were ideal in helping to concoct a special mixture of biblical and medical studies.

My story ends in 1612 with the publication of Portaleone's encyclopedia. It does so for several reasons. For one thing, *Shiltei HaGibborim* marks the culmination of a half century of studying the Bible from a natural philosophical perspective – both within Jewish circles and in Italian culture more broadly. That approach to the Bible evolved from straightforward philological analysis to creative reconstruction of

also the sources gathered by Toaff in his *The Jews in Umbria*, 3 vols. (Leiden: Brill, 1993). A few medical contracts between Jews and Christians survive, some extremely detailed. For fifteenth-century Pisa, see Michele Luzzati, "Il medico ebreo e il contadino: un documento pisano del 1462," *La Rassegna mensile di Israel* 45 (1979): 385–92.

119 Biblioteca Laurenziana pluteus 88,12: 21r–63r. Some of these letters have been published in Yaakov Boksenboim, *Iggrot Yehudei Italya* (Tel Aviv: Tel Aviv University Press, 1994). The letters are briefly mentioned in Natascia Danieli, "Sull'epistolografia ebraica in Italia nei secoli XVI–XVIII," *Annali di Ca' Foscari, serie orientale* 42:3 (2003): 29–56, 44.

120 The cardinal, though not named explicitly, was Franciotto Orsini. Solomon declined the invitation, citing, in a letter to his former teacher, the predicted diminution of his business, a great part of which depended on peasant clients. See Biblioteca Laurenziana pluteus 88,12, 58r. This letter is reproduced in Boksenboim, *Iggrot Yehudei Italya*, 56–7. For information on the Orsini family, see Pompeo Litta, *Famiglie celebri italiane*, 11 vols. (Milan: presso l'autore, 1819–85), 9: tav. 113–18.

121 Giuseppe Celata, "Gli ebrei in una società rurale e feudale: Pitigliano nella seconda metà del Cinquecento," *Archivio storico italiano* 138 (1980): 197–255, 210. In sixteenth-century Pitigliano, Jews were also permitted to own land. See p. 241.

biblical products. In a way, little remained to be done after scholars began to build models of the biblical stories;[122] the ideas set in motion in the mid-sixteenth century had run their course and reached their fruition. Furthermore, to seventeenth-century scholars throughout Europe, excessive hands-on experimentation with religious texts could weaken faith in miracles.[123] Additionally, the seventeenth and eighteenth centuries witnessed the institutional and intellectual isolation of natural philosophy from medicine.[124] Around the same time, theology faculties moved from their place at the periphery of Italian intellectual society – Jesuit schools – to the center, universities.[125] Biblical scholars retreated into the protective confines of university theology faculties, and once there their writings disengaged from other disciplines and became more specialized.[126] Physicians, in turn, narrowed their range of inquiry and ceased to study the Bible seriously.[127] For a fleeting moment at the end of the sixteenth and beginning of the seventeenth century, medical doctors had the knowledge, the desire, and the professional flexibility to study both nature and scripture.

Other factors contributed to the extinguishing of this movement in the first third of the seventeenth century. Demographic and political realities in the 1620s and 1630s halted the bilateral Jewish-Christian effort to integrate biblical studies and natural philosophy. The ambitious Duke Carlo Emanuele I of Piedmont Savoy, in annexing the Marquisat of Saluzzo, a French enclave on the Italian side of the Alps, provoked

122 For a later parallel, consider Jacob Judah Aryeh Leon's (Judah del Templo's) model of Solomon's temple, which he designed and assembled in mid-seventeenth-century Amsterdam. See A. Offenberg, "Bibliography of the Works of Jacob Jehudah Leon (Templo)," *Studia Rosenthaliana* 12:1–2 (1978): 111–32; Offenberg, "Dirk van Santen and the Keur Bible: New Insights into Jacob Judah (Arye) Leon Templo's Model Temple," *Studia Rosenthaliana* 37 (2004): 401–22.

123 See, for example, Thomas Browne, *Religio medici* (London: J. M. Dent & Sons, 1906 [orig. 1643]), 23–24. On Browne and the Bible, see Kevin Killeen, *Biblical Scholarship, Science and Politics in Early Modern England: Thomas Browne and the Thorny Place of Knowledge* (Burlington, VT: Ashgate, 2009).

124 Ogilvie, *Science of Describing*.

125 Grendler, *The Universities of the Italian Renaissance*, chap. 10.

126 François Laplanche, *L'écriture, le sacré et l'histoire: érudits et politiques protestants devant la Bible en France au XVIIe siècle* (Amsterdam: APA-Holland University Press, 1986).

127 On scientific culture in the seventeenth century, see Christoph Lüthy, "What to Do with Seventeenth-Century Natural Philosophy? A Taxonomic Problem," *Perspectives on Science* 8.2 (2000): 164–95.

a destabilizing war with France. Carlo Emanuele also laid claim to Monferatto and machinated to bring all of the Mantovano under his control. Those actions led to numerous skirmishes with Spanish and Austrian forces and eventually all-out war in the region.[128] A devastating plague in 1630, whose ill effects extended to Venice and claimed the life of the Venetian rabbi Leon Modena's son-in-law, further ravaged the northern part of the peninsula and sapped the energies of Italian intellectuals. Finally, the fall of Mantua to Austrian invaders, followed by the temporary displacement of Mantua's Jewish community, badly damaged the delicate conditions in which figures like Portaleone, Cavallara, and Magno could pursue their related researches.[129]

The Natural Philosophy of the Biblical World does not present a grand narrative of intellectual change. Instead, it explains how the adherents of one learned tradition shed light on another. As Amos Funkenstein observed, true novelty often consists "not in the invention of new categories or new figures of thought, but rather in a surprising employment of existing ones."[130] Similarly, as Salo Baron pointed out, Azariah de' Rossi's contribution to intellectual history does not lie in the originality of his thought or method but rather in his synthesis of diverse sources and his application of those sources' methods to different historical problems.[131] The same may be said of the physicians and naturalists examined here: by applying methods of natural philosophy to a reenergized scrutiny of the Bible, sixteenth-century Italian scholars drew on the creative energies and novel methods of their profession to change the way the Bible was studied.

Although Aldrovandi, de' Pomi, and Portaleone may have inadvertently passed on their methods to seventeenth- and eighteenth-century scholars who labored to dethrone the Bible from its exalted position atop the Western canon, their original goals were pious. To the extent that

[128] Domenico Sella, *Italy in the Seventeenth Century* (New York: Longman, 1997), 3–4.

[129] For a Jewish perspective on the fall of Mantua, see Catalano, *Olam Hafukh*. On the looting of art in Mantua, see Hugh Trevor-Roper, *The Plunder of the Arts in the Seventeenth Century* (London: Thames and Hudson, 1970), 27–36.

[130] Amos Funkenstein, *Theology and the Scientific Imagination: From the Middle Ages to the Seventeenth Century* (Princeton: Princeton University Press, 1986), 14.

[131] Salo Baron, "Azariah de' Rossi's Historical Method," in *History and Jewish Historians: Essays and Addresses* (Philadelphia: Jewish Publication Society of America, 1964), 205–39, 225–6.

they wished to revise scriptural translations or create new applications for the Bible, they did so to deepen their devotion, not to nurture their skepticism. Although I suggest that the body of work this book presents had an afterlife in later centuries,[132] the project's primary goal is to narrate the history of a symbiosis between natural philosophy and scriptural study. Strictly speaking, the creative combination of medical and religious learning that characterized the lives of a conspicuous group of naturalists in late Renaissance Italy did not survive the tumultuous end of the first third of the seventeenth century; it died. The pages before you attempt an autopsy. But, as the emphasis of this book makes plain, the details of this phenomenon's life teach us more than the causes of its death do.

Later biblical criticism – including the high criticism of the nineteenth century – depended on critical distance between biblical history and the present day. In the works of Ulisse Aldrovandi, David de' Pomi, and Abraham Portaleone, that distance was collapsed. In different ways all three wanted to project themselves back into the world of the Bible; or, perhaps more accurately, wished to transport the Bible into their everyday lives. Their efforts constitute a lost chapter of Jewish and Renaissance history, and this book endeavors to reconstruct that history.

[132] Portaleone had readers in the seventeenth and eighteenth centuries. See, for example, Blasio Ugolini, *Thesaurus antiquitatum sacrarum*, 34 vols. (Venice: J. G. Herthz, 1744–69), 11: cclvij to dxlviij and herein Chapter 1. David de' Pomi's dictionary was one of the seven that Edmund Castell relied on. See his *Lexicon Heptaglotton hebraicum, chaldaicum, syriacum, samaritanum, aethiopicum, arabicum* (London: Thomos Roycroft, 1669), sig. b2r. De' Pomi is also a consistent presence in Samuel Bochart's *Hierozoicon sive bipertitum opus de animalibus s. scripturae cuius pars prior libris IV* (Frankfurt: Balthasar Christoph Wüsten, 1675).

1

"This Is What King David Meant"

Amatus Lusitanus and Ulisse Aldrovandi on the Natural Science of Scripture

During the second half of the sixteenth century, when religious authorities wanted to understand the natural world of the Bible, they sometimes asked medical doctors to help them. Few physicians were as besieged by requests for help as Ulisse Aldrovandi, a professor of natural philosophy at the University of Bologna.[1] In particular, various members of the influential Paleotti family who held powerful positions in the church solicited information from Aldrovandi about the natural world they encountered in the Bible.[2] On 17 February 1577, for example, Aldrovandi reported that Alfonso Paleotti, a local priest, had asked him the previous evening to write a history of the nine gemstones mentioned in chapter 28 of Ezekiel. Aldrovandi obliged, but not without noting that if he were to do this thoroughly, "the book would swell into a massive volume."[3]

[1] In 1561 Aldrovandi assumed the chair he would occupy until his death: Lectura philosophiae naturalis ordinaria de fossilibus, plantis et animalibus (professor ordinarius of natural philosophy in fossils, plants, and animals). On Aldrovandi, see Paula Findlen, *Possessing Nature: Museums, Collecting, and Scientific Culture in Early Modern Italy* (Berkeley: University of California Press, 1994); on the naturalist's unpublished writings, see Lodovico Frati, *Catalogo dei manoscritti di Ulisse Aldrovandi* (Bologna: N. Zanichelli, 1907); and, more recently, Maria Cristina Bacchi, "Ulisse Aldrovandi e i suoi libri," *L'Archiginassio* 100 (2005): 255–366.

[2] On the Paleotti family in sixteenth-century Bologna, see Paolo Prodi, *Il Cardinale Gabriele Paleotti (1522–1597)*, 2 vols. (Rome: Edizioni di storia e letteratura, 1959).

[3] BUB Ms. Aldrovandi 91, "Ulyssis Aldrovandi Historia novem gemmarum de quibus fit mentio in Ezechiele (cap. 28). Reverendissimo ac summa religione praedito Excellentissimoque jurisconsulto D. Alphonso Palaeoto S. Petri Ecclesiae Cardinalis Canonico Prestantissimo, Ulysses Aldrovandus philosophus et medicus s.p.d.," 383r–409r. "Cum a me, Reverende Alphonse, superioribus diebus petieris, ut illarum novem gemmarum, de quibus meminit Ezechiel cap 28, historiam omnem ac facultatem breviter enodarem, non potui non tibi morem gerere ... quam quidem [historiam] si uno fasce totam comprehendere vellem, mihi

Even so, he took up his pen to address the topic the very next day. Eight years later Alfonso's brother Gabriele, a cardinal and the archbishop of Bologna, would press Aldrovandi further on the issue of nature in the Bible:

> When September drew to a close I made my way to Croara, to see the most illustrious and revered Cardinal Paleotti, having been summoned there by him for a few days of recreation.... During lunch we took up conversation of various matters, and by good fortune we fell upon the passage in book 2 of Augustine's *De doctrina christiana*, where he argues that it was necessary for some Christian to undertake the task of interpreting the Old and New Testaments when they speak about plants, stones and metals, herbs and trees, animals and other things that pertain to geography, since in them there are many difficult passages. Impelled by that authority, the illustrious Cardinal tried by many means to persuade me.[4]

Understanding the natural world of the Bible and demonstrating its relevance was a serious intellectual challenge, one Aldrovandi deemed an "immense labor, arduously placed on my shoulders."[5] In spite of the task's difficulty, Aldrovandi explained, Saint Augustine thought it essential.[6] For Augustine, it was a Christian duty to be expert in knowledge of

crede, in magnum volumen excresceret," 383v. Dated (409r) "Bononiae 13 kal. Martii MDLXXVII."

4 BUB Ms. Aldrovandi 54, *Theatrum biblicum naturale* (2 vols.): 1:5v–6r: "Cum mense septembri elapso me contulissem ad Crovariam montem ad Illustrissimum et Reverendissimum cardinalem Paleottum, cum ab eo accersitus essem ibique per aliquot dies recreationis causa cum Amplitudine eius moram traxissem et cum a prandio in varios incidissemus sermones, forte fortuna incidimus in locum D. Augustini lib. 2 *De doctrina christiana*, ubi persuadet necesse fore Christianum aliquem suscipere laborem interpretandi in ea parte Testamenti Veteris atque Novi, in qua sermo habetur de plantis, nempe de lapidibus atque metallis, herbis atque arboribus, animalibus et aliis, quae ad ipsam geographiam spectant, cum multae difficultates in eis sint. Unde hac authoritate impulsus Illustrissimus Cardinalis multis rationibus conatus est mihi persuadere, praesente etiam D. Antonio Gigante Forosemproniensi viro undequaque doctissimo, ego autem aperte cognoscens hoc onus impar esse humeris meis excusavi me ab hoc labore, sed tandem ab Illustrissimo convictus non potui nisi morem gerere Amplitudini suae." A portion of this passage is quoted in Prodi, *Il Cardinale Gabriele Paleotti* 2:543 n. 56. On *villeggiatura* and Bolognese culture at this time, see Nadja Asksamija, "Architecture and Poetry in the Making of a Christian Cicero: Giovanni Battista Campeggi's Tuscolano and the Literary Culture of the Villa in Counter-Reformation Bologna," *I Tatti Studies* 13 (2010): 127–91.

5 BUB Ms. Aldrovandi 54, *Theatrum biblicum naturale*, 1:2r. "hunc laborem licet immensum ... arduum humeris meis imponere."

6 Aldrovandi makes this point at various places in his writings. See, for example, his letter to the (unnamed) *protettore* of the Collegio di Spagna, in BUB Ms. Aldrovandi 66, 355r–367r,

natural things such as "the places of the earth, animals, herbs, and trees, unknown stones and metals, and other things mentioned in the Holy Scripture."[7] Aldrovandi described how Paleotti would "admonish, even exhort me to take up this task as my vocation, as my very own profession."[8] Paleotti prevailed: Aldrovandi, who attained worldwide fame for his extensive collection of natural objects, his far-reaching correspondence, and his learned writings on all branches of natural philosophy, would go on to scrutinize the Bible as a scientific text. He did so not only in his unpublished two-volume *Theatrum biblicum naturale* (Natural theater of the Bible) but also in many other works.[9]

AMATUS LUSITANUS: MEDICAL COMMENTARY AND THE BIBLE

A generation before Ulisse Aldrovandi began to explicate the role of nature in the Bible, a work of medical science appeared that greatly influenced him. In 1553 Amatus published at Venice a commentary on an ancient Greek medical text: Dioscorides' first-century *De materia medica*.[10] Like Aldrovandi, Amatus integrated biblical commentary into his medical work. Numerous later sixteenth-century scholars with medical backgrounds who wrote about the Bible would do the same;

esp. 362v: "come dice santo Augustino nel secondo libro della dottrina Christiana al Capitolo 16 dove prova la cognitione delli Animali, Pietre, Herbe esser molto necessaria al Christiano." See also BUB Ms. Aldrovandi 54, *Theatrum biblicum naturale*, 1:1r–1v.

7 BUB Ms. Aldrovandi 54, *Theatrum biblicum naturale*, 1:1v. For the relevant passages of Saint Augustine, see *PL* 34:46–9.

8 BUB Ms. Aldrovandi 54, 1:1r–1v: "Quapropter res naturales in sacris Bibliis commemoratas alacri spiritu interpretandas suscepi, tum quod D. Augustini verbis in libro de Doctrina Christiana ad huiusmodi munus excipiendum excitarer – ubi Christiani viri in rerum cognitione versati officium fore innuit quoscunque terrarum locos quaeque animalia vel herbas atque arbores sive lapides vel metalla incognita, alias species commemorat Sacra Scriptura generatim digerere solaque exposita literis mandare – tum etiam quod Illustrissimus et Reverendissimus Cardinalis Paleotus saepius me admonuit exhortatque, ut huiusmodi provinciam susciperem tamquam vocationi meae professionique propriam."

9 Findlen, *Possessing Nature*, 66–7; Giuseppe Olmi and Paolo Prodi, "Art, Science, and Nature in Bologna c. 1600," in *The Age of Correggio and the Carracci: Emilian Painting of the Sixteenth and Seventeenth Centuries* (Washington, DC: National Gallery of Art, 1986), 213–36, 224–5; Bacchi, "Ulisse Aldrovandi e i suoi libri," 345. Although Findlen has noted Aldrovandi's interest in biblical studies, she has not explored his study of natural philosophy in the Bible in detail. Additionally, there are scattered mentions of Aldrovandi's interest in the Bible in Frati, *Catalogo dei manoscritti*.

10 Amatus Lusitanus, *In Dioscorides Anazarbei de materia medica libros quinque enarrationes eruditissimae Amati Lusitani* (Lyon: apud viduam Balthazari Arnoletti, 1558).

there were earlier exponents of this trend, too.[11] Amatus, however, was perhaps the first to fuse analysis of the Bible and natural philosophy in a medical treatise.

Amatus was a Portuguese physician born in 1511 to New Christian parents in Castelo Branco and baptized as João Rodrigues.[12] He was educated at the University of Salamanca, where in 1530 he took his degree in medicine and philosophy. In the sixteenth century, Spanish medical faculties, like Italian ones, offered their students broad training in the *studia humanitatis* and classical philology. Amatus put that training to good use: in addition to his medical writings, he also translated classical Latin texts into Castilian.[13] Spanish medical faculties also emphasized hands-on training in practical medicine.[14] In or around 1530, Amatus took his medical degree and, after a brief interlude in Portugal, accepted an offer in 1533 to practice medicine in Antwerp – a haven for *conversos* and Jews alike.[15] Even though Amatus was born in Portugal, educated in Spain, employed briefly in the Low Countries, and died in the Ottoman Empire, his professional life took wing in Italy, and he spent his most

[11] See, for example, Abraham Farissol's commentary on Job, *Perush al Iyov*, published in the first edition of the *Biblia Rabbinica* (Venice: Bomberg, 1518). It was also published in the second edition (Venice: Bomberg, 1524–5).

[12] Maximiano Lemos, *Amato Lusitano: a sua vida e a sua obra* (Porto: Eduardo Tavares Martins, 1907); Harry Friedenwald, *The Jews and Medicine*, 2 vols. (Baltimore: Johns Hopkins University Press, 1944), 1:332–80. On Amatus's *curationes* especially, see Gianna Pomata, "Sharing Cases: The *Observationes* in Early Modern Medicine," *Early Science and Medicine* 15 (2010): 193–236, 206–15.

[13] See Eleazar Gutwirth, "Amatus Lusitanus and the Location of Sixteenth-Century Cultures," in David B. Ruderman and Giuseppe Veltri, eds., *Cultural Intermediaries: Jewish Intellectuals in Early Modern Italy* (Philadelphia: University of Pennsylvania Press, 2004), 216–34, 219.

[14] For general information on the University of Salamanca, see Manuel Fernández Álvarez, ed., *La Universidad de Salamanca*, 3 vols. (Salamanca: Universidad de Salamanca, 1989). On the breadth and diversity of contemporary medical education, see Luis S. Granjel, "Los estudios de medicina," in ibid., II: *Átmósfera intelectual y perspectivas de investigación*, 97–117. On the importance of training in classical languages, see Andrés Gallego Barnés, "Humanidades renacentistas," in ibid., 211–35. For humanism in sixteenth-century Spanish universities, especially Salamanca, see Katherine Elliot Van Liere, "Humanism and Scholasticism in the Sixteenth-Century Academy," *Renaissance Quarterly* 53:1 (2000): 57–84; Richard L. Kagan, "Universities in Castile 1500–1700," *Past and Present* 49 (1970): 44–71. For a student's (rather melancholy) perspective on life at Salamanca in the sixteenth century, see Luis E. Rodríguez-San Pedro Bezares, *Vida, aspiraciones, y fracasos de un estudiante de Salamanca: el diario de Gaspar Ramos Ortiz, 1568–9* (Salamanca: Ediciones Universidad de Salamanca, 1987).

[15] Jonathan I. Israel, *Diasporas within a Diaspora: Jews, Crypto-Jews and the World Maritime Empires (1540–1740)* (Leiden: Brill, 2002), 14–16.

productive years on the Italian Peninsula. In 1540 Amatus was invited to Ferrara by Duke Ercole II to lecture at the University of Ferrara in medicine; he remained in that position until 1547.[16] From 1547 to 1555 Amatus lived and worked in Ancona, while spending brief interludes in Rome between 1550 and 1555, having been summoned there to treat Pope Julius III. Amatus proudly recounts one such visit in the third volume of his medical case studies.[17] In fact, Amatus saw several volumes of his medical case studies into print at Venice. Later in life Amatus emigrated to Salonika, where he died in 1568.[18]

Writing about the Bible, or saying unflattering things about the church and its dependents, could get sixteenth-century writers into serious trouble. Amatus was no exception. In fact, according to two accomplished scholars of the Inquisition, only Girolamo Cardano and Leonhart Fuchs exceeded Amatus as medical authors whose works were most frequently targeted for censorship by church authorities.[19] In the Spanish Indexes of 1583 and 1584, Amatus's work was to be corrected; in the Roman Indexes

[16] On the University of Ferrara in the fifteenth and sixteenth centuries, see Paul Grendler, *The Universities of the Italian Renaissance* (Baltimore: Johns Hopkins University Press, 2002), 102, 347; on Jewish medical students in Ferrara, see Adriano Franceschini, "Privilegi dottorali concessi ad ebrei a Ferrara nel sec. XVI," *Atti e memorie della Deputazione provinciale ferrarese di storia patria* 3:19 (1975): 163–95.

[17] See his letter "illustrissimo et sapientissimo viro, domino D. Alphonso Alencastrensi, supremo apud Lusitanos Commendatario, Amatus Lusitanus medicus, felicitatem et perpetuam salutam optat," published between *centuriae* two and three in *Curationum medicinalium Amati Lusitani medici physici praestantissimi tomus primus continens centurias quator* (Venice: apud Balthesarem Constantinum, 1557), 340. The letter is dated "Anconae Idibus Aprilis Millesimi Quingentesimi Quinquagesimi quarti," or 13 April 1554. Ibid., 342 [*sic*: 341]. Alphonso Alencastrensi, or Alphonso of Lancaster, was a friend of Amatus with whom he lodged in Rome. See Paul Rieger and Hermann Vogelstein, *Geschichte der Juden in Rom* (Berlin: Mayer & Müller, 1895), 2:257.

[18] Older bibliography on Amatus is listed in David B. Ruderman, *Jewish Thought and Scientific Discovery in Early Modern Europe* (New Haven: Yale University Press, 1995), 307 n. 113. Also see Eleazar Gutwirth, "Jewish Bodies and Renaissance Melancholy: Culture and the City in Italy and the Ottoman Empire," in Maria Diemling and Giuseppe Veltri, eds., *The Jewish Body: Corporeality, Society, and Identity in the Renaissance and Early Modern Period* (Leiden: Brill, 2009), 57–92; Giuseppe Veltri, "Jüdische Einstellung zu den Wissenschaften im 16. und 17. Jahrhundert: Das Prinzip der praktisch-empirischen Anwendbarkeit," in Gerd Biegel and Michael Graetz, eds., *Judentum zwischen Tradition und Moderne* (Heidelberg: Universitätsverlag C. Winter, 2002), 149–59; Veltri, "Il *lector prudens* e la biblioteca della sapienza antica: Pietro Colonna Galatino, Amato Lusitano e Azaria de' Rossi," in Giancarlo Lacerenza, ed., *Hebraica hereditas: studi in onore di Cesare Colafemmina* (Naples: Università degli studi di Napoli "L'Orientale," 2005), 369–86.

[19] Ugo Baldini and Leen Spruit, *Catholic Church and Modern Science: Documents from the Archives of the Roman Congregations of the Holy Office and the Index*, 4 vols., in *Fontes*

of 1590, 1593, and 1596, his work was to be expurgated. The Portuguese Index was the most stern: in 1581 his medical writings were prohibited outright.[20] The most offensive portions of Amatus's oeuvre were not those in which he commented on the Bible or emended the Vulgate's translation; they were those in which he described Catholics in disrespectful language or wrote about them in compromising medical situations.[21] Though his work on Dioscorides was not considered to be threatening, it did contain critical remarks about the accuracy of the Vulgate.

But the portions of Amatus's medical writings that seriously engaged biblically literate naturalists later in the sixteenth century had little to do with anti-Catholic sentiment; they concerned scriptural descriptions of nature. For example, the sixty-sixth *enarratio*, or exposition, of Amatus's commentary on Dioscorides examines *stacte*, otherwise known to Renaissance readers by its Latin names *gutta* and *pinguissimus flos myrrhae*. Amatus's analysis of this natural product afforded him the chance to show off his botanical expertise, demonstrate his linguistic facility, and challenge one of the early sixteenth century's most celebrated Christian Hebraists: Sebastian Münster.[22] The impression Amatus strove to create was that Münster was unqualified to analyze scriptural botany; only a naturalist could accurately read and appropriately render scientific language in the Bible. Skilled as both a Hebraist and a naturalist, Amatus used his knowledge of natural science to correct a common reading of the Bible.

Amatus directed his critical acumen at Jerome's Vulgate translation of the Bible, a frequent object of criticism in sixteenth-century Italian culture, both Jewish and Christian.[23] Amatus pointed out that "many

archivi sancti officii romani series documentorum archivi Congregationis pro Doctrina Fidei. Vol. 1:1, *Sixteenth-Century Documents* (Rome: Libreria editrice vaticana, 2009), 744.

20 Ibid., 744–68.

21 An example is provided later in this chapter. See the section "The Vulgate Bible in the Sixteenth Century."

22 For older bibliography on Münster, see Karl Heinz Burmeister, *Sebastian Münster: eine Bibliographie mit 22 Abhandlungen* (Weisbaden: G. Pressler, 1964). On Münster as a Hebraist, see Stephen G. Burnett, "Reassessing the 'Basel-Wittenberg Conflict': Dimensions of the Reformation-Era Discussion of Hebrew Scholarship," in Alison Coudert and Jeffrey Shoulson, eds., *Hebraica Veritas? Christian Hebraists and the Study of Judaism in Early Modern Europe* (Philadelphia: University of Pennsylvania Press, 2004), 181–201.

23 See Eugene Rice Jr., *St. Jerome in the Renaissance* (Baltimore: Johns Hopkins University Press, 1985), 115–76. Profiat Duran, Abraham Farissol, Abraham Portaleone, and others all

think that the psalmist indeed called [the spice] in Psalm 44 [45:8–9] *gutta* or 'tear,' as the verse reads: 'Therefore God, thy God, hath anointed thee with the oil of gladness above thy fellows, all thy garments smell of myrrh, and aloes, and cassia.'"[24] Showing his knowledge of the Hebrew scriptures as well as his botanical expertise, Amatus protests that "the truth is that the Davidic text does not have it as such, as the true Hebrew shows."[25] Amatus's commentary then presents the Hebrew words of the psalm in question. It is one of only two appearances of Hebrew characters in Amatus's printed oeuvre.[26]

But Amatus was not content merely to criticize an ancient work; he also took on a contemporary analysis by the renowned Hebraist Sebastian Münster. Amatus's first words about Münster were favorable: he lauded him as "a most learned man of our time, extremely skilled in many languages," and then cited Münster's version of Psalm 45:9, which renders the three spices in question as "myrrh, aloe, and keiam." Münster's translation of *mor* as "myrrh" remained faithful to the Vulgate, but he replaced *gutta* with "aloe" and *cassia* with "keiam."[27] As such, Münster's translation presented Amatus the opportunity to criticize the Vulgate alongside Münster. Since Jerome had a full command of Hebrew and Greek and was widely respected in the Renaissance, Amatus criticized the Vulgate while suggesting that Jerome was not responsible for it.

did the same. For Duran, see *Kelimat HaGoyim*, chap. 12; for Farissol, see *Magen Avraham*, chap. 29; for Portaleone, see *SG*, 87v.

24 Amatus Lusitanus, *De materia medica*, book I, enarratio 66, p. 91. "Apud vero Psalmistam, ut multi putant, psalmo 44 gutta, sive lachrima nominatur, quum legitur: 'propterea unxit te deus, Deus tuus oleo laetitiae, prae consortibus tuis, myrrha et gutta et casia.'"

25 Ibid., 91–2: "At re vera textus Davidicus non ita habet, ut Hebraica veritas indicat, quae sic habet: אהבת צדק ותשנא רשע על כן משחך אלהים אלהיך שמן ששון מחבריך: מור ואהלות קציעות כל בגדתיך

26 I have not had the opportunity to examine Amatus's autograph manuscript of this text, held in Lisbon's Biblioteca nacional de Portugal. The other instance of Hebrew characters appearing in Amatus's work is when he is examining several contradictory translations of Avicenna; he quotes an Arabic version of the text in Hebrew characters to show that Jacob Mantino's translation is the most accurate. See Amatus Lusitanus, *Curationum medicinalium centuria sexta* (Venice: apud Vincentium Valgrisium, 1556), curatio 53, p. 94.

27 Amatus Lusitanus, *De materia medica*, book I, enarratio 66, p. 92: "Quae ita ad verbum Munsterus Germanus, vir hac nostra aetate doctissimus et linguarum multarum peritissimus, vertit psalmo 45 sponsis dicato dicens: 'dilexisti iustitiam et odisti impietatem, propterea unxit te deus, deus tuus, oleo laetitiae prae consortibus: myrrham, aloen, et keiam (redolent) omnia vestimenta tua.' Hactenus Munsteri interpretatio." Amatus's source was most likely Münster's אצר ישע *Veteris Instrumenti tomus secundus, prophetarum oracula atque Hagiographa continens* (Basel: Michel Isengrin and Heinrich Petri, 1535), 590v.

"That inept imitator," Amatus interjected, "who was not really Jerome, whoever he was, had *gutta* for *ahalod* … the word itself clearly indicates aloe wood."[28] The Vulgate Bible that sixteenth-century readers were using was beset by two problems: some translations were infelicitous, or even inaccurate, and scholars could not be sure that the text truly represented Jerome's efforts.

But Amatus also criticized his contemporary Münster. About the German scholar Amatus lamented that "he translated *ahalod* with aloe, but the truth of the matter is that he should have translated it as lignum *aloes*, and not aloe."[29] Amatus's comment indicates that Münster's botanical expertise, as well as his knowledge of Hebrew, was limited since he omitted the important correction aloe *wood* from the translation. Showing his talent for both biblical exegesis and botanical identification, Amatus pointed out that "aloe is a type of sap, which the Hebrews call in their language aloe. *Ahalot*, on the other hand, is aloe wood. As such, Münster would have been more correct to say 'myrrh, aloe wood, and keza.'"[30]

In the final tally, Amatus criticized not only the Latin Vulgate but also Sebastian Münster. The renowned Christian Hebraist, according to Amatus, was correct when he translated *ahalot* as aloe rather than accepting the Vulgate's rendering of *gutta*. Still, Amatus castigated Münster for neglecting to call *ahalot* aloe wood as opposed to simply aloe. More forcefully criticizing Münster, Amatus prefers the Vulgate's rendering of קציעות as *cassia,* as opposed to Münster's unaltered transliteration. Amatus's learned glosses on this verse in Psalm 45 create the impression that Amatus saw within himself the ideal marriage of skill as a Hebraist with proficiency in botany. Amatus was accustomed to analyzing classical Greek texts and considering all possible Latin translations

[28] Amatus Lusitanus, *De materia medica*, book I, enarratio 66, p. 92: "In qua mea sententia optime verbum 'redolent' suplet, et ex ea satis constat, quam inepte personatus ille et non vere Hieronymus, quisque ille fuerit, guttam pro ahalod, interpretatus fuerit, quum vox ipsa clamet ahalod agallochum Graecorum esse, Romanorum vero lignum aloes."

[29] Ibid., 92: "unde Munsterus emendandus a me quoque venit, quum verbum aholod, aloen verterit, cum re vera lignum aloes, et non aloen dicere debuisset."

[30] Ibid., 92: "nam aloe succus herbae est, quem Hebraei sua voce Aloe appellant, ahaloth vero lignum Aloes est, quamobrem Munsterus rectius sic interpretaretur, dicendo: 'Myrrham, lignum aloes et keizam (redolent) omnia vestimenta tua.'"

of them – his medical training conditioned him to do that.[31] What is surprising in this passage is that Amatus did the same for a Hebrew text from the Bible. Because of his unique skill set, Amatus viewed his own glosses on the Psalms as more faithful than Jerome's or Münster's.

The context of Amatus's remarks about the accuracy of the Vulgate, the competence of contemporary Christian scholars of Hebrew, and the usefulness of natural philosophy in explicating the Bible is of paramount importance. Amatus embedded his observations in a collection of detailed essays on a major classical author, Dioscorides. Generally speaking, Renaissance commentaries on classical texts – literary, philosophical, or scientific – offered their authors the opportunity to display their extensive erudition. From childhood on, pupils who received strong Latinate educations were accustomed to a method of instruction in which teachers proceeded slowly through canonical authors such as Virgil and Horace and took each phrase, and sometimes each word, as stimulus for digression and expansive analysis that drew upon a wide array of other ancient texts.[32] The Bible was one of those texts. Medical works were just as likely to encourage wide-ranging discourses as literary or philosophical ones. As such, reflections on the Bible occasionally found their way into scientific commentaries. The character of medical commentary in the middle years of the sixteenth century, and especially the state of scholarship on Dioscorides, explains the motives for Amatus's creative associations.

By the middle of the sixteenth century, most major medical and scientific texts such as those of Galen, Hippocrates, Theophrastus, and Dioscorides had been established in bilingual Greek and Latin editions.[33] In some cases, vernacular translations existed for these texts. In the years after 1530, by which time many classical medical texts were available in Greek and Latin, the challenge for European scholars shifted from

[31] Grendler, *The Universities of the Italian Renaissance*, 243–4, 352.

[32] Kristine Louise Haugen, "A French Jesuit's Lectures on Vergil, 1582–1583: Jacques Sirmond between Literature, History and Myth," *Sixteenth Century Journal* 30:4 (1999): 967–85; Anthony Grafton, "On the Scholarship of Politian and Its Context," *Journal of the Warburg and Courtauld Institutes* 40 (1977): 150–88.

[33] Grendler, *The Universities of the Italian Renaissance*, 325. See also the articles in Paul Oskar Kristeller, ed., *Catalogus commentariorum et translationum: Medieval and Renaissance Latin Translations and Commentaries* (Washington, DC: Catholic University of America Press, 1960–).

establishing accurate editions and readable, faithful translations. Their mission, instead, was to flesh out cryptic statements, expand truncated descriptions, and make the text of these canonical authors more relevant to modern-day medical life.[34]

This was especially the case for Dioscorides. A survey of scholarship on his *De materia medica* is illustrative of broader trends in sixteenth-century medical humanism. Dioscorides' first-century work had survived in Greek throughout the eastern Mediterranean. Because of its comprehensive nature and its medical utility, manuscripts circulated widely. Occasionally, these manuscripts presented opportunities for illustrators and patrons to display, respectively, their diligence and their largess. One conspicuous example is the so-called Vienna Dioscorides, an illustrated codex from 512 that was originally a wedding gift for Anicia Juliana, daughter of the emperor Flavius Olybrius.[35] This particular manuscript was a magnet for multilingual glosses; scribes have affixed Arabic equivalents to nearly all of the plant names, and a medieval Greek hand elaborates on the names, etymologies, and descriptions of the plants. Curiously, a Byzantine scribe has translated each of the plant names into Hebrew in a minuscule, careful script. This polyglossia came to be associated with Dioscorides in particular and adumbrated the later fascination with polylingual appellations that is so characteristic of the Renaissance.

In the Latin West, a partial translation of *De materia medica* was available from the sixth century onward. In spite of this, Dioscorides' text was little used. Around 1085 Constantinus Africanus revised this translation, and the text, as a result, achieved a marginally broader circulation. Still, Dioscorides languished in obscurity until Ermolao Barbaro completed a new translation in 1481; however, it was not published until 1516. At the same time, Greek editions of Dioscorides were being printed in the Western world, chiefly in Italy. Aldus Manutius put out the first Greek edition in 1499, and that text was revised by Girolamo Rossi and Francesco Torresani and printed, again by Aldus, in 1518. Still, these editions were not useful to practicing physicians and active botanical

[34] Grendler, *The Universities of the Italian Renaissance*, 352.

[35] Vienna Nationalbibliothek Ms. med. gr. 1. For a modern reprint, see *Der Wiener Dioskurides: Codex medicus graecus 1 der Österreichischen Nationalbibliothek*, 2 vols. (Graz: Akademische Druck u. Verlagsanstalt, 1998–9).

scholars. As an expert on sixteenth-century medical humanism put it, scholars like Ermolao Barbaro and Marcello Vergilio were "more adept at philological subtleties than botany, and more willing to enter into polemics than into the fields in search of plants."[36] While early translators and commentators interpreted Dioscorides literally – their professional orientation was philological and their stated aim was to defend Dioscorides' accuracy – later scholars such as Franciscus Frigimelica and Benedictus Textor, and eventually Otto Brunfels, Valerius Cordus, and Conrad Gesner, were more concerned with the botanical application of Dioscorides' text. The proliferation of vernacular translations of his work is a good sign of Dioscorides' popularity by midcentury. Seventy-eight editions of Piero Andrea Mattioli's commentary on Dioscorides – the most read scientific book in the sixteenth century, according to one expert – were published in the second half of the sixteenth century, in both Italian and Latin.[37] Similarly, the Spanish physician Andreas Laguna published four editions of his work on Dioscorides in Castilian between 1563 and 1586 alone.[38]

Once Dioscorides' work had been established in reliable editions, scholars shifted their focus away from philological debate and toward different sorts of applications. Botanical gardens were proliferating throughout northern Italy just as Dioscorides was becoming more popular. The text and the novel gardens had a reciprocal impact on one another: Dioscorides was consulted to identify new plants in Italian gardens, and pharmacists, botanists, and physicians cultivated and circulated plants thought to be the equivalents of items in Dioscorides' *De*

[36] Jerry Stannard, "P. A. Mattioli: Sixteenth-Century Commentator on Dioscorides," *University of Kansas Library Bibliographic Contributions* 1 (1969): 59–81, 67. Also see Sara Ferri, ed., *Pietro Andrea Mattioli, Siena 1501–Trento 1578: La vita, le opere* (Ponte San Giovanni: Quattroemme, 1997).

[37] Paula Findlen, "The Formation of a Scientific Community: Natural History in Sixteenth-Century Italy," in Anthony Grafton and Nancy Siraisi, eds., *Natural Particulars: Nature and the Disciplines in Renaissance Europe* (Cambridge, MA: MIT Press, 1999), 373–4. I have used Pietro Andrea Mattioli, *I discorsi di M. Pietro Andrea Matthioli nelli sei libri di Pedacio Dioscorides Anazarbeo della materia medicinale* (Venice: Vincenzo Valgrisi, 1568). On Mattioli, see Ferri, *Pietro Andrea Mattioli*; Brian Ogilvie, *The Science of Describing: Natural History in Renaissance Europe* (Chicago: University of Chicago Press, 2006); Karen Meier Reeds, "Renaissance Humanism and Botany," *Annals of Science* 33 (1976): 522–7; Reeds, *Botany in Medieval and Renaissance Universities* (New York: Garland, 1991).

[38] Andrés de Lagunas, *Pedacio Dioscorides Anazarbeo, acerca de la materia medicinal y de los venenos mortiferos* (Salamanca: Mathias Gast, 1563).

materia medica. The prefatory epistles to Mattioli's Dioscorides provide proof of both tendencies. In his dedicatory letter to Johanna of Austria, Mattioli lauds the work of recent scholars, such as Barbaro, Leoniceno, and Manardo, who have "rediscovered and experimented with a considerable number of plants" that could be found in Dioscorides.[39] In that same epistle Mattioli boasted that Francesco Calceolari, the Veronese apothecary, had sent him "ever more rare plants" that he could put to good use in his commentary on Dioscorides.[40] Additionally, in these years courses on medical "simples" became more widespread, and doctors sought to deepen their knowledge of the classical botanical corpus as well as incorporate new medicinals into their practices.[41] Dioscorides helped them to do that. Finally, and most relevant to our purposes, Dioscorides' text, like many Greek and Latin classics, came to be the subject of antiquarian exegesis: scholars interested in the history of ancient medicine or the material life of the first-century Mediterranean read *De materia medica* as a work that furnished rare and important examples of the quotidian life of an ancient culture. It is from this matrix of plant collecting, pharmaceutical innovation, and antiquarian research that Amatus's commentary emerged. Eventually, philological establishment of "true" Greek scientific texts paved the way for various sorts of analyses – including the combination of botanical research and biblical studies. Seeking an ever-wider range of ancient texts to clarify Dioscorides, Renaissance scholars turned to the Bible as well. At the same time, Dioscorides illuminated obscure biblical passages.

Amatus used Dioscorides to amplify the Bible more than once. For example, in a concise essay entitled "On the Genitals of the Male Deer," Amatus explained the simple meaning of a verse from Psalm 42.[42] His aim was to improve his readers' understanding of a biblical passage in

39 Mattioli, *Discorsi* (Venice: Vincenzo Valgrisi, 1568), sig *6v. The letter begins on sig *2r and is entitled "alla serenissima principessa Giovanna archiduchessa d'Austria, etc., Principessa eccellentissima di Fiorenza, et di Siena, etc., mia clementissima signora." Johanna of Austria was the daughter of Emperor Ferdinand I. She married Francesco of Tuscany in 1565. Mattioli was a stark critic of Amatus, and wrote a short work that accused Amatus not only of poor scholarship but also of Judaizing. For more on this episode, see Friedenwald, *The Jews and Medicine*, 1:341–9.

40 Mattioli, *Discorsi*, sig **2v. Calceolari's name is spelled Calceolario here.

41 Ogilvie, *The Science of Describing*, 33.

42 Amatus Lusitanus, *De materia medica*, book II, enarratio 39, pp. 269–71: "De cervi masculi genitale."

order to strengthen its spiritual impact. Though the topic was technical, the effect of his exposition was anything but: it made sense of a vague natural metaphor in the Psalms.

Amatus's analysis of the medicinal value of a male deer's bodily discharges explained the behavior of deer. Notably, a classical Roman author was his main guide. Following Pliny's *Natural History*, Amatus observed that stags are deadly to serpents, which hide away in caves but are eventually eaten by them.[43] Turning his mind to the Bible, Amatus immediately added that "this is what King David, the prophet, meant in his Psalm, when he said 'as the hart longs for water streams, so does my soul long for you, O God.'"[44] Pliny's zoological observations taught Amatus how deer voraciously pursue their prey, and Psalm 42 provided an example. That knowledge helped him understand the meaning of the psalmist's metaphor. Not content with generalizations about deer behavior, Amatus supplemented his gloss on the feeding habits of that animal with geographic precision. He added that "in the regions of the east, where serpents customarily grow to be very large, deer often lurk around stagnant waters to find serpents to eat."[45] In other words, King David, living "in the regions of the East," would have had the opportunity to see keen deer give chase to large serpents that hide in mountain streams. Geographic specificity lent greater precision to Amatus's explanation of biblical deer.

Amatus consulted diverse sources of geographic knowledge. For example, accounts about the New World by Iberian explorers were conspicuous. In "On the Genitals of the Male Deer," Amatus observed that "a certain jewel is gaining popularity these days, which was first brought from India to the Portuguese ... many people call this stone deer's tear,

[43] Ibid., 270. "Nam cervi ut testatur Plinius capite 32. libri octavi, cum serpentibus habent pugnam, ita ut investigent cavernas, et eas narium spiritu extrahant, renitentes: quod libro xxviii. cap. 9. prope finem confirmavit, dicens: 'exitio iis (hoc est serpentibus) esse cervos nemo ignorat ut si quae sunt, extractas cavernis, mandentes.'" See Pliny, *Natural History* 28:39.

[44] Amatus Lusitanus, *De materia medica*, book II, enarratio 39, 270: "Hoc innuit Regius Propheta David in psalmo, cum dicat: 'sicut cervus desiderat ad fontes aquarum ita anima mea desiderat ad te domine.'" I have used the Jewish Publication Society version of the Bible in my translation above. Psalm 42:1.

[45] Amatus Lusitanus, *De materia medica*, book II, enarratio 39, 270: "Nam post esum serpentium, in orientalibus regionibus, ubi praegrandes reperiri solent, tunc vero ea infestus siti, cervus praesto ad stagnantes aquas confluit."

and some others call it *belzahart*. It is an exceptional and divine antidote, proven to work against all sorts of poisons."[46] For a practicing physician of the mid-sixteenth century, medical expertise necessitated firsthand experience with a variety of medicaments, including exotic ones. In the case of a medicinal product as rare and desirable as a deer's tear, Amatus was compelled to describe his initial acquaintance with it. In Venice, one of sixteenth-century Europe's thriving seaports, precious stones were avidly sought and easily found.[47] Amatus recounts a tale about meeting Beatriz de Luna, "an extremely wealthy woman who, arriving in Venice, had one of those [i.e., deer's tear] stones that came from animals of the Indies, brought back by some noble Portuguese [sailor]."[48] Amatus included this anecdote to prove that he had seen and handled this stone. To later natural philosophers such as Ulisse Aldrovandi, passages such as this one were especially apposite and were explicitly flagged.[49]

Medical inquiry led Amatus to meditate on the meaning of a natural metaphor in the Psalms. But before his mind wandered to the psalmist's strategies, he began his study of a medicinal product that originated in an animal's body with a description of that animal's behavior and,

[46] Amatus Lusitanus, *De materia medica*, 269–70: "circumfertur hodie lapillus quidem ex India ad Lusitanos primo advectus, ut plurimum magnitudine et figura glandis colore cineritio ad cyaneum inclinante, multis compositus laminis, quem 'cervi lachrymam' quidam, alii vero 'lapidem belzahart' appellant, et illum, tanquam praestantissimum ac divinum antidotum, contra omne genus veneni approbant." Deer's tears (*lacrimae cervi*) were mineral substances excreted by male deer which, in the Renaissance, were thought to possess curative powers. See Lynn Thorndike, *History of Magic and Experimental Science*, 8 vols. (New York: Columbia University Press, 1941), 4: 311.

[47] See Jacqueline Herald, *Renaissance Dress in Italy, 1400–1500* (London: Bell & Hyman, 1981), 173–5.

[48] Amatus Lusitanus, *De materia medica*, 271: "nunc quum haec literis commendabamus, illustris Domina Beatrix à Luna, mulier opulentissima, Venetiis agens, lapillum unum ex iis quos describimus ab Indiae animali extractum a quodam nobili Lusitano, qui apud Indos Prorex fuerat." Lusitanus went on to give the price that the noblewoman paid for the stone – 130 golden ducats – and describes its ovular shape and impressive size: "centum et triginta aureis ducatis emit: erat enim lapillus ille, ut hoc quoque dicamus ovalis fere magnitudinis." Beatriz de Luna, also known as Doña Gracia Nasi, lived in Venice between 1544 and 1549, when she relocated to Ferrara. For information on her movements, see José Emilio Burucúa, "Les enjeux culturels du texte biblique dans l'Europe du XVIe siècle," *Annales: Histoire, Sciences Sociales* 58:6 (November–December 2003): 1347–66, 1350. On Beatriz de Luna, see Maria Giuseppina Muzzarelli, "Beatriz de Luna, Viuda de Mendes, llamada doña Gracia Nasi: una hebrea influyente (1510–c. 1569)," in Ottavia Niccoli, ed., *La mujer del Renacimiento* (Madrid: Alianza Editorial, 1993), 115–47.

[49] See subsequent discussion in this chapter's section "Ulisse Aldrovandi and Biblical Studies."

eventually, the properties of deer's tears themselves. That was common practice in sixteenth-century natural philosophy.[50] Still, Amatus's leap to biblical exegesis was anything but common, and his intense interest in the language of the Psalms requires explanation.

THE VULGATE BIBLE IN THE SIXTEENTH CENTURY

Of all the biblical books, the Psalms were perhaps the most popular in sixteenth-century Italy. Because of their centrality to religious worship, their proper translation was hotly debated, and new editions of the Psalms rolled off European presses in Latin and various vernaculars from the 1530s on. Furthermore, establishing an accurate and readable biblical text was a preoccupation of European clergymen and scholars throughout the sixteenth century. And that preoccupation grew in scale and scope after midcentury. Even though the Council of Trent upheld the authenticity of the fifth-century Latin Vulgate, dissatisfaction with that text was growing, and Hebraists – Jewish and Christian – had much to do with promoting that dissatisfaction.[51] Additionally, from the perspective of textual criticism the Psalms were especially problematic. The text of the Psalms found in the Vulgate Bible was based not on the Hebrew but rather on a revision of the *Vetus Latina* against the Septuagint column of Origen's Hexapla.[52] Amatus expressed his dissatisfaction with the Vulgate's rendering of the Psalms so boldly because he was steadfast in his belief that translations ought to be based on the Hebrew text of the Bible.

Criticism of the Vulgate Bible was not new in the sixteenth century. Nor did natural philosophers play a conspicuous role in promoting it. Indeed, vociferous criticism of the Vulgate may be traced back to the

[50] See Laurent Pinon, "Conrad Gesner and the Historical Depth of Renaissance Natural History," in Nancy Siraisi and Gianna Pomata, eds., *Historia: Empiricism and Erudition in Early Modern Europe* (Cambridge, MA: MIT Press, 2005), 241–59.

[51] On the status of the Vulgate in post-Tridentine Italy, see G.-M. Vosté, "La Volgata al Concilio di Trento," *Biblica* 27 (1946): 301–19; Edmund F. Sutcliffe, "The Council of Trent on the Authentia of the Vulgate," *Journal of Theological Studies* 49 (1948): 35–42; Hildebrand Höpfl, *Beiträge zur Geschichte der Sixto-Klementinischen Vulgata* (Freiburg im Breisgau: Herder, 1913), esp. 1–43; Gigliola Fragnito, *La Bibbia al rogo: la censura ecclesiastica e i volgarizzamenti della Scrittura (1471–1605)* (Bologna: Il Mulino, 1997), esp. 75–109.

[52] Ernst Würthwein, *The Text of the Old Testament: An Introduction to the Biblia Hebraica*, trans. Erroll F. Rhodes (London: S.C.M. Press Ltd., 1980), 91–5.

late fifteenth and early sixteenth centuries and prominent figures such as Lorenzo Valla (1406–57), Desiderius Erasmus (1466–1536), and Jacques Lefèvre d'Étaples (1455–1536). As early as 1444 Lorenzo Valla pointed out errors in the Vulgate in his work on the Greek New Testament. But he did not correct them.[53] Other scholars, such as Sante Pagnini (1470–1536), doubted that Jerome was its author. For how could such an authority, the argument went, compose such a problematic translation? While direct criticism of the Vulgate originated in the late fifteenth century, scholars had expressed doubts concerning its veracity and fidelity to the Hebrew Bible in the Middle Ages. Raymondus Martinus (d. 1286) and Nicholas of Lyra (ca. 1270–1349) pointed out places where the Vulgate text did not square with the Hebrew version. Additionally, they observed how the language of the Vulgate frequently diverged from the Latin that Jerome quotes in his commentaries.[54] Though criticisms of the Vulgate Bible were frequent, critics did not question the text's inerrancy. A common way of reconciling the Vulgate's inaccuracies with the esteem in which the Western church held that text was to argue, as the Spanish commentator Johannes Driedo did, that while Jerome may have made mistakes in his translation, he was irreproachable on doctrinal issues and on the portions of the Bible upon which those doctrinal formulations rest.[55] In other words, linguistic details mattered less than doctrinal ones. The censor and Hebraist Bellarmine made the same argument years after Driedo.[56] As the foregoing evidence suggests, the doctrinal portions of the Bible were not the only ones that mattered to natural philosophers such as Amatus and Ulisse Aldrovandi; to them, scripture's natural terminology was at least as important, since it could augment their knowledge of natural philosophy.

Besides the overall accuracy of Jerome's Vulgate, another closely related topic that engaged sixteenth-century Bible scholars was the status of Hebrew and Greek versions of scripture. The Complutensian

[53] Charles Trinkaus, *In Our Image and Likeness: Humanity and Divinity in Italian Renaissance Thought*, 2 vols. (Chicago: University of Chicago Press, 1970), 1:223.

[54] Eugene Rice Jr., *St Jerome in the Renaissance* (Baltimore: Johns Hopkins University Press, 1985), 175.

[55] Ibid., 181.

[56] X.-M. LeBachelet, *Bellarmin et La Bible Sixto-Clémentine: études et documents* (Paris: G. Beauchesne, 1911), 107.

Polyglot, published in the early years of the sixteenth century, held a dim view of Greek texts of the Bible. For example, the editors tailored the Greek text to correspond more cleanly to the Vulgate.[57] In the Old Testament section of the Complutensian Polyglot, the Latin text of the Vulgate was set in the middle of the page, flanked by Greek and Hebrew on either side. A prologue to the text remarks that the Vulgate lay innocently between two thieves, calling to mind for early sixteenth-century readers how Jesus himself was crucified between two thieves.[58] At the century's beginning, the reigning assumption was that the Vulgate was the superior biblical text: discrepancies between it and its Greek and Hebrew sources could be attributed to faulty manuscripts and improper readings of those sources.

By the end of the sixteenth century, Catholic authorities reversed their views. The prefatory material to the 1592 Clementine/Sixtine Bible conceded that a revision of Jerome's Vulgate was necessary. More to the point, it admitted that recourse to Greek and Hebrew texts was essential to establishing a dependable biblical text.[59] In seventy-five years, the Catholic Church radically shifted its views to recognize the value of Hebrew and Greek. As José Emilio Burucúa has shown, the publication of this particular Bible provoked crises all over the Catholic world, and not just in the offices of learned philologists: since parish priests in far-flung communities continued to read from previous editions of the Bible in church, the authority of the Clementine/Sixtine text was very slowly established.[60]

This reorientation toward the value of Greek and Hebrew was facilitated by the persistence and vehemence of attacks on Jerome's Vulgate translation, to which Amatus lent his voice. Although the Council of Trent mandated in a decree of 8 April 1546 that the "Old Latin Vulgate" was the only authorized version of the Bible, scholars in Italy and beyond

57 Trinkaus, *In Our Image and Likeness*, 1:101.

58 *Biblia Polyglotta* (Alcalá de Henares, 1514–17), 6 vols: vol. 1, sig. + iii v: "mediam autem inter has latinam beati Hieronymi translationem velut inter Synagogam et Orientalem Ecclesiam posuimus: tamquam duos hinc et inde latrones medium autem Iesum, hoc est Romanam sive latinam Ecclesiam, collocantes."

59 Giancarlo Pani, "Un centenaire à rappeler: l'édition Sixtine des Septante," in Irena Backus and Francis Higman, eds., *Théorie et pratique de l'exégèse* (Geneva: Droz, 1990), 413–38, 417.

60 Burucúa, "Les enjeux culturels," 1365–6.

expressed their dissatisfaction with Jerome's Latin.[61] Valla initiated a trend and did not serve as its sole bearer. Desiderius Erasmus, Marsilio Ficino, and Giles of Viterbo all took issue with Jerome's translation and preferred that of Sante Pagnini.[62] Neither Jews nor *conversos*, as we have seen, refrained from lambasting the Vulgate, either.

Amatus stood at the confluence of two traditions: Hebrew biblical scholarship and Latinate humanism. Born to Jewish parents and the beneficiary of early instruction in Hebrew, he knew the language well enough in his middle age to make piquant comments on proper translation from Hebrew to Latin. In his medical case studies he also alludes to reading Hebrew manuscripts, as when he discusses the *Alphabet of Ben Sira* in his *consilium* about an unfortunate nun who found herself with child.[63] And he knew contemporary European biblical scholarship. Amatus's commentary on Dioscorides' *De materia medica* presented an opportunity for him to use natural philosophic knowledge to clarify the Bible.

When it came to using research in natural philosophy to deepen scholars' knowledge of the Bible and the biblical world, Amatus's future readers were just as devoted to these matters as he was. No mere eccentric, Amatus's interests can be understood within and traced back to a distinct moment in Italian cultural, intellectual, and institutional history. The combination of medical training and biblical literacy enabled Amatus's discussion of the Bible in the context of a scientific work. And the impact of this approach was significant: future readers of Amatus's *consilia* and his commentaries displayed similar tendencies and combined botanical research with scriptural observations. Ulisse Aldrovandi was one such reader.

[61] For the decree, see F. Schulte and A. L. Richter, eds., *Canones et decreta concilii Tridentini* (Leipzig: Bernhardus Tauchnitii, 1853), 12.

[62] On Pagnini, see T. M. Centi, "L'attività letteraria di Santi Pagnini (1470–1536) nel campo delle scienze bibliche," *Archivum Fratrum Praedicatorum* 15 (1945): 5–51; Giorgio Spini, *Tra rinascimento e riforma: Antonio Brucioli* (Florence: La Nuova Italia, 1940), 204–5; David B. Ruderman, *The World of a Renaissance Jew: The Life and Thought of Abraham ben Mordecai Farissol* (Cincinnati: Hebrew Union College Press, 1981), 83.

[63] *Curationum medicinalium Amati Lusitani medici physici praestantissimi tomus primus continens centurias quator* (Venice: apud Balthesarem Constantinum, 1557), *centuria* IV, 36, p. 562: "hodie extant non pauca egregia documenta et dicteria elegantissima Hebraica lingua conscripta." This case study received unfavorable attention from church authorities. See Girolamo Rossi's expurgatory *Censura* of *Centuriae* from Ravenna, 1597 in ACDF, Index, *Protocolli*, O (II.a.13), fols. 626r, 627r–628v, 629v; reproduced in Spruit and Baldini, *Catholic Church and Modern Science*, 751–5, 752.3333.

ULISSE ALDROVANDI AND BIBLICAL STUDIES

The prominent Bolognese naturalist Ulisse Aldrovandi was, like Amatus, a close reader of the Bible and an accomplished natural philosopher. Furthermore, Aldrovandi knew that Amatus wrote about the Psalms in his commentary to Dioscorides. He shared Amatus's interest in the acquisition of a rare medicinal product, deer's tears, and brought the Bible into his discussion of it. As we saw, a discourse on stones believed to function as antidotes – known as deer's tears – provided Amatus an opportunity to discuss a natural metaphor in Psalm 42. Aldrovandi knew this work and openly acknowledged his debt. The Bolognese naturalist penned a five-folio essay called "On Deer's Tears" that may be found within an unwieldy manuscript volume entitled *Miscellanea de animalibus et plantis* (Miscellany concerning animals and plants). Their similar educational backgrounds and consistent approach toward the study of nature led both Amatus and Aldrovandi, though separated by a generation, to intermingle medical commentary and scriptural exegesis.

Ulisse Aldrovandi knew Hebrew. Hebrew words appear frequently in works such as his *Pandechion epistemonicon* and throughout his writings.[64] He wrote several short paragraphs about the word *arov*, a word meaning various types of wild beasts, and lengthier ones on the Hebrew terms for fermentation and yeast.[65] In fact, his study of the language was serious enough that he composed a short tract entitled *Rudiments of Hebrew Grammar*.[66] Furthermore, he also addressed the role Hebrew played in his intellectual worldview, and such comments illuminate his view of the Hebrew language. "Among the seventy-two languages that were born from the seventy-two nations of the house of Israel," Aldrovandi wrote, "only three were always held in greatest veneration among all the others: Hebrew, Greek, and Latin. In those languages,

[64] BUB Ms. Aldrovandi 105 (83 volumes). See, for example, ALIM–ANET 71v; A–AM 286v, 288r, 296r; FER–FIN 114v; GLAPH–GYRI 103v; UNI–ZYR 515v. This list is far from exhaustive and reflects a perusal of a portion of the eighty-three volumes of *Pandechion epistemonicon*.

[65] For *arov*, see BUB Ms. Aldrovandi 21, 4:531r: "Arob quid apud Hebreos." For Aldrovandi's remarks on fermentation, see "Ulyssis Aldrovandi Historia περὶ τῆς Ζυμῆς, seu de fermento ad Illustrissimum et Reverendissimum Cardinalem Palaeotum Bononiensem Episcopum vigilatissimum," in BUB Ms. Aldrovandi 6, 3:57r–79r, esp. 60r–61v.

[66] *Hebraicae linguae rudimenta*, in BUB Ms. Aldrovandi 97, 128r–133r.

writings on divine and indeed human things were preserved."[67] The order in which Aldrovandi listed those languages is indicative of how he felt about them: Hebrew held a primary position. And the fact that Hebrew preserved "human things" was alluring to the Bolognese naturalist. To emphasize Hebrew's importance beyond theological investigation, Aldrovandi maintained that "Hebrew has something to do with every sort of human talent." He elaborated that "in it there is a profound abyss of secrets, impossible to penetrate, in which the more progress extremely learned men make, the more they confess their ignorance."[68] The notion that Hebrew contained or provided access to secrets was a belief Aldrovandi shared with his medical colleague and fellow lexicographer David de' Pomi.[69]

But Aldrovandi was especially fervent in his cultivation of Hebrew letters: he suggested that the language might displace other tools of scientific learning. In his essay "How the Hebrew Language Perfectly Expresses the Nature of Things," Aldrovandi asserted that "this holy and divine language is useful not only for knowing divine things but also for gaining knowledge of the human sciences. As such, he who diligently considers the virtues of [its] words and knows the power of their etymologies will progress further in the knowledge of natural things than if he had memorized all of Aristotle, Theophrastus, Pliny, Dioscorides, and other similar authors."[70] For Aldrovandi, Hebrew was the holiest language.

[67] BUB Ms. Aldrovandi 83, *Bibliologia*, 1:438–9: "Tra le settantadue lingue che dalle 72 natione della casa d'Israel son nate, sole tre sono state tenute sempre in grandissima veneratione fra tutte l'altre lingue cioè l'Hebrea, Graeca, et Latina. Sì perchè in quelli sono state conservate le scritture delle cose divine et parimente humane."

[68] Ibid., 1:443: "perche lì si trova un profundo abisso de' secreti, che mai si può penetrare nello quale quanto più gran progresso fanno gli huomini literatissimi, tanto più confessano la sua ignoranza."

[69] For more on de' Pomi and the belief that Hebrew provided access to "secrets," see Chapter 3.

[70] BUB Ms. Aldrovandi 83, *Bibliologia*, 1:445: "questa santa et divina lingua non solo è utilissima a fare conoscere le cose divine ma ancora per conseguire le scienze humane. Periochè chi considerarà diligentemente la virtù delle parole et saprà la forza della lor etimologia farà più gran progresso in la cognitione delle cose naturali, che se egli havesse a memoria tutta la dottrina d'Aristotele, Teofrasto, Plinio, Dioscoride, et altri autori simili." These ancient natural philosophers were not randomly chosen; they were the dominant figures in and sources for sixteenth-century natural philosophy. For an introduction to sixteenth-century natural philosophy, see William A. Wallace, "Traditional Natural Philosophy," in Charles B. Schmitt and Quentin Skinner, eds., *Cambridge History of Renaissance Philosophy* (Cambridge: Cambridge University Press, 1988), 201–35.

However, its holiness derived not from its instantiation in the Bible but rather from the fact that it corresponded more closely to nature than either Latin or Greek did.[71]

Very little is known about how Aldrovandi learned Hebrew. In his voluminous writings, he never mentions a Jewish teacher, nor does he comment on the genesis of his Hebrew knowledge or his progress in learning the language. The Jewish banker, biblical commentator, and educator Ovadiah Sforno lived mere meters from Aldrovandi's home.[72] Though there is no firm evidence of intellectual contact between the two men, it is possible that Aldrovandi may have sought Sforno's help on matters Hebraic. The Bolognese naturalist did, however, possess Hebrew

[71] On the standard view of Hebrew as a divine language, see Jean Ceard, "Le 'De originibus' de Postel et la linguistique de son temps," in M. L. Kuntz, ed., *Postello, Venezia e il suo mondo, Atti del II Convegno internazionale su Postel (Venezia, 5–9 settembre 1982)* (Florence: L. S. Olschki, 1988), 19–44, 24. For more on the idea that Hebrew expresses natural things, see Paolo Simoncelli, *La lingua di Adamo: Guillaume Postel tra accademici e fuoriusciti fiorentini* (Florence: L. S. Olschki, 1984), 67. Two sixteenth-century sources that predate Aldrovandi are worthy of mention here. Théodor Bibliander, in his *De ratione communi omnium linguarum et literarum commentarius* (Zurich: C. Frosch, 1548), argued that Hebrew "was the most perfect of all languages; its words explain natural things [illa perfectissima esset omnium, cujus verba rerum naturas explanarent]." Postel, in his *De Etruriae regionis … commentatio* (Florence: Torrentini, 1551), argued that Hebrew came the closest to natural things, followed by other Semitic languages such as Arabic, Aramaic, and Syriac. See p. 59: "sic inter omnes linguas mundi opus est esse unam primariam rerumque veritati proximam, in qua ante omnes vocabulorum elucescat veritas. Volo autem mihi ex sola authoritate illorum, qui hoc asseverarunt, concedi, quod sit ipsa Hebraica, et quae illi sunt proximae, ut est Arabica, Chaldaicae duae, Syriaca Maroniticave et Ethiopica." See also Chevalier's *פתח אהל מועד Rudimenta hebraicae linguae* (Paris: Stephanus, 1567), particularly his letter to Theodor Beza of December 1559, unnumbered pages: "confido fore ut huius linguae studia tanto omnium maxime necessaria, quanto pietas omni humana eruditione praestat, cum caeteris bonis artibus ac disciplinis tandem penitus ex densissimis tenebris emergant." For medieval antecedents to this view among Jewish scholars, see Moshe Idel, *Language, Torah, and Hermeneutics in Abraham Abulafia* (Albany: State University of New York Press, 1988), 1–28; in the sixteenth century, see Azariah de' Rossi, *Me'or Enayim*, chap. 57 (Vilna, 1866 [1572]), 453–66; Azariah de' Rossi, *The Light of the Eyes*, trans. and ed. Joanna Weinberg (New Haven: Yale University Press, 2001), 672–90; Judah Moscato, *Kol Yehudah*, 2:68.

[72] Sforno's address (no. 80 il Vívaro, at the corner of Piazza Santo Stefano) is listed in Guidicini, *Cose notabili della città di Bologna,* 5 vols. (Bologna: tipografia delle scienze di Giuseppe Vitali, 1868–73), 5:99. See also Mario Fanti, ed., *Gli schizzi topografici originali di Giuseppe Guidicini per le cose notabili della città di Bologna* (Bologna: Arnaldo Forni, 2000), 342, illustration no. 506 for the location of Sforno's home; for the proximity of Aldrovandi's home, see ibid., 291, illustration no. 416. Information about the location and sale of Ovadiah Sforno's home may be found in his will of 1 February 1549. See Archivio di Stato di Bologna, Notarile Pietro Zanettini 7/0 filza 26 (2496). When Sforno died in 1550, Aldrovandi was twenty-eight years old.

grammars and other works concerning Hebrew philology, including books by Johannes Reuchlin, Antoine Rodolphe Chevalier, Johannes Drusius, and Robert Bellarmine.[73] One of his manuscripts presents evidence of Aldrovandi repeatedly copying out the Hebrew alphabet, as a beginning student might.[74] Given the large number of Hebrew grammars he owned, and absence of any mention of an instructor, it would appear that Aldrovandi learned Hebrew autodidactically.

As information regarding Aldrovandi's study of Hebrew is rare, evidence of his use of that language is abundant. One of the many ways he displayed his knowledge of Hebrew was by arguing that a deer's tear is different from Bezar, or Belzar, "as it is called by the Jews."[75] After reviewing several standard, published Latin accounts of the properties of this stone written by Marsilio Ficino, Tomasso Cospi, and Julius Caesar Scaliger, Aldrovandi informed his friend and patron, the bishop Gabriele Paleotti, that he could buy one for himself.[76] As he encouraged the powerful bishop to acquire such a stone, he also told Paleotti – and future readers as well – where he came upon a description of this stone. "Most revered father," Aldrovandi writes, "you could see one for yourself if you were able to buy it with money. Amatus testifies to having seen a honey-colored deer's tear." Aldrovandi also explained that his description of

[73] Of the Hebrew grammars Aldrovandi owned, Bologna's Biblioteca Universitaria still possesses the following: Johannes Reuchlin, *De accentibus, et orthographia, linguae hebraicae ... libri tres* (Haguenau: Anshelm, 1518); Reuchlin, *De rudimentis Hebraicis ... libri tres* (Pforzheim: Anshelm, 1506); Johannes Drusius, *Ebraicarum quaestionum, sive, quaestionum ac responsionum libri duo* (Lyon: Elsevier, 1583); Reuchlin, *Drusii animadversionum libri duo. In quibus praeter dictionem Ebraicam plurima loca Scripturae, interpretumque veterum explicantur, emendantur* (Leiden: Iohannes Paetsius, 1585); Wigand Happel, *Linguae sanctae canones grammatici* (Basel: Thomas Guerinus, 1561); Nicolas Clénard, *Tabulae in grammaticam hebraeam ... ad haec literarum, quas serviles nominant, potestates adiectae sunt, itemque Psalmi aliquot ad verbum redditi* (Cologne: Birckman, 1567); Luiz de Sao Francisco, *Globus canonum, et arcanorum linguae sanctae, ac diuinae Scripturae* (Rome: Bartholomeus de Grassis, 1586); Roberto Bellarmino, *Institutiones linguae hebraicae ex optimo quoque auctore collectae* (Rome: Dominicus Basa, 1585). BUB Ms. Aldrovandi 147 contains an inventory of the naturalist's library. Dr. Maria Cristina Bacchi of Bologna's Biblioteca universitaria is currently preparing an edition of this manuscript for publication. I wish to thank her for her private correspondence with me on this matter.

[74] BUB Ms. Aldrovandi 21, 4:23r–25r.

[75] BUB Ms. Aldrovandi 97, 514r.

[76] I have not been able to identify Thomasso Cospi. Of him Aldrovandi writes that he composed a "luongo trattato" on deer's tears. See Ms. Aldrovandi 97, 514v. Perhaps Thomasso Cospi was a progenitor of Ferdinando Cospi, the seventeenth-century Bolognese naturalist whose collection became the Museo Cospiano in Bologna.

the stone comes from Amatus, and a marginal annotation makes this explicit, stating the precise location in Amatus's *De materia medica* where he opined about what "King David meant."[77] But Aldrovandi was not merely a reader of Amatus; he followed in his footsteps. Many passages in his immense corpus of naturalistic writings display a conscious effort to try to understand the Bible better by using natural philosophy – and to understand natural philosophy better by using the Bible. For Aldrovandi, as for Amatus, philology was the foundation upon which his biblical commentary rested.

Aldrovandi's debt to Amatus is not always obvious. In another, very different work, Aldrovandi reveals himself to be a reader of Amatus but not an acknowledged one. His definition of *agolochum* (aloe wood), which may be found in his unpublished three-volume, trilingual Latin-Hebrew-Syriac dictionary, indicates that he was reading Amatus. Furthermore, it shows that he sided with Amatus against Münster. Most importantly, it demonstrates how seriously Aldrovandi took philology. An analysis of Aldrovandi's lexicographical work allows us to see how powerful and pervasive the combination of Hebraic knowledge and natural expertise was in sixteenth-century Italy.

Ulisse Aldrovandi's *Lexicon latino-hebraico et syro-chaldaicum rerum quae in Sacris Bibliis leguntur* (Latin-Hebrew and Syriac-Chaldean lexicon of things read in Holy Scriptures) is not a work of original scholarship but largely a series of extracts from two major sources: Sante Pagnini's *Thesaurus linguae sanctae* and Benito Arias Montano's *Lexicon hebraicum et chaldaicum* that constitutes part of the apparatus to the Antwerp Polyglot.[78] Although most entries in Aldrovandi's sprawling lexicon – it extends to three volumes, each more than one thousand folios – are admitted borrowings from these two popular lexicographical works, a few entries display originality of thought. Conspicuously, terms touching upon natural matters receive Aldrovandi's fullest attention.

The woods of the biblical world were one of Aldrovandi's consuming interests. Much of his two-volume vernacular study of the cross upon which Jesus was crucified is an extended analysis of woods of the ancient

[77] Ibid., 516r–516v: "potrebbe Vostra Illustrissima vedere se per danari la potesse comprar da qual Reverendissimo Padre. Testifica Amato Lusitano haver veduto una lagrima di cervo, di color di mele." The marginal note "lib. 2 in Enar. Dios. c. 39" is on 517v.

[78] *Biblia sacra hebraice, chaldaice, graece, latine* (Antwerp: Plantin, 1568–73), 8 vols.; vol. 7.

Near East.[79] In his prolix work, Aldrovandi penned two entries for *agalochum*. Both mention specific biblical books, and both display the combination of botanical expertise and biblical fluency that Amatus also exhibited in his work a generation earlier. Aldrovandi's first entry treats *agalochum* as a geographic place; his second examines it as a botanical product. In the preliminary entry, Aldrovandi defines the term with the Hebrew word *egel* and speculates that *agalochum* might be the name of a region where aloe wood – the featured product in Amatus's debate with Münster – comes from. He also notes that it is a "most celebrated" medicinal product and posits that "agallim," a cognate term, is a place mentioned in Isaiah, "whence perhaps aloe wood is brought to us."[80] In his subsequent entry Aldrovandi pushes his analysis further and moves beyond geographic into philological matters. Once again he reveals his debt to Amatus.

Aldrovandi, echoing Amatus's gloss on *ahalot*, or aloe wood, draws an equivalence between *agalochum*, *lignum aloes*, *ahalot*, *aksila leavan*, and *stacte*. The precise association of like terms in Latin, Hebrew, Aramaic, and Greek that Amatus had advocated, and which was a feature of Renaissance botany, is upheld by Aldrovandi.[81] "In the Nebiensis Heptaplus," Aldrovandi observes, *agalochum* "is discovered to be *aksila leavan*. In Hebrew it is *ahalot*, and in Greek *stacte*."[82] For Aldrovandi, this substance is "aloe wood, or storaceis" and is found in the "Venetian Bible, Psalm 45."[83] Psalm 45, of course, is the same psalm that Amatus scrutinized in his commentary to Dioscorides' *De materia medica*. Though Aldrovandi neither explicitly acknowledges Amatus as his

[79] BUB Ms. Aldrovandi 51, *De cruce* (2 vols.).

[80] BUB Ms. Aldrovandi 50, *Ulyssis Aldrovandi Lexicon latino-hebraico et syro-chaldaicum rerum quae in Sacris Bibliis leguntur*, 1:15r. "Agalochum, אגל egel, stella, gutta, vel emanatio unde fortasse lignum aloe Agalochum nuncupatur quod exemanat et stillat succus in medicina celeberrimus. Agallim etiam est proprium nomen loci in Esaia, unde fortasse pretiosissimum hoc genus ligni ad nos advehitur."

[81] On polyglossia in Renaissance botanical texts, see Ogilvie, *The Science of Describing*, 44, 173.

[82] Aldrovandi is referring to Agostino Giustiniani's 1516 polyglot psalter: *Psalterium, hebraeum, graecum, arabicum, et chaldaeum* (Genoa: Impressit Petrus Paulus Porrus, 1516). Known as the Nebiensis Heptaplus (because Giustiniani was the bishop of Nebbio on Corsica), it contained seven versions of the Psalms: Hebrew, Greek, Arabic, and Aramaic, as well as three Latin versions. Psalm 45 is on Sig. H iiv. There are no scholia on this psalm.

[83] Aldrovandi is referring to the *Biblia Rabbinica*, or *Miqra'ot Gedolot* (Venice: Daniel Bomberg, 1516–17).

source nor takes on Münster directly, he emphasizes that this substance is "*aksila*, which comes from the Greek *ksulon*." And if his readers could not understand Aramaic or Greek, Aldrovandi puts it quite plainly and adds that this is "wood." If there were any doubts at this point about the fact that this natural ingredient is not a leaf or a resin but something more durable, Aldrovandi notes, "I believe that this cannot be understood as stacte or *storax*, since stacte is a fresh, scented type of myrrh. And the storax plant comes from *xyloaloë*, that is, Hebalogho. So we cannot understand the aloe herb here."[84] From a manuscript catalog of his library that was completed shortly before Aldrovandi's death in 1605, we know that he owned and signed Amatus's commentary on Dioscorides with his usual autograph "Ulisse Aldrovandi and friends."[85] More importantly, these two entries, especially the second one, provide additional evidence of how interconnected natural knowledge and biblical competence were in this Italian community of natural philosophers. An important key to reading the Bible accurately was a thorough knowledge of natural science – in this case, expert acquaintance with trees and their leaves, resins, and woods.

Aloe was not the only type of wood to appear in the Psalms that engaged Aldrovandi's attention. He was just as interested in cedar wood and wrote about it extensively in another unpublished manuscript composition. Those remarks establish that Aldrovandi's approach to biblical natural history was empirical: once he was satisfied with his definition of a biblical term, his next priority was to experience it.[86] With the help of several of his correspondents, Aldrovandi was able to hold in his hand what he deemed to be biblical cedar wood.

Like many naturalists of his time, Aldrovandi desired to see and touch the natural products he wrote about. Empiricism, after all, was a hallmark

[84] BUB Ms. Aldrovandi 50, *Ulyssis Aldrovandi Lexicon latino-hebraico et syro-chaldaicum rerum quae in Sacris Bibliis leguntur*, 1:15v: "Agalochum. In exemplari Nebiensis Heptaplo reperitur אסקילא ליאוון askila leavan. Ubi est in Hebraeo אהלות ahaloth, in Graeco στακτή. Lignum Aloës, seu storacis, Psal. 45 in Bibliis venetianis et Chaldaice scribitur אקסילא aksila a Graeco ξύλον. Lignum. Credo autem nequaquam intellegi posse stacte nec storax, quoniam stacte est pinguedo recentis myrrhae et storax planta est ab xyloaloë id est Achalocho, hic autem non possemus intelligere de alöe herba."

[85] "Ulyssis Aldrovandi et amicorum."

[86] On the importance of "experience" for early modern Italian naturalists, see Findlen, *Possessing Nature*, 194–240.

of natural philosophy in the later sixteenth century.[87] But the yearning to see, smell, and touch natural elements from the biblical world was something new in the second half of the sixteenth century. To bolster his faith and deepen his reading of the Bible, Aldrovandi applied the same expectations to its woods, gemstones, and animals as he did to those described in Pliny, Theophrastus, or Dioscorides. Cedar wood is mentioned frequently in the Bible. It was also the type of wood, Aldrovandi maintained, that was used to construct important objects in scripture, such as Aaron's staff and the musical instrument David played to ease Saul's spirit.[88] Most important, it was a type of wood that Europeans of his own day could experience firsthand.

Aldrovandi introduced the topic of cedar wood in *De cruce,* his two-volume natural history of Jesus' cross. The Bolognese naturalist's discussion of this wood comes in the context of a wide-ranging antiquarian investigation of the physical properties of the cross, including its length and its materials.[89] In these pages, Aldrovandi hails two other natural philosophers who had an equivalent interest in biblical botany, and in cedar specifically: Melchior Guilandinus and Luca Ghini.[90] Guilandinus, the curator of Italy's most celebrated botanical garden in Padua, made a special effort to correspond with Aldrovandi about a rare type of cedar believed to have been the very species mentioned in the Bible. And, most importantly, Luca Ghini, who established the botanical garden at Pisa and maintained it, went so far as to send Aldrovandi a specimen of this tree.

Aldrovandi's writings show how fascination with biblical woods extended far beyond a circle of precocious naturalists; clergymen and political figures sought to have specimens of that same wood and construct objects meant to remind them of its biblical origin. For example, this same section of *De cruce* observes about cedar wood that "the

[87] See Gianna Pomata and Nancy Siraisi, eds., *Historia: Empiricism and Erudition in Early Modern Europe* (Cambridge, MA: MIT Press, 2005), 30. See also my discussion in Chapter 5.

[88] See Exodus 7:9ff.; and 1 Samuel 16:23, respectively. On contemporary European interest in that biblical episode, especially among medical men, see Werner Kümmel, "Melancholie und die Macht der Musik: Die Krankheit König Sauls in der historischen Diskussion," *Medizinhistorisches Journal* 3–4 (1968–9): 189–209.

[89] BUB Ms. Aldrovandi 51, *De cruce*, 1:99v et seq. "lunghezza della croce," 100r et seq. "legni della croce."

[90] For more on Guilandinus, see Chapter 2. Little is known of Ghini's life. See Findlen, *Possessing Nature*, esp. 6, 164–9. On Aldrovandi's relationship with Ghini, see ibid., 368–9.

posts of the room of the Council of Ten in Venice are made from it." Reminders of biblical products abounded even in the halls of power. And that same passage informs readers that Cardinal Paleotti was equally enthused about this wood, going so far as to build a tabernacle out of it. "If I remember correctly," Aldrovandi wrote, "the illustrious Monsignor Paleotti made an effort to have some of this wood to create a tabernacle for the most holy sacrament on the altar."[91] As these quotations attest, an interest in identifying the natural elements of the biblical world was widespread in Italian culture in the later sixteenth century. Aldrovandi's reflections about cedar wood indicate his eagerness to relate to biblical realia in contemporary terms and his desire to share his experiences with like-minded individuals.

That same community, consisting of political figures, clergymen, and naturalists, may have received stimulus to deepen its knowledge of the Bible – and investigate the Bible's natural world on empirical grounds – from the mid-sixteenth century's most celebrated religious event: the Council of Trent. Aldrovandi reminisces about hunting for biblical *manna* during odd moments of the Council of Trent in 1562:

> And speaking of that same *agarico*, and heavenly *manna*, it is harvested in the midst of common Larch [*Larix decidua*], which I believe is a species of great cedar, as I show in my histories.[92] It is certainly not the Larch of Vitruvius, or of Pliny, or of Julius Caesar in his *Commentaries*, since it has flowers and fruit and it burns in fire. These observations are entirely opposed to the description given of the Larch by the ancients. This noble tree grows abundantly in the mountains of Pergine above Trent, where there are mines. I can testify to this, having seen it, and having picked *agarico* with my own hands in 1562 during the first session of the holy Tridentine Council, being in the company of Monsignor Cardinal Paleotti and his brother Signor Camillo and Pope Urban VII.[93]

[91] BUB Ms. Aldrovandi 51, *De cruce*, 1:109v: "mi scrisse la pia memoria di Melchiore Guilandino già prefetto dell'horto di Padova, che oltre il cedro tanto celebrato, del quale sono fatte le porte della sala de capo di dieci in venetia, et se bene mi ricordo Monsignore Illustrissimo Paleotti fece diligegnza d'havere di questo legno per fare un tabernacolo del santissimo sacramento dell'altare me ne mandò un ramo il Ghini con frutti, osservò ancora in quello molte piante non conosciute da moderni."

[92] I have not been able to locate the precise passage Aldrovandi refers to here.

[93] BUB Ms. Aldrovandi 51, *De cruce*, 1:4v–5r: "avvertendo ancora che il medesimo agarico et mana celeste si raccoglie alcuna volta nel larice commune, il qual larice credo, che sia

Not only does this passage demonstrate how Aldrovandi combined rigorous textual research and active engagement with Italian wildlife to dispute the findings of ancient botanists; it also shows the shared interest that Aldrovandi and highly placed clergymen held in one of the Bible's most magical and elusive foods. It was only after being sure that the *larice* that he and the Paleotti brothers saw in Trentino was not the *larice* described by Vitruvius, Pliny, or Caesar that Aldrovandi felt comfortable enough to pronounce this plant *manna*. This reminiscence also indicates that during the Council of Trent there was another type of religious study taking place in addition to debates concerning church doctrine. Clergymen and laymen alike were sallying into the hills around Trent to find natural products from the Bible. Paleotti's modern biographer notes that "as soon as he was free from his conciliar duties, and very often at the end of each session, Paleotti would wander the nearby mountains collecting botanical simples to transplant into a botanical garden in Bologna."[94] With the help of Ulisse Aldrovandi, Cardinal Paleotti and Pope Urban VII found tangible evidence of the Bible in the Dolomite foothills.

Aldrovandi's research as a naturalist conditioned him to look for overlaps between sacred history and natural history. In another section of *De cruce*, Aldrovandi used a passage from Dioscorides' *De materia medica* not only to explain the Bible – much as Amatus had a generation before – but also to expound upon the Jewish custom of interment, which was of considerable interest to other scholars of the time, notably Isaac Casaubon.[95] In doing so, Aldrovandi blended biblical and medical

una specie di cedro maggiore, come provo nelle mie Istorie, non essendo in alcun modo il larice di Vitruvio, e di Plinio, et Giuglio Cesare nei Commentarii, per haver fiori, e frutti, e brusciando nel fuoco, le quali note sono tutte contrarie alla descrittione data del Larice degli antichi e questo nobile albero nasce copiosamente nei monti di Pergeni sopra Trento nel luogo, dove sono le minere de metalli, come posso fare fede havendolo veduto, et cavatone con le proprie mani l'agarico, essendo in compagnia di Monsignore Illustrissimo Card. Paleotti, et il Sig. Camillo suo fratello, et Papa Urbano settimo l'anno 1562 nella prima sessione del sacro Concilio Tridentino." For classical references to *agaricum*, which often grows on larch trees, see Gigliola Maggiulli, *Nomenclatura micologica latina* (Genoa: Istituto di Filologia Classica e Medievale, 1977), 84–96. Dr. Maggiulli identifies *agarico* as either *Fomes officinalis*, or *Boletus laricis*, both of which are common fungi that grow on larch trees throughout Northern and Central Europe, especially in forests and mountainous regions. Many types of Larch agaric have medical properties. Ibid., 90.

94 Prodi, *Il Cardinale Gabriele Paleotti*, 1:130 n. 24.

95 See Isaac Casaubon, *De rebus sacris et ecclesiasticis exercitationes XVI* (Frankfurt: Ruland, 1615), exercitatio XVI, § XCVIII: "de forma sepulchorum Iudaicorum observationes

commentary. Burial and specifically the burial customs of the Jews were topics Aldrovandi developed elsewhere in his writings.[96] In *De cruce*, Aldrovandi's remarks on cedar wood clarify its symbolic value to the prophets as well as its curative and salubrious powers.

Cedar wood was a subject that led Aldrovandi to add a new dimension to his writing: sociological observation. Aldrovandi pointed out that poorer Jews around the time of Jesus' life used a product called *cedria*, a resin obtained from cedar trees, to enclose cadavers and slow decomposition. Having established this fact, Aldrovandi proceeded to clarify the architectural, symbolic, and medical value of the resin. Aldrovandi posited that "Noah's Ark was made of it, and Solomon's temple constructed of it." The first testimony to the power of cedar wood came not from a scientific text but rather from the Bible. This wood was "lauded greatly by Ezekiel the prophet in the thirty-first chapter." Among the verses Aldrovandi cites is Ezekiel 31:3, which reads "therefore its height was exalted above all the trees of the field, and its boughs were multiplied, and its branches became long because of the multitude of waters when it shot forth."[97] This description of the cedar's majesty is vague on the specific curative properties of that wood. But for Aldrovandi that was not the sort of datum the Bible was supposed to supply; he merely wished to find a verse that cast the cedar in a majestic light. For specific information about its medicinal value, Aldrovandi turned to a trusted source: Dioscorides.

e scriptis Iudaeorum"; and § XCIX: "an mos sepeliendi in lateribus cryptarum ortus sit è sepulchro Domini," pp. 470 and 471, respectively. Casaubon's remarks about Christ's burial, composed in response to Cardinal Cesare Baronio's *Annales ecclesiastici* (Cologne: sumptibus Ioannis Gymnici et Antonii-Hierati, 1609), are discussed in Anthony Grafton and Joanna Weinberg, *"I Have Always Loved the Holy Tongue": Isaac Casaubon, the Jews, and a Forgotten Chapter in Renaissance Scholarship* (Cambridge, MA: Harvard University Press, 2011), 281–3. I thank Joanna Weinberg for bringing this passage to my attention.

[96] See BUB MS. Aldrovandi 30, *De ritu sepeliendi*, where he states in an essay entitled "On the Preservation and Interment of Corpses" (De sepeliendis et condiendis cadaveribus, 39r), dedicated to Gabriele Paleotti, that "it seems necessary that it be explained how the Jews preserved and buried their dead" (Necesse videtur explicandum esse modum, quo Hebrei condiebant sua cadavera ac sepeliebant).

[97] BUB Ms. Aldrovandi 51, *De cruce*, 1:4v: "Era ancora un secondo modo di condire per quelli, che non volevano fare tanta spessa, come i primi. La onde usavano d'empire il cadavero di cedria, che è una sorte di resina, che nasce nel cedro maggiore, del quale fu fatta l'Arca di Noe, e constrotto il tempio di Salomone, celebrato grandimente da Ezekiel profetta nel trigesimo primo capitolo dove dice: Ecce Assur quasi cedrus in Libano pulcher ramis, et frondibus nemorosus, excelsusque altitudine, et inter condensas frondes elevatum

Dioscorides furnished proof for Aldrovandi that the cedar tree was an effective retardant of decomposition. Of Jews in first-century Palestine, Aldrovandi observed that "they used this to embalm the deceased, since it has the ability to protect them from putrefaction. Dioscorides, in the 106th chapter of book 1, calls it *vita mortuorum*, when he says: 'It has a power that conserves deceased bodies and decomposes living ones. For this reason some call it *Life of the Dead*.'"[98] Aldrovandi was not the only sixteenth-century naturalist to note Dioscorides' praise of cedar resin as a preservative for corpses. In his *On the Admirable Works of the Ancients*, the French traveler and naturalist Pierre Belon did so as well.[99]

For Aldrovandi, scrutinizing cedar's medicinal value led to yet another biblical meditation, this one on the magical food *manna*. Pondering cedar's other medicinal uses, Aldrovandi pointed out that "this cedar has great power with various sicknesses, and wherever it grows one also finds *agarico* and the heavenly *manna* celebrated by the Jews, which, in my opinion is called *cedromeli* [cedar honey] by Hippocrates and is truly *mel cedarinum* [honey of cedars]."[100] Cedar is not only important as a tree possessing symbolic power, as the verses from Ezekiel indicate. It is also an effective medical product, especially insofar as it facilitates burial. Finally, the power of the cedar tree extends far beyond its symbolic value or its direct medical application. It nourishes the soil around

est cacumen eius. Aquae nutrierunt illum, abyssus exaltavit illum: flumina eius manabant in circuitu radicum eius et rivos suos emisit ad universa ligna regionis. Propterea elevata est altitudo eius super omnia ligna regionis: et multiplicata sunt arbusta eius, et elevati sunt rami eius prae aquis multis" (emphasis in the original).

[98] BUB Ms. Aldrovandi 51, *De cruce*, 1:4r–4v: "et imbalsamando con quella i cadaveri per haver facoltà di conservarli dalla putrefattione, è chiamata da Dioscoride nel capitolo centisimo sesto del primo libro vita mortuorum, quando dice: δύναμιν δὲ ἔχει σηπικὴν [μὲν τῶν εμψύχων, φυλακτικήν] δὲ τῶν νεκρῶν σωμάτων ὅθεν καὶ νεκροῦ ζωήν τινες αὐτὴν ἐκάλεσαν cioè: Cui ea vis inest, ut defuncta corpora conservet, et viventia corpora corrumpat, qua ex causa aliqui mortuorum vitam appellavere (emphasis in the original).

[99] Pierre Belon, *De admirabili operum antiquorum et rerum suspiciendarum praestantia liber primus. De medicato funere, seu cadavere condito, et lugubri defunctorum eiulatione liber secundus. De medicamentis nonnullis servandi cadaveris vim obtinentibus liber tertius* (Paris: Guglielmo Cavellat, 1553), 2.3, 24v–25v. I am grateful to Nancy Siraisi for this reference.

[100] BUB Ms. Aldrovandi 51, *De cruce*, 1:4r–4v: "La qual cedria ha gran facoltà in diversi morbi e dove ella nasce, si ritrova ancora l'agarico, et la mana celeste tanto celebrata da gli Ebrei, la quale al mio giudicio è chiamata da Ippocrate cedromeli id est mel cedarinum, et da Galeno eomeli id est Mel aereum, et drosomeli id est mel rosidum."

it and enables fungi like *agarico*, which Aldrovandi believed to be the equivalent of *manna*, to thrive. Aldrovandi's remarks call to mind a vivid tableau of tall, stately cedar trees shading the ancient Near East, while its branches preserved deceased bodies and provided solace to families in mourning, and its roots fertilized surrounding terrain, creating the conditions necessary for fungi such as *agarico* to grow. The implication of Aldrovandi's research is clear: biblical events thought to be miraculous are explicable by research into natural history. As early as the fifth century BCE, ancient medical writings strove to explain things in natural terms and minimize supernatural intervention.[101] Early modern medical scholarship continued that tradition and amplified it. According to Aldrovandi, Jesus' body was preserved for several days in the tomb because, like other impecunious Jews of his time, he was entombed in a wood – cedar – that slowed decomposition. And *manna* was an especially nourishing type of mushroom that was fertilized by the cedar tree.

Aldrovandi's investigations of biblical woods typically contain fewer flights of fancy than his studies of *manna* and cedar. It is in his more subdued writings that we are able to chart the reciprocal relationship between natural science and biblical studies. His philological observations are the essence of his work on the Bible. Aldrovandi's comments on oak wood, for example, reveal how his botanical expertise qualified him to translate the Bible more accurately. Additionally, the Bible's comments about oak and its various species accomplish far more than Ezekiel's homily about cedar: they describe the wood in naturalistic language and enrich Aldrovandi's acquaintance with a common, rather than a rare, type of wood.

Aldrovandi occasionally contradicted himself, or at least offered evidence that challenged his prior assertions. For example, after arguing that Jesus' cross was made of cedar, he stated that the cross was made from oak, or *ayla* in Hebrew. But finding the precise term was another matter entirely. As he often did, Aldrovandi opened Benito Arias Montano's polyglot Bible for assistance and informed his readers that "some, as Arias Montano says in his *Sacra Bibia*, interpret it as *olmo*, and still others as *ilice*, which seems to me to be the best translation." Aldrovandi

[101] Arnaldo Momigliano, "La storia tra medicina e retorica," in *Tra storia e storicismo* (Pisa: Nistri-Lischi, 1985), 11–24, 12.

went on to display his knowledge of the differences between these two plants. "For we should not say that it is *olmo*, being the living type of oak, bearing acorns, as does the *querza*. This [oak] is included among the great and durable plants, of considerable age. Ordinarily its leaves fall as is normal; I have never seen any type that is always green."[102] Once again his firsthand experience is crucial, but only insofar as it is paired with textual learning. Oak trees are deciduous, Aldrovandi points out, and "the nature of the oak, whose leaves fall, is to extend its branches far and wide, whence derives an argument that this tree denotes prosperity." Two scriptural quotations buttress his argument: "as Isaiah shows in chapter four, when he [Isaiah] says 'as the terebinth tree, and as an oak, whose substance is in them, when they cast their leaves [Isaiah 6:13]'"; Aldrovandi also invokes Amos: "by the testimony of the prophet Amos, the *querza* shows great strength and robustness 'yet I destroyed the Amorite before them ... he was strong as the oaks.'"[103] In Aldrovandi's reading, the Bible contains not only metaphorical insight into the oak's power but also accurate descriptions of its deciduous nature.

Aldrovandi's analysis of oak in the Bible demonstrates his knowledge of Hebrew etymology and celebrates the ability of the Bible to clarify the nature of plants. "What else does the *basan* signify," Aldrovandi avers, "if not the richest and most powerful? For the very name *ayla* or *alon* in Hebrew means power and influence."[104] Aldrovandi quotes

[102] BUB Ms. Aldrovandi 51, *De cruce*, 1:112r: "Havendo di sopra parlato della querza del cui legno credo sia stata fatta la S. Croce, chiamata dagli ebrei אלה ancorche alcuni come dice l'Arrio Montano nella Sacra Bibia, interpretano olmo, altri ilice, il che pare ancora a me essere molto megliore interpretatione, che non è a dire olmo, essendo l'elce specie di querza et glandifera, come quella; la qual querza è annoverata fra le piante grande e dure et di lunga età le cui foglie cascano la vernata per ordinariamente, ancora che io n'habbi osservato una sorte, che perpetualmente verdeggia."

[103] Ibid., 112r–112v: "la natura della querza, le cui foglie cadono, è di stendere in larghezza i rami suoi, onde hanno pigliato argomento di denotare prosperità, amplificatione di fameglia e populi, come mostra Esaia al capo quarto, quando dice: et erit in ostentionem sicut terebinthus et sicut quercus quae expandit ramos suos. Gran forza, e robustezza mostra la querza per testimonio del Profeta Amos al capo secondo ego autem exterminavi Amorrheum à facie eorum cujus altitudo cedrorum altitudo ejus, et fortis ipse quasi quercus" (emphasis in the original).

[104] Ibid., 112v–113r: "La querza Basan che altro significa se non i piu potenti e richi percioche il nome stesso hebraico אלה over אלון significa potenza, et estensione." I have not been able to find a definition of אלה or אלון in any fifteenth- or sixteenth-century Hebrew dictionary that translates either term as "power" or "influence."

Isaiah (2:13 and 1:30) and Zechariah (11:12) before observing that "the *querza* [oak], losing its leaves, alludes to the people of a republic, being ornamental and luxurious and filled with divine grace as Isaiah says in the first chapter: 'when you were like an oak tree losing its leaves.'" Still, Aldrovandi was interested in nature in the Bible, and he quoted scripture to inform his readers about the natural world, not politics. "See how this prophet expresses the nature of our *querza*," Aldrovandi states, "whose properties and strength are very easily seen in the wood of the holy cross, as we said above."[105] For Aldrovandi accurate readings of scripture derived from a synthesis of natural philosophy and biblical studies. To Aldrovandi's mind, the contributions of Hebraists like Sebastian Münster and Benito Arias Montano were of scholarly value. But only a natural philosopher who held plants in his hand, considered their medical use, and pondered their meanings in a variety of languages could truly assess the biblical text.

CONCLUSION

Ulisse Aldrovandi was motivated to investigate the natural world of the Bible by a series of conversations with bishops and priests in his native Bologna. Like his predecessor Amatus had done a generation before, Aldrovandi used his expertise in natural philosophy to scrutinize the Bible. Amatus, in his explication of Dioscorides, and Aldrovandi, in his reflections on various topics in natural philosophy, sharpened their reading of the Bible and brought its natural world to life. Medical commentaries in the second half of the sixteenth century, with their digressive tendencies and propensity to supplement knowledge of one classical author with selections from a wide variety of others, occasionally embraced the Bible as an alternative source. In that process, the Bible itself was subjected to closer readings. Sixteenth-century naturalists viewed scripture as a source not only for theological and doctrinal positions but

[105] Ibid., 112r: "Però disse Esaia al capo secondo: super omnes quercus Basan: et Zacaria al capo undecimo ululate quercus Basan. La querza, cascate, che lascian le foglie che cosa significa se non il popolo della repubblica essere d'ornamenti e commodi et divina gratia abbandonato, come ben mostra Esaia nel capo primo, quando disse cum fueritis veluti quercus defluentibus foliis. Ecco come da questo Profetta si esprime la natura della nostra querza. Le proprietà della quale, e fortezza si vede molto bene convenire al legno della Santa Croce come habbiamo detti di sopra" (emphasis in the original).

for historical and natural philosophical information as well. Amatus's *Enarrationes* on Dioscorides' *De materia medica* is a fitting example of this. Furthermore, just as the character of medical commentaries welcomed biblical analysis, debates regarding biblical translation and the establishment of a reliable scriptural text inspired closer study of Holy Writ and motivated those with linguistic facility to learn its original languages and put them to use in their natural philosophic pursuits. Ulisse Aldrovandi, well known as a naturalist but unknown as a Hebraist, exemplifies this trend. Commentaries on Dioscorides and miscellaneous scientific investigations penned by Amatus and Aldrovandi embraced biblical analysis. Aldrovandi's studies of Pliny's *Natural History*, in turn, demonstrate how Hebraism facilitated scientific research.

2

Pliny, Papyrus, and the Bible

Several scholars in sixteenth-century Italy investigated writing practices in the ancient Mediterranean world. To comprehend the nuances of writing technologies in the distant past, early modern scholars looked for information in a variety of texts, including the Bible.

One aspect of scribal culture in the Bible that attracted Italian naturalists such as Ulisse Aldrovandi and his peers was the provenance, cultivation, and use of papyrus. For Melchior Guilandinus, for example, the prefect of Padua's botanical garden, papyrus became the subject of an entire book.[1] For the Bolognese naturalist Ulisse Aldrovandi, that plant assumed a prominent role in his unpublished history of ancient libraries, books, and writing technologies.[2] Renaissance humanists besides Guilandinus and Aldrovandi were particularly interested in paper, papyrus, and ancient forms of writing. Years ago, Charles Perrat explored how fifteenth- and sixteenth-century humanists, mostly French and Italian, scrutinized mentions of papyrus in classical texts, collected samples of it, and flocked to libraries, museums, and botanical gardens that possessed papyrus specimens.[3] More recently Anthony Grafton has written about divergences of opinion among sixteenth-century philologists on

1 *Melchioris Guilandini Papyrus, hoc est commentarius in tria C. Plinii maioris de papyro capita. Accessit Hieronymi Mercurialis repugnantia, qua pro Galeno strenue pugnatur. Item Melchioris Guilandini assertio sententiae in Galenum a se pronunciatae* (Venice: M. Antonio Ulmus, 1572).

2 BUB, Ms. Aldrovandi 83 (2 vols.), *Bibliologia*.

3 Charles Perrat, "Les humanistes amateurs de papyrus," *Bibliothèque de l'école des chartes* 109 (1951): 173–92.

the subject of papyrus in classical texts.[4] These contributions underscore the fascination ancient scribal culture held for humanists in Renaissance Europe.

We know less, however, about the overlapping fascination with the material aspects of ancient scribal culture and biblical natural history in early modern Europe. That fascination had roots in late antiquity. The Mishnah, which was compiled in the second century and quickly became one of rabbinic Judaism's foundational texts, emphasizes the importance of and the magic inherent in the Bible's writing implements. At several key points in the biblical narrative, God communicates by means of inscription, and aspects of that writing process attracted scholarly interest in late antiquity. The Mishnaic tractate Avot, for example, states that ten things were created at twilight on the eve of the Sabbath. Of those ten items, three concerned writing: writing itself, the script of the Ten Commandments, and the tablets upon which they were written.[5] The traditional belief that the stone upon which the Ten Commandments were inscribed was diaphanous and its script legible from either side was of special interest to many scholars. And not only early modern Jews, who traditionally studied tractate Avot every year between the festivals of Passover and Shavuot, were familiar with this particular rabbinic tradition; Christian scholars had access to it as well. Avot was included in Paul Fagius's 1541 Latin translation of the Mishnah.[6]

[4] Anthony Grafton, "Rhetoric, Philology and Egyptomania in the 1570s: J. J. Scaliger's Invective against M. Guilandinus's *Papyrus*," *Journal of the Warburg and Courtauld Institutes* 42 (1979): 167–94.

[5] Mishnah Avot, 5:6.

[6] *Pirke Avot. Sententiae vere elegantes, piae, mireque, cum ad linguam discendam tum animum pietate excolendum utiles, veterum sapientum Hebraeorum, quas* פרקי אבות *id est Capitula, aut si mavis Apophthegmata Patrum nominant: in Latinum versae, scholiisque illustratae: per Paulum Fagium in gratiam studiosorum linguae sanctae* (Isny: Paul Fagius, 1541). Twelve Hebrew books were printed in Isny during the sixteenth century. See Stephen G. Burnett, "Christian Hebrew Printing in the Sixteenth Century: Printers, Humanism and the Impact of the Reformation," *Helmantica* 51:154 (January–April 2000): 13–42, 18. For more on Fagius's interests in postclassical Hebrew, see Burnett, *From Christian Hebraism to Jewish Studies: Johannes Buxtorf (1564–1629) and Hebrew Learning in the Seventeenth Century* (Leiden: Brill, 1996), 134–68; for Fagius and his press at Isny, see Burnett, "Christian Hebrew Printing in the Sixteenth Century," 26. There were at least two other Latin editions of Pirke Avot available before 1570: one by Sebastian Lepusculus and one by Paul Weidner. Lepusculus's translation was appended to *Iosippus de Bello Iudaico deinde decem Iudaeorum captivitates* (Basel: Henrichus Petri, 1559); see Joseph Prijs, *Die Basler hebräischen Drucke 1492–1866* (Olten: Urs Graf-Verlag, 1964), 151–3, for a description of

But Aldrovandi and Guilandinus were not concerned with magic and miracles; they were interested in history and material culture. In the 1570s, Aldrovandi and Guilandinus probed the Bible for evidence of papyrus's origins and early purposes. Their analyses of papyrus indicate a larger, more complicated intellectual project: using biblical verses, removed from their context and stripped of their liturgical and theological significance, to clarify and emend other ancient writings, in this case Pliny's *Natural History*. There are numerous disputes about Pliny in the unpublished writings of Ulisse Aldrovandi and in the published, but rarely studied ones of Melchior Guilandinus. The prominent role of the Bible in those disputes illuminates connections between biblical studies and natural philosophy. For Aldrovandi and Guilandinus, using the Bible to adjudicate disputes about the *Natural History*'s accuracy led them to assess not only an august pagan authority but translations of the Bible itself.

In the sixteenth century, many commentaries were written on Pliny's *Natural History*, an encyclopedic work from the late first century CE. In the 1570s and 1580s, papyrus and its use in the ancient world commanded the attention of several Italian naturalists. Since Pliny's *Natural History* offered sixteenth-century scholars key information about papyrus, it was a fitting subject for analysis and an appropriate point of departure for a study of that plant.

Renaissance natural philosophers asked two sorts of questions about Pliny's work: lexical and evaluative. From the late fifteenth century onward, scholars worked to edit and publish the *Natural History*. To do so, they had to ensure that they understood the words Pliny used and recognized the objects in nature to which they referred. They also strove to evaluate the quality and accuracy of the information Pliny provided. For example, Pliny claimed that papyrus was first cultivated at a precise point in the history of the ancient Mediterranean: during the reign of Alexander the Great (fourth century BCE). Additionally, Pliny stated that paper was not commonly used until the reign of Ptolemy Philadelphus, in the middle of the third century BCE. According to Aldrovandi and Guilandinus, Pliny was wrong on both counts. Indeed, the stated goal

this text. For Weidner, see *Mishnah Pirke Abot sententiae hebraicae ad vitae institutionem perutiles breviter explicatae et praeclarissimis dictis tam Sacram quam aliarum Scripturarum illustratae a Paulo Weidnero* (Vienna: Michaël Zimmerman, 1563). I would like to thank Professor Burnett for this last reference.

of Guilandinus's book was to persuade the "stiff-necked reader" and "refute Varro," Pliny's original source, who proposed that nothing was written on paper before Ptolemy Philadelphus.[7]

One of the ways in which Aldrovandi and Guilandinus assessed the accuracy of statements like these was to compare Pliny's account of papyrus's early cultivation to that contained in the Bible. For those who were versed not only in booklore and natural philosophy but also in biblical languages, the antiquarian study of ancient writing technologies came to embrace the Bible as a source. In his *Bibliologia*, Aldrovandi used the Bible to write a definitive history of book culture in the ancient world. And in his commentary on Pliny, Guilandinus carefully examined scripture to gather as much information as possible about papyrus. Using the Bible in this manner meant treating it as an auxiliary text: they scrutinized its language and narrative in order to evaluate ancient pagan works of natural philosophy. When Aldrovandi and Guilandinus studied the Bible in Hebrew and Greek, their intention was not to perform biblical analysis; it was to understand Pliny's *Natural History* and the ancient world it described. To write a definitive natural history of papyrus, Aldrovandi and Guilandinus needed access to the Bible in its original languages. They knew that translations, especially the Vulgate, introduced inaccuracies when rendering the natural terminology of scripture into other languages.

These investigations into the natural world of the Bible had a secondary result. They did more than help Aldrovandi and Guilandinus understand the cultivation and applications of papyrus in the ancient Mediterranean; they clarified difficult terms in the Bible itself. Discussions of Pliny's reliability widened the scope of biblical studies and multiplied the applications of sacred learning at the end of the sixteenth century. In effect, Aldrovandi and Guilandinus helped expand the classical canon to include the Bible. They pioneered new, nontheological ways of reading scripture. In turn, the admission of biblical knowledge into scientific texts changed natural philosophy as well. It broadened the horizons of scientific writing at this time and created another venue in which biblical commentary could develop and diversify in the late Renaissance.

[7] Guilandinus, *Papyrus*, 129: "Ut vel unus hic locus sufficere possit non moroso et obstipa cervice lectori, ad refellendum Varronem, fidem suam interponentem non ante Ptolemaeum Philadelphum in chartis esse scriptitatum."

MELCHIOR GUILANDINUS

Melchior Wieland, or Guilandinus as he was known south of the Alps, was a botanist of international reputation. Shortly after his death, Luigi Lollino, a learned cleric of Belluno, penned a laudatory biography of him, which remains unpublished.[8] Though many details of his life are sketchy, a few basic facts are beyond dispute.[9] Born in Königsberg around 1520, Guilandinus began his studies in that city before moving to Rome as a young man. Eventually he relocated to Padua, where he made the acquaintance of Gabriele Fallopia, one of that university's most accomplished physicians. Under Fallopia's supervision, he "diligently and ingeniously made progress in all areas of learning."[10] Having earned the financial support of Marino Cavalli, a reformer of Padua's curriculum, he traveled throughout the Near East, including Palestine and Egypt, to study botany.[11] During his return journey he was captured by pirates and had to be ransomed by the Venetian authorities.[12] In September 1561, he succeeded Luigi Anguillara as the director of Padua's botanical garden. At that time he was appointed to a chair of "lecture and demonstration of medicinal herbs" at the University of Padua. Apart from a few practical inventions, including an irrigation machine that he developed

[8] Aloysio (Luigi) Lollino, "Melchior Guillandinus stirpium medicarum in Gymnasio Patavino Nomenclator," in his *Vite di Francesco Piccolomini, Jacopo Zabarella, Tommaso Peregrino, Melchiore Guillandino, Antonio Riccobono, Girolamo Mercuriali, Guido Pancirola, Faustino Sommo, Giuseppe Molezio, Bastesiano Monticolo, Professori nell'Univ. di Padova.* Belluno, Biblioteca civica, Ms. 505, 55v–60v. On Lollino, see *DBI* 65:449–53.

[9] The following is based partly on Loris Premuda's entry "Melchior Wieland," in *Dictionary of Scientific Biography* 14: 335–6. See also R. de Visiani, *L'orto botanico di Padova* (Padua, 1842), 9–12; and G. B. de Toni, "Melchiorre Guilandinus," in A. Mieli, ed., *Gli Scienziati Italiani I* (Rome: Casa Editrice Leonardo da Vinci, 1933), 73–6, which has the most thorough list of older scholarship on Guilandinus (esp. 76). In addition, see G. E. Ferrari, "Le opere a stampa del Guilandinus," in Giuseppe Bellini, ed., *Libri e stampatori in Padova* (Padua: Tipografia Antoniana, 1959), 377–463. None of these scholars mentioned Lollino's biography.

[10] Lollino, "Melchior Guillandinus stirpium medicarum in Gymnasio Patavino Nomenclator," 55v: "Italiam pervenit ad Gabrielem Falopium, medicorum sui aevi principem, apud quem sedulitate et ingenio in omni litterarum genere adeo profecit, ut brevi homo exterus scythicumque adhuc nescio quid olens, veluti Anacharsis alter, inter praesantes eruditione viros, quibus tunc Academia florebat, inclaresceret hospitis sui artes aemulatus."

[11] Ibid.: "quod dum agit, cupido illum, ut erat laboris inexhausti, incessit balsami, casamique et iunci odorati noscendi causâ Palaestinam, et Solis orientis conscia loca peragrare."

[12] Ibid., 55v–60r.

in 1575, Guilandinus published very little.[13] In 1557 a collection of letters entitled *De stirpibus … epistolae* was published.[14] The next year he wrote a short *Apologia* against Mattioli, and in 1572 he published *Papyrus*, a commentary on the chapters in Pliny's *Natural History* that describe that plant.[15] He also wrote two brief works that were published posthumously: a list of synonyms of plant names in the Paduan botanical garden and a report on the plants of the wealthy Venetian Pietro Antonio Michiel.[16] Guilandinus died on 18 January 1589.

Modern evaluations of Guilandinus have not been favorable; nevertheless, his career and writings merit further study. Loris Premuda, writing in the *Dictionary of Scientific Biography*, summed up scholarly consensus on Guilandinus when he opined that Guilandinus "left no writings of particular value."[17] Owing to the influence of comments like these, very little modern scholarship treats Guilandinus in any depth. But Guilandinus was a well-respected botanist at Italy's leading university. Lollino's biography of him is included in a collection of reminiscences about illustrious Paduan professors, including Francesco Piccolomini, Jacopo Zabarella, Antonio Riccoboni, and Girolamo Mercuriale.[18]

[13] Premuda, "Melchior Wieland." Premuda does not specify what those inventions were.

[14] *De stirpium aliquot nominibus vetustis ac novis, quae multis iam saeculis vel ignorarunt medici, vel de eis dubitarunt … epistolae II* (Basel: apud Nicolaum Episcopus Juniorem), 1557. It was reprinted in P. A. Mattioli's *Epistolarum libri V* (Lyon: apud Cesarem Farinam, 1564). The collection of letters was also published in 1558 under the title *De stirpibus aliquot epistolae V* (Padua: Gratiosus Perchacinus, 1558).

[15] *Apologia adversus Petrum Andream Mattiolum liber primus, qui inscribitur* Theon (Padua: Gratiosus Perchacinus, 1558).

[16] Johann Georg Schenck, *Hortus Patavinus, cui accessere Melchioris Guilandini coniectanea synonymica plantarum* (Frankfurt: Johann Theodor de Bry, 1608); *Judicium Melchioris Guilandini de quibusdam plantis horti Petri Ant. Michaelis*, published in G. B. de Toni, "Contributo alla conoscenza delle relazioni del patrizio veneziano Pietro Antonio Michiel con Ulisse Aldrovandi," *Memorie dell'Accademia di scienze, lettere ed arti Modena* (series 3) 9 (1908): 21–70.

[17] Premuda, "Melchior Wieland," 336.

[18] For information on Piccolomini and Riccobono, see N. Jardine, "Keeping Order in the School of Padua: Jacopo Zabarella and Francesco Piccolomini on the Offices of Philosophy," in Daniel A. di Liscia, Eckhard Kessler, and Charlotte Methuen, eds., *Method and Order in Renaissance Philosophy of Nature: The Aristotle Commentary Tradition* (Aldershot: Ashgate, 1997), 183–209; Heikki Mikkeli, "The Foundations of an Autonomous Natural Philosophy," in ibid., 211–28. Riccobono was the author of perhaps the best-known early modern work on the University of Padua. See his *De gymnasio patavino … commentariorum libri sex* (Padua: apud Bolzetam, 1598). On Zabarella, see Charles B. Schmitt, *Aristotle and the Renaissance* (Cambridge, MA: Harvard University Press, 1983), 10. On Mercuriale, see *DBI* 73:620–5.

Furthermore, Guilandinus maintained relationships with prominent physicians such as Gabriele Fallopia and learned theologians such as Girolamo Vielmi. He discussed the natural world of the Bible with both and seamlessly integrated biblical analysis into his examinations of natural history. Guilandinus's work is a complement to Aldrovandi's and shows that Aldrovandi's tendency to read the Bible alongside pagan natural philosophy was not exceptional; it was representative of a broader trend in the late Renaissance.

ALDROVANDI, GUILANDINUS, AND PLINY'S *NATURAL HISTORY*

The debate about Pliny's *Natural History* that Aldrovandi and Guilandinus entered into in the 1570s and 1580s was not new. Beginning at the end of the fifteenth century, European naturalists debated the merits of Pliny's encyclopedia and its proper application to humanist learning and medical science.[19] In the fifteenth century the *Natural History* was known as a text valuable for its many Latin words: because of its immense topical range, it provided rich vocabulary for Renaissance humanists to assimilate into their writings. In the late fifteenth and early sixteenth centuries, scholars tried to establish its scientific accuracy, or lack thereof. Nearly everybody agreed that new and more reliable editions of Pliny were needed. But they disagreed on the problem with existing texts. Some thought generations of editors and copyists had distorted Pliny's original intention.[20] Others argued that Pliny himself did not understand science as well as he might have.[21] Ultimately the debate centered on whether Pliny's book should be understood as a linguistic or a scientific resource. Some scholars – chiefly linguists and philologists – felt that the copiousness and diversity of *Natural History*'s vocabulary

[19] Charles G. Nauert Jr., "Humanists, Scientists, and Pliny: Changing Approaches to a Classical Author," *American Historical Review* 84:1 (February 1979): 72–85.

[20] The chief proponent of this argument was Pandolfo Collenuccio. See M. Santoro, "La polemica pliniana fra Leoniceno e Collenuccio," *Filologia Romanza* 3 (1956): 162–205; G. Pozzi's introduction to *Hermolai Barbari Castigationes Plinianae et in Pomponium Melam* (Padua: Antenore, 1973), cxxvii–cxxviii; F. Kudlien, "Zwei medizinische Polemiken am Ende des 15. Jahrunderts," *Gesnerus* 22 (1965): 85–92.

[21] The main advocate of this line of thinking was Niccolò Leoniceno. See, in addition to Nauert, "Humanists, Scientists, and Pliny," Vivian Nutton, "The Rise of Medical Humanism: Ferrara, 1464–1555," *Renaissance Studies* 11:1 (1997): 2–19.

was its chief virtue. Physicians and botanists, on the other hand, held that the book's identification and analysis of medicinal products was its best asset. Whatever their position, scholars could agree with Guilandinus's observation that there are "many very obscure places in Pliny" that came down to sixteenth-century scholars "not in the [true] words of Pliny but in the words of many other authors."[22] Whichever side of these battle lines a Renaissance scholar stood on, he agreed that it was necessary to draw from other works to understand Pliny.

Another point of agreement that united sixteenth-century students of Pliny was their belief that it was possible to restore the text, as Guilandinus put it, to its "old dignity." They disagreed only on the method of doing so. Guilandinus contended that other scholars may "not without due cause substitute one [word] for another or one topic for another topic by using another Greek or Latin writer."[23] Guilandinus's model for doing this was Niccolò Leoniceno (1428–1524), a physician and philologist from Ferrara who dominated Italian medical scholarship, especially its philo-Hellenic fields, in the late fifteenth and early sixteenth centuries.[24] Guilandinus, as well as others who attended Italian medical faculties in the 1540s and 1550s, was steeped in Leoniceno's writings and sympathetic to his intellectual perspectives. Though he never openly acknowledged Leoniceno's importance, Aldrovandi was one of his followers, too. Leoniceno's influence on sixteenth-century medical scholarship, which has been duly noted and traced by historians of medicine, also extended into the realms of classical philology and biblical studies.

More than any other scholar, Niccolò Leoniceno instigated the acrimonious debate about Pliny's reliability. In his *On the Errors of Pliny and Many Others in Medicine*,[25] he insisted that Pliny erred in his use

[22] Guilandinus, *Papyrus*, sig**r.

[23] Ibid., *4v: "Tamen non idem etiam protinus iudicium faciendum erit de Plinio, Solino, et caeteris id genus scriptoribus, qui quod res in natura existentes non carmine, sed soluta oratione, nec fabulose sue ficte, sed historica fide, et ut sunt, persequuti fuerunt, possunt non inepte alter per alterum, et alii multi per illos, et vicissim illi per alios multos cum Latinos, tum Graecos, qui idem argumentum tractavere, instaurari, atque in Veterum dignitatem, integritatemque restitui."

[24] The best introduction to Leoniceno's work is Daniela Mugnai Carrara, "Profilo di Nicolò Leoniceno," *Interpres* 2 (1979): 169–212.

[25] Niccolò Leoniceno, *De Plinii et aliorum in medicina erroribus* (Ferrara: Laurentius de Rubeis, 1492). I have used *De Plinii et plurium aliorum medicorum in medicina erroribus*,

of medicinal products for two reasons: he did not understand the Greek authors he read, and he lacked firsthand knowledge of the materials he was writing about. Ermolao Barbaro, whose position was contrary to Leoniceno's, blamed errors in Pliny's text on his commentators and editors, not on Pliny himself. Leoniceno's lasting contribution to this debate was to insist that Pliny's text should be emended with evidence from other ancient scientific texts – especially Dioscorides, Galen, and Paul of Aegina. The belief that scholars could improve their knowledge of unreliable ancient texts by consulting other, more reliable ones would have a significant impact on biblical studies. Followers of Leoniceno throughout the sixteenth century applied two of his scholarly tenets – that things are more important than words and that classical texts could reinforce each other – to their reading of the Bible. Because of Leoniceno and his influence, Aldrovandi and Guilandinus felt justified in borrowing from other classical texts to amplify the meaning of the Bible, as well as in their use of biblical passages to illuminate other ancient texts, such as Pliny's *Natural History*.

For Leoniceno, to study ancient botany, and natural science more broadly, was to focus on things rather than on words. "To philosophize truthfully seems to me," Leoniceno intoned, "to battle with barbarians not on the subject of words but on things that pertain to the health of many men."[26] Peter Dilg has articulated how Leoniceno's primary goal was not to restore the text of Pliny to a pristine, uncorrupted state but rather to discover the truth about actual substances used by ancient physicians.[27] That was a sentiment that Aldrovandi and Guilandinus could embrace. In fact, Guilandinus went so far as to say that he rejected and dismissed quibbles about "vain opinions" and instead preferred to "seek the truth about things." And one of Leoniceno's later followers,

libri quator, in *Nicolai Leoniceni Vicentini, philosophi et medici clarisssimi, opuscula* (Basel: Cratandrum, 1532), 1–61.

[26] See "Nicolaus Leonicenus Hieronymo Menochio Lucensi philosopho ac medico praestantissimo s. d.," in Leoniceno, *De Plinii … erroribus libri quator*, book 4, in *Opuscula*, 53v: "hoc sane mihi videtur vere philosophari, non de vocabulis, sed de rebus ad hominum salutem plurimum necessariis cum barbaris decertare."

[27] Peter Dilg, "Die botanische Kommentarliteratur italiens um 1500 und ihr Einfluss auf Deutschland," in August Buck and Otto Herding, eds., *Der Kommentar in der Renaissance* (Boppard: Boldt, 1975), 225–52, esp. 236–9.

the French physician Jacques Daléchamps, gave voice to this sentiment in his 1587 introduction to Pliny's *Natural History*:

> My mind has a natural proclivity to give precedence to those things that contribute to the understanding of the material rather than to those that are investigated and determined concerning the beauty and eloquence of speech, because I think that an understanding of the inner meaning of things is more useful for a wise man than vigor of expression and eloquent beauty.[28]

Throughout this debate, and especially in the language that Leoniceno and his followers used, the word *res*, or things, echoes in readers' ears.[29]

The emphasis of Leoniceno and his followers on *res* as opposed to *verba* is important in and of itself. But equally if not more important was his belief that the sorts of investigations he undertook should be applied to other fields of study. "It would not be an arduous task," Leoniceno insisted in his work on Pliny, if "known things [*familiaria*] were applied not only to medicine but to some other uses as well."[30] And, in fact, those "familiaria," or things known to be true, do really exist; they are not irretrievable ghosts of a distant past. "Things that exist in nature," Leoniceno's follower Guilandinus reflected, "are not employed by means of incantation, or set loose by speech, fable, or fiction, but exist according to faith in history, and, as such, may be employed."[31] Guilandinus insisted that the natural products that Pliny and his contemporaries wrote about could be identified and used in the medical practice of his own day.

[28] Jacques Daléchamps, *C. Plinii Secundi historiae mundi libri XXXVII* (Lyon: Bartholomeaus Honoratus, 1587), 3r: "primum igitur, ex quo studia humaniora degustavi, ea mihi fuit ingenita mentis propensio, ut quae ad rerum cognitionem faciunt iis anteponerem, quae ad ornatum et copiam orationis quaeruntur ac comparantur, quod arbitrarer interiorem literarum scientiam homini cordato magis convenire, quam dicendi vim ac facundam venustatem." I have used the translation in Nauert, "Humanists, Scientists, and Pliny," 85.

[29] On this theme, see Eckhard Kessler and Ian Maclean, eds., *Res et verba in der Renaissance* (Wiesbaden: Harrassowitz in Kommission, 2002).

[30] Leoniceno, *De Plinii ... erroribus libri quator,* book 1, in *Opuscula*, 5v: "neque enim impendio arduum esset, si non omnia, saltem earum pleraque cognoscere, quae adeo familiaria sunt ut non modo ad medicinam, sed ad alios quoque usus aliquando adhibeantur."

[31] Guilandinus, *Papyrus,* *4v: "qui quod res in natura existentes non carmine, sed soluta oratione, nec fabulose seu ficte, sed historica fide, et ut sunt, persequuti fuerunt." On *fides historica*, see Anthony Grafton, "The Identities of History in Early Modern Europe: Prelude to a Study of the *Artes Historicae*," in Gianna Pomata and Nancy Siraisi, eds., *Historia: Empiricism and Erudition in Early Modern Europe* (Cambridge, MA: MIT Press, 2005), 41–74, 41, 49.

Given this emphasis on the medical application of Pliny's writings, Leoniceno's quest to understand the Roman natural philosopher was not an empty intellectual exercise; it was a pressing concern undertaken for the benefit of others. Guilandinus said as much when he gushed that he was "extremely desirous for the public good."[32] Because the *Natural History* mentioned scores of medicinal products, it was advantageous for doctors to read Pliny closely.[33] Long before Guilandinus took up the topic, Leoniceno lamented that "there are very few who read Pliny for his medical teachings; more read him for his vocabulary and – it cannot be denied – his divine eloquence."[34] Since doctors prescribed items listed in Pliny's book without knowing the text, it was of utmost importance that they know which medicaments the author actually referred to. "It is not without great danger," Leoniceno wrote, that doctors prescribe medical products from ancient writings without knowing precisely what they are. To have full control over those products, many doctors grew herbs in their own botanical gardens. As Leoniceno put it, "There is no one who does not have [those drugs] in their botanical garden, and who does not use them frequently."[35] Pliny's text had clear medical applications, and those applications demanded precise identification of its terminology.

For Leoniceno, in order to correct Pliny it was necessary to seek out other classical texts. Leoniceno believed that, because Pliny was a venerated writer, the stakes were high in criticizing him. Writing to Angelo Poliziano, the dedicatee of his *De Plinii ... in medicina erroribus opus*, he noted that he did not approach Pliny "with rash judgment" but rather with "most firm reasons."[36] And he insisted in a letter to Poliziano that

[32] Guilandinus, *Papyrus*, sig**r: "quoniam quidem mihi publicae utilitates cupidissimo non aggrediendi voluntas defuerit, sed perficiendi facultas."

[33] Between books 20 and 34 of the *Natural History* alone, more than nine hundred medical products are listed, more than in Dioscorides or Galen. See Giovanna Ferrari, *L'esperienza del passato: Alessandro Benedetti filologo e medico umanista* (Florence: L. S. Olschki, 1996), 177.

[34] Leoniceno, *De Plinii ... erroribus libri quator,* book 3, in *Opuscula*, 22v: "paucissimi enim sunt qui Plinium propter medicinas legant, plures propter vocabula et divinam, quod negari non potest, elocutionem."

[35] Ibid., 5v: "quum tamen nemo sit qui illa in horto suo non habeat, ac non eisdem frequentissime utatur."

[36] Ibid., 2v: "pauca tamen e multis hoc in loco censui aperienda, ut intelligas me non temerario iudicio sed certissimis rationibus adductum, ut existimarem Plinium ita in haederae descriptione, quemadmodum in multis aliis ad medicinam pertinentibus aberrasse."

the way to do this properly was to find complementary passages in other classical authors. Leoniceno explained that Pliny was often mistaken, as he was in his description of *marubio*.[37] "Dioscorides, Galen, and Paul," Leoniceno observed, "wrote about many herbs and stalks with leaves similar to *marubio*, which Pliny rendered [incorrectly] as *prasso* rather than *prassio*."[38] Elsewhere Leoniceno bemoaned the fact that "many [things] lie hidden from us, and if we thus endeavor to read the books of the ancients ... in this manner, we ought not to ignore other authors who show much ostentation but little utility."[39] In other words, even when a topic seemed irrelevant, it was important for Niccolò Leoniceno to seek out other authors who might amplify his understanding of a given topic, regardless of their other merits or demerits. For example, Leoniceno lambasted Pliny for confusing the plants *hedera* and *cithon*. In his remarks on *hedera*, Pliny distinguished between the male and female forms of the plant and stated that both had a flower "like a wild rose." That description of *hedera* did not correspond to the works of "Theophrastus, Dioscorides, or any man of weighty authority." But, Leoniceno argued, that distinction did apply to *cithon*. Pliny erred because the Greek words for *hedera* and *cithon* (*kissos* and *kisthos*, respectively) were so similar that the Roman naturalist simply mixed them up.[40] Leoniceno used his encyclopedic knowledge of ancient botanical texts, and his skills as a Hellenist, to point out one of Pliny's egregious mistakes.

[37] On *marubio* in pre-Linnean nomenclature, see Caspar Bauhin, *Pinax theatrum botanicum* (Basel: Impensis Johannis Regis, 1671 [1623]), 229 and 236, where *marubio*, or *marrubium*, is a translation of πράδιον. Dioscorides discusses this plant in book 3, chaps. 119–20.

[38] Leoniceno, *De Plinii ... erroribus*, book 1, in *Opuscula*, 2r: "multas herbas ac frutices foliis marubio similibus scribunt Dioscorides, Galenus ac Paulus, quas omnes Plinius non prassio, id est marubio, sed prasso, id est porro, folia tradit habere similia." According to Leoniceno, the correct translation for *marubio* is *prasio*, which comes from the Greek πράσιον, or white horehound, an herb. See Lewis and Short, *A Latin Dictionary* (Oxford: Oxford University Press, 1991 [1879]), s.v. *prasion*. The "Paul" Leoniceno refers to is Paul of Aegina, a seventh-century Byzantine physician whose works were available in several editions by the late fifteenth century.

[39] Leoniceno, *De Plinii ... erroribus libri quator*, book 1, in *Opuscula*, 5r–v: "multa nos latent, quae si veterum libros ita legendos censeremus, sicuti Calculatores, Iacobos, Conciliatores, Plusquam commentatores reliquosque huiuscemodi autores, in quibus plurimum ostentationis, minimum utilitatis, non ignoraremus."

[40] Ibid., 13r–15r. Brian Ogilvie discusses this passage from Leoniceno in his *The Science of Describing: Natural History in Renaissance Europe* (Chicago: University of Chicago Press, 2006), 127–8.

For Leoniceno and his followers, a reliable way to ensure accuracy in reading Pliny was to be an expert in Greek philology, especially that branch concerned with medicine. Since Pliny had borrowed many terms from Greek texts, it was essential for the student of Pliny to know the sources from which he drew. Vivian Nutton has described the crucial importance Leoniceno assigned to Greek, and Daniela Mugnai Carrara has documented the many Greek manuscripts in Leoniceno's library.[41] Leoniceno insisted that one had to know Greek in order to study Pliny:

> What they should do in this matter, since they have never pored over medical studies, nor the authoritative works of Greek physicians, to which I adhere in my opinions worthy of confirmation, or if they at last began to read them, since they do not know Greek, indeed they cannot understand one word unless those things which were impudently edited under their name were taught them by other people. Even though they do not seem to have composed anything for themselves, they fight over Pliny with quarrels and reproaches.[42]

Insistence on the importance of Greek underlay not only Leoniceno's work but that of Melchior Guilandinus and Ulisse Aldrovandi.

FROM PLINY TO THE BIBLE: LEONICENO'S LEGACY IN THE LATER SIXTEENTH CENTURY

By the end of the sixteenth century, finding complementary passages to supplement an understanding of Pliny meant not only seeking out other texts of pagan origin but also exploring the Bible as well as patristic and rabbinic literature. Melchior Guilandinus's work on Pliny provides a good example of this tendency. At one point in his *Papyrus*, Guilandinus cites

41 Nutton, "The Rise of Medical Humanism"; Mugnai Carrara, "Profilo di Nicolò Leoniceno."

42 Leoniceno, *De Plinii … erroribus libri quator*, book 2, in *Opuscula* 13v: "Quid enim ipsi agerent, quum neque medicinae studiis unquam incubuissent, neque graecorum medicorum autoritates, quas ego in meis sententiis confirmandis adhibueram, unquam legissent, aut si nunc demum legere inciperent, quoniam graecas litteras ignorarent, nec unum quidem verbum possent intelligere nisi ab aliis illa docerentur, quae sub suo nomine erant impudenter aedituri et, ne nihil de suo interseruisse viderentur, iurgiis atque conviciis pro Plinio contenderent."

passages in Cicero and Livy concerning the use of writing implements in the classical world. And then, seamlessly, Guilandinus quotes the Deuterocanonical Bible: "In the first book of Maccabees, in chapters 8 and 14, we read that he rewrote [the epistle] on brass tablets, first to the Romans and then to the Spartiates, which they sent to Jerusalem in order to establish friendship and fellowship with them."[43] For Guilandinus, the canon of classical sources included the Bible: he commented on biblical paraphernalia as comfortably as he did on pagan writing implements. Moreover, Guilandinus invoked the Bible not as an inerrant authority that stood apart from and above the rest of classical literature but as a source simultaneously sacred and historical that could confirm his contention about the antiquity of writing.

Italian natural philosophers who sought out biblical support for their arguments were not satisfied to quote the Latin Bible; they consistently reached for Greek, Hebrew, and Aramaic versions. Melchior Guilandinus and Ulisse Aldrovandi personify this tendency to reach past the Vulgate and toward the Septuagint and the Hebrew original when they looked for biblical proof texts. Though not a Hebraist, Guilandinus in his discussion of the word *byblus* sought out a Greek word and a rabbinic interpretation to understand a biblical verse, which in this case has nothing to do with the topic of books or writing. "We read in Ezekiel chapter 8," Guilandinus noted, "'Behold, the women sat there crying for *Adonidis*.' [Scripture] wants to say that it was idolatry celebrated in honor of Adonidis. For Adonidis, the Septuagint has *Thammous*, which is a Hebrew term." Guilandinus sought out a Greek version of scripture to understand the particulars of this biblical verse. But he was not content to know that Thammous was a Hebrew term; he wished to know what its precise associations were. So he turned to Maimonides.

[43] Guilandinus, *Papyrus*, 60–1: "M. Tullius scribens in Catilinam ait aera legum in Capitolio fuisse tacta de coelo, et liquefacta. Livius quoque decadis quartae libro 3 memorat consulta olim fuisse relata in aedem Cereris ad aediles, et decadis primae libro 2 faedus ictum cum Latinis fuisse insculptum in aenea columna. Sed et in primo Machabaeorum capitibus 8 et 14 legimus tum Romanos, tum Spartiatas rescripsisse Iudaeis tabulis aereis, quas Hierosolymam miserunt de stabilienda cum eis amicitia et societate." One such passage may indeed be found in 1 Maccabees 8:22, "Et hoc rescriptum est quod rescripserunt in tabulis æreis, et miserunt in Hierusalem, ut esset apud eos ibi memoriale pacis et societatis." The other is from chapter 12, not 14. See 1 Maccabees 12:1–2, "et vidit Ionathas quia tempus eum iuvat, et elegit viros, et misit eos Romam statuere et renovare cum eis amicitiam. Et ad Spartas, et ad alia loca misit epistolas secundum eandem formam."

"Rabbi Moses of Corduba" informed Guilandinus that Thammous was a prophet of the Zabites.[44] Recourse to a Greek Bible translation and then to a medieval Jewish commentator helped Guilandinus understand a biblical verse with greater accuracy.

Guilandinus's colleague Ulisse Aldrovandi was even more explicit about the problems inherent in consulting the Latin Bible. The Bible was "finally translated into the Latin language much later," Aldrovandi reminded his readers. He also informed them that Latin was the least elevated of the ancient tongues.[45] When studying scripture, he suggested, it was best to go back to Greek and Hebrew if at all possible. In order to truly know what the Bible said, it was imperative to read it in its original languages. Aldrovandi often sent his readers back to the Hebrew and Greek versions of scripture, as he did in a passage in which he wanted to emphasize that the Ten Commandments were given to Moses on stone tablets.[46] And in a related comment about engraving and writing, Aldrovandi quoted the book of Job [19:23], which mentions books "sculpted in stone." The Vulgate Bible has "flint" for stone, but Aldrovandi quoted the Greek, which has "lead or stone"– a more faithful rendering to Aldrovandi's mind.[47] Emphasizing that the Vulgate did not accurately convey the true meaning of the biblical verse, Aldrovandi quoted the Septuagint to support his point about engraving practices in the ancient world.

It was a short jump from bypassing the Vulgate and seeking out earlier, more authoritative versions of scripture to criticizing the Vulgate's

[44] Guilandinus, *Papyrus*, 32: "Unde apud Ezechielem prophetam capite VIII legitur: Ecce sedebant ibi mulieres plangentes Adonidem. Ubi intelligi vult fuisse idololatriam celebratam in honorem Adonidis. Septuaginta ibi pro Adonide habent Θαμμούζ vocem Hebraicam." See ibid., 33, for mention of Maimonides. For Maimonides' remarks about Tammuz as a prophet of the Sabeans, see *Guide for the Perplexed,* part 2, chap. 29.

[45] See his essay "Quali lingue tra l'altre siano state sempre li più nobili," in *Bibliologia* 1:438–42, 441.

[46] Ibid., 36: "Il capitolo 22 in Essodo dove Iddio parla à Mose, volendo dare gli dieci commandamenti dice: 'Ascende ad me in montem et esto ibi daboque tibi את לחות האבן tabulas lapideas etc.' in greco τὰ πυξία τὰ λίθινα, si che si vede che in tutti i testi cioè questa voce lapidea, come anco nel Caldeo לוחין אבנא [*sic*: לוחי אבנא] luche abna."

[47] Ibid., 8: "vel sculpantur in silice? Le quali parole dalli Settante Interpreti sono scritto in greco in questo modo: τίς γὰρ ἄν δοίη γραφῆναι τὰ ρήματά μου, τεθῆναι δὲ τὰ αυτὰ εν βιβλίῳ εἰ̂ς τὸν αἰῶνα ἐν γραφείῳ σιδηρῷ και μολίβδω [*sic*: μολίβῳ] ἢ ἐν πέτραις ἐγγλυφῆναι quis enim utique det ut scripta sint verba mea, ut posita sint autem ea in libro in seculuum in stylo ferreo et plumbeo aut in petris isculpta est." See Job 19:23–4.

translator, Jerome. Indeed, for Aldrovandi and Guilandinus, as well as for scholars who desired accuracy in their reading of the Bible, Jerome's Vulgate translation did not suffice. It was not that Jerome was always wrong; on the contrary, Aldrovandi occasionally praised him. In an extended essay on papyrus, he approvingly cited Jerome's translation of the Hebrew term "in the reeds" (*betoch hasuph*) as "in papyrus." In that particular instance, the Greek text was less helpful: the Septuagint had "in the swamp" (*en to helei*).[48] But commendation of Jerome was frequently paired with criticism of his translation of the Bible's naturalistic language. In an essay entitled "De volumine," Aldrovandi remarks, "In Exodus chapter 22 [*sic*: 24:7] Jerome translates *volumen federis* [volume of the covenant] where the Hebrew text has the word *sepher*, which means book. Almost everywhere else he translates this word as book [*liber*] but here he translates it as *volumen*."[49] Significantly, the portion of this phrase that mentioned "covenant" was less important to Aldrovandi than the part that mentioned "book"; his interest lay in the realm of physical bibliography rather than theology.

Aldrovandi's keen interest in ancient scribal culture drew him to passages in the Bible that mentioned writing implements and the materials from which they were made. Upon examining those biblical verses, Aldrovandi recognized Jerome's limitations as a translator and his inability to depict the Bible's natural world with accuracy. He reflected that

> in the second chapter of Exodus Jerome translated this word *suph* as reed grass, which is a place abundant in fronds. When scripture says "when she saw a wicker basket in the papyrus," [the Hebrew word] *basuph* [might mean] reed grass by the shore of the river; some explain this word to mean algae. We read in Jonah 2:6 "the water surrounded me to my very soul; an

48 Aldrovandi, *Bibliologia*, 1:2: "sarà ben da avertire che in quel loco dove S. Girolamo traduce 'in papyrione' che 'l testo hebreo ha בתוך betoch che vuole dire in mezzo; et certamente S. Girolamo ha detto bene dicendo 'papyrione' essendo che quel fiume era pieno di papyro, come dalle parole di sopra si comprende dove la Scrittura dice: 'et exposuit eum בסוף bassuph in carecto,' perchè 'suph' apresso gli Hebrei si piglia per un luoco pieno di gronchi et papiri et significa ancora propriamente un gronco. Gli Settanta interpreti non hanno questa parola 'scirpeam' ma solamente 'θήκην' cio cistello, et dove S. Girolamo dice 'papyriones' loro hanno 'ἐν τῶ ἕλει' cio nella pallude."

49 Ibid., 35: "In essodo al capito 22 S. Girolamo traduce volumen federis dove il testo Hebreo ha parimente quella voce ספר sepher, che significa libro; la quale in quasi tutti gli altri luoghi della bibia traduce libro: et nondimeno traduce qui volume" (emphasis in the original).

> abyss opened to me." [Could we translate] *suph habush leroschi* as "algae came up to my head?" Because *suph* also means the depth of the sea and the deep sea, Saint Jerome translated it as such: "The deep sea overcame my head."[50]

If Aldrovandi admits that Jerome was correct to translate *suph* in the book of Jonah as simply "the deep sea" and not "algae," there is a subtler point here: Jerome was mistaken about the name and nature of the Sea of Reeds. A few lines later, Aldrovandi adds, "For *suph* Jerome says red."[51] Because of Jerome's rendering in the Vulgate, centuries of readers had understood the Sea of Reeds to be the Red Sea. By comparing different uses of the word *suph*, Aldrovandi showed that while the term had a figurative meaning in the book of Jonah, its meaning in Exodus was unambiguous: it meant reed.

And Aldrovandi was not alone in his criticism of Jerome. Guilandinus also maintained that the Vulgate could not supply the precision he was looking for. In a letter to the Polish botanist Stanislao Rosario, who was then employed in the botanical garden in Padua, Guilandinus wrote that in Genesis 6 God commanded Noah to build an ark from *gopher* wood. For Guilandinus, *gopher*, an ambiguous Hebrew term, should be translated as cedar. The Vulgate, incorrectly, had it as pine.[52]

[50] Ibid., 905: "Girolamo in Essodo al secondo capitolo tradusse questa parola 'suph' pro iunceto, che è un luogo ove nasce gran copia di frondi. Quando dice: 'quae cum vidisset fiscellam in papyrione' et v. 3: 'et possint בסוף basuph' id est in iunceto 'iuxta ripam fluminis' alcuni expongono questa voce per alga, come si legge in Jonah 2.6: 'circumdiderunt me aquae usque ad animam, abyssus aperuit me סוף חבוש לראשי suph chabusch le roschi id est alga alligata est capiti meo' et perchè 'suph' significa ancora il profondo del mare et il pelago, però S. Girolamo ha tradotto: 'pelagus operuit caput meum.'"

[51] Ibid., 905–6. "Questo è una sorte de gronchi che nasce nelle rive de' fuimi et ne' lidi del mare, et però il mar Rosso per nascer ivi gran copia de gronchi, pappiri et simile piante è chiamato 'Iam suph' che si può interpretare algosum come leggemo in Essodo 10.19: 'infixit eam ימה in mare סוף algoso,' che san Gerolomo dice Rubro."

[52] Melchior Guilandinus Borussus R. Stanislao Rosario Polono S.P.D. *Plinii et Dioscoridis error demonstratus. Cedrum magnam, Laricem esse probatur. Ghopher apud Moysen quid. Item Agaricum non nisi in Laricum truncis gigni. Inibi duo Plinii loci emaculati* in *De stirpibus aliquot, epistolae V: Melchioris Guilandini* (Padua: Gratiosus Perchacinus, 1558), 8r: "siquidem in libro divini Pentateuchi primo capite sexto refers Deum Optimum Maximumque mandasse Nöae ante supremum illum cataclysmi diem, quo universum genus humanum, atque cuncta animalia terrena delere voluit, uti arcam eximiae magnitudinis ex lignis Gopher, hoc est cedri construeret, qua se suosque et animalia pauca ab imminenti clade interituque erueret. Nec obstat quod in Vulgata aeditione ex lignis pineis fabrefactam legimus."

Though Guilandinus does not explicitly state that the Vulgate erred, the implication is clear: the Vulgate, at least in its references to natural phenomena, is an unreliable source for one who desires an accurate rendering of scripture. For all his learning, Jerome did not possess the expertise of Pliny in matters of natural philosophy.

In spite of this considerable skepticism regarding the Vulgate's accuracy, natural philosophers believed that knowledge of the geographic and naturalistic details of scripture was possible. As Guilandinus assured his readers, "I shall state [matters] in the most accurate Greek, Latin, and Hebrew words, so that the reader might understand that nothing is about to be pronounced rashly regarding the names that pertain to geography in the Old Testament."[53] And for scholars such as Guilandinus and Aldrovandi, accurately defining biblical terms was not a theological challenge. They sought to use biblical words and phrases as elements in their natural historical arguments. When its precise meaning was accurately understood, the Bible was a text that could furnish historical proof.

One reason the Bible was valued as a historical source was its antiquity. In his work *Papyrus*, Guilandinus attempted to identify the biblical city Tanis. His sources were the biblical books Psalms, Isaiah, and Numbers, as well as Josephus's *Antiquities*. Since Moses lived six hundred years before Homer, Guilandinus asked rhetorically, why turn to Homer for geographic data about biblical cities when the Bible itself provides it?[54] Guilandinus informed his readers that biblical information is more reliable than Greek wisdom primarily because it is older. His stated source for this notion was Josephus. The Greeks' knowledge of antiquity is "to be laughed at," Guilandinus intoned, citing Josephus's *Against Apion*.

[53] Guilandinus, *Papyrus*, 78: "Adscribam ipsissima verba Graece, Latine, Hebraice, ut intelligat lector, nihil temere esse pronunciandum de nominibus, quae ad geographiam in vetere instrumento pertinent." For an excellent discussion of early modern efforts to understand the Bible's geography, see Zur Shalev, "Sacred Geography, Antiquarianism and Visual Erudition: Benito Arias Montano and the Maps in the Antwerp Polyglot Bible," *Imago Mundi* 55:1 (October 2003): 56–80; and *Sacred Worlds and Words: Geography, Religion, and Scholarship, 1550–1700* (Leiden: Brill, 2012).

[54] Guilandinus, *Papyrus*, 75: "Tanim autem, in qua Moyses sexcentis amplius annis Homero antiquior praeclara illa, et stupenda miraculorum facinora edidit, etiamne Homero iuniorem dicemus? David Psalmo 77: coram patribus eorum fecit miracula in terra Aegypti in campo Taneos. Esaiae 20: Stulti principes Taneos, sapientes consiliarii Pharaonis dederunt consilium insipiens. Tanta vero est civitatis istius antiquitas, ut Moyses Numerorum 13 septem tantummodo annis recentiorem faciat Hebrone, quam Hebronem inhabitavit Abraham patriarcha referente Iosepho libro 1 antiquitatum Iudaicarum, capite 8."

Josephus, Guilandinus explained, taught that "historical knowledge of ancient things is to be sought not from the Greeks but from the Egyptians and Chaldeans." Even though the Greeks have a reputation for their historical prowess, they should be considered "adolescents" and not "adults" in world history. Guilandinus accepted Josephus's argument: the further back one could go, and the farther east one could reach, the more accurate the knowledge one could obtain.[55] Guilandinus stated the maxim with even greater clarity when he suggested that "he who desires to know the truth of ancient history ... should inquire into [the works of] the Egyptians, Tyrians, and Chaldeans."[56]

Guilandinus's faith in the Bible's ability to provide accurate information concerning natural knowledge was strong. It was so strong, in fact, that he took it upon himself to correct other biblical translations in addition to the Vulgate. In a notable display of bravado, Guilandinus went so far as to propose a correction to the Septuagint text. The basis for his dissatisfaction was not textual corruption or philological proof; it was natural knowledge. In his discussion of a passage in Isaiah 18 (18:2), which mentions ships made of papyrus transversing water, he notes that the Vulgate has "papyrus vessels" for these ships. Upon examination, the Septuagint's text was even less helpful. Guilandinus told his readers that "for 'papyrus vessels' the Septuagint has *epistolas biblinas*, whereas I might translate it as *entolas biblinas*, that is, sent forth on paper."[57]

But the most compelling reason to use the Bible as a historical document was that it debunked Pliny's and Varro's theory about the history of

55 Ibid., 79: "Quam Graecorum circa cognitionem antiquitatis ridendam infantiam, copiose prosequitur sacrificulus ille eodem in loco, et magnopere post eum elevat Iosephus in principio statim operis, quod contra Appionem condidit. In quo docere volens non a Graecis antiquarum rerum historiam requirendam esse, sed ab Aegyptiis, et Chaldaeis, quorum fuit institutum, ut eorum sacerdotes, et philosophi circa scribendam historiam versarentur, mirari sese inquit eos, qui tantum Graecis tribuunt in historia, cum ipse docere paratus sit Graecos non modo adulto iam mundo, ut ita dicam, sed etiam propemodum senescente natos, eorumque inventa omnia esse recentia."

56 Ibid., 80: "proinde qui vetustae historiae veritatem nosse cupiat, hunc oportere dicit ab Aegyptiis, Tyriis, et Chaldaeis exquirere."

57 Ibid., 129: "Malo quoque spineo, et velis ex biblo utuntur. Proinde Esaias propheta interminaturus Aegypto, exorditur caput XIIX his verbis: Vae terrae cymbalo alarum, quae est trans flumina Aethiopiae, quae mittit in mare legatos, et in vasis papyri super aquas. Ubi Septuaginta pro vasis papyri habent ἐπιστολὰς βιβλίνας, quas ego interpretor ἐντολὰς βιβλίνας, id est mandata in chartis descripta." See Isaiah 18:2.

papyrus cultivation in the ancient Mediterranean. For both Aldrovandi and Guilandinus, the Bible contained numerous passages that testified to the cultivation and use of papyrus long before Hellenistic times, the period to which Varro, and subsequently Pliny, dated papyrus's emergence. For example, quoting both the Vulgate and the Septuagint, Guilandinus observed that Moses was placed in the Nile protected by a "papyrus basket." Guilandinus observed that the Hebrew word here is *gome*, which he knew meant papyrus. He supplemented his assertion by quoting David Kimḥi, the twelfth-century Jewish exegete and lexicographer, who, Guilandinus pointed out, explained that *gome* was a "very light plant, from which ships were made."[58] And Ulisse Aldrovandi was even more explicit in connecting the Bible's statements about papyrus to Pliny's argument about its recent cultivation. "On the strength of Varro's statement," Aldrovandi explained, "Pliny says that paper was found during the victory of Alexander the Great.... But in truth it seems to me that Marcus Varro greatly deceives us, since paper was used before Alexander the Great." In fact, Aldrovandi continued, "the use of paper or papyrus is much older than what Varro says, for here [Isaiah 18] one should understand papyrus vessels to mean ships or, more precisely, an oblong galley ship." For Aldrovandi, the Aramaic paraphrase of this portion of scripture made the association between "papyrus vessels" and ships explicit.[59]

As enthusiastic as Aldrovandi and Guilandinus were about biblical sources, they were just as enthralled with other ancient Jewish writings,

[58] Guilandinus, *Papyrus*, 129–130: "Illustravit etiam naves papyraceas Moysis ad huc infantis in aquam abiectio, quem ἐν θὶβῃ παπύρου, id est in fiscella papyracea, vel, ut vulgata editio habet, stirpea [*sic*: scirpea], ad Nilum Aegypti fluvium expositum fuisse, legitur Exodi secundo. Cumque iam celare non posset, inquit propheta, sumpsit fiscellam scirpeam, et linivit eam bitumine, ac pice, posuitque intus infantulum, et exposuit eum in carecto ripae fluminis. Vocabulum Hebraicum ibi est GOME, quod Rabi David Kimḥi exponit plantam levissimam, unde fiunt naves." The phrase ἐν θὶβῃ παπύρου does not appear in Exodus 2. The noun πάπυρος is not to be found here.

[59] Aldrovandi, *Bibliologia*, 4: "vuole Plinio per sentenza di Marco Varone che la charta fosse trovata nella vittoria di Alessandro Magno, essendosi edificata Alessandria in Egitto, et vuole, che avanti non si usasse la charta nell'uso della quale principalmente consiste l'humanità e la memoria della vita; ma mi pare in verità che Marco Varrone di gran longa s'inganna essendo stato l'uso della charta avanti Alessandro Magno." See also ibid., 3: "Perchè l'uso della charta over papiro è molto più antico di quello scrive Marco Varrone. Che in questo luoco per 'vasi di papira' si debba intendere gli navigii, et principalmente una nave oblonga over galera si coglie dal testo caldeo che ha in questo luogo ובדגוגין ubidgugejan id est 'in

notably Philo and Josephus. The two sixteenth-century naturalists liberally drew on those Greek Jewish thinkers and used their writings to debate Pliny's merits and demerits. Even though neither Philo nor Josephus was a contemporary witness to biblical events, and neither was reputed to be an expert on Near Eastern flora, their exposition of the Bible was of considerable interest to Aldrovandi and Guilandinus. In their quest to understand the natural terminology of the Bible, and to use that terminology to clarify other ancient texts, Philo and Josephus were trusted authorities.

Josephus was especially popular in the sixteenth century.[60] Guilandinus turned to his *Antiquities* when he wanted to know more about the basket Moses' mother used to place him in the Nile. "In book 2, chapter 5, of the *Antiquities* Josephus describes the basket in which Moses was deposited into the Nile. And he calls it *plegma biblinon empheres tei kata skeuei koitidi*, that is, papyrus material similar to that which is used to bind together birds' nests." Guilandinus, often prone to quibble with translations, pointed out that Gelenius's rendering of this passage "was hardly competent."[61] And Aldrovandi referred to Josephus, too. On the subject of the material on which the translators of the Septuagint wrote, Aldrovandi noted that "we have, on the testimony of Josephus in book 12 of the *Antiquities* that the books of the Jews which Eleazar sent to Ptolemy were written on vellum."[62]

trieribus' come ha la translatione della paraphrase chaldea." A *trieris* is a galley ship with three banks of oars; the Aramaic דגוגא (pl.: דגוגין) simply means a small fishing vessel. See Targum to Isaiah 18:2.

60 For an introduction to studies of Josephus in the Middle Ages and Renaissance, see Peter Burke, "A Survey of the Popularity of Ancient Historians, 1450–1700," *History and Theory* 5:2 (1966): 135–52.

61 Guilandinus, *Papyrus*, 130: "Iosephus libro II archeologias, capite V describens arculam, in qua Moyses in Nilum depositus fuerat, vocat eam πλέγμα βὶβλινον ἐμφερὲς τῇ κατα σκευῇ κοιτίδι, id est texturam papyraceam similem compagi cunae. Quem locum Gelenius, qui libros eos in Latinum vertit haud bona fide reddidit." See Josephus, *Antiquities*, 2:220. Gelenius translated the relevant passage thusly: "lectulo e papyro contexto, quantus infantulum commode capere poterat, bitumineque illito, ne aqua penetrare posset, indiderunt puerum." *Flavii Iosephi Opera, in sermonem Latinum iam olim conversa* (Basel: Froben, 1567), 46. On Sigismundus Gelenius (ca. 1498–1554), see Peter G. Bietenholz, ed., *Contemporaries of Erasmus: A Biographical Register of the Renaissance and Reformation*, 3 vols. (London: University of Toronto Press, 1985), 2:84–5.

62 Aldrovandi, *Bibliologia*, 7: "Habbiamo per testimonio de Giuseppe nel 12 lib dell'antichità che i libri degli Hebrei mandati da Eleazaro a Tolomeo erano scritti in pelli."

Though not as well known to sixteenth-century scholars, Philo was an important source, too.[63] Although the *Biblical Antiquities* had been falsely attributed to Philo, as Guillaume Budé showed in the sixteenth century, many scholars, Jewish and Christian alike, read that work and considered it authentic.[64] The Pseudo-Philonic *Biblical Antiquities* aided Guilandinus's investigation of *gopher* – a wood so mysterious that the translators of the King James Bible could not find an English equivalent. Guilandinus's proof that *gopher*, the Hebrew word used in the book of Genesis, meant cedar and not pine came from Jewish sources rather than pagan or Christian ones. He wrote that "Philo Judaeus, a most serious author, wrote in his book called *Biblical Antiquities*, that [the ark] was 'made from cedar.' The most erudite of the Jews confirms this, since all of the Talmudists and the Targum[im], Rabbi Nathan [ben Yeḥiel of Rome], Rabbi Yehoshua the son of Karah [*sic*: Korha], and others as well, state unanimously that *gopher* is cedar."[65] For Melchior Guilandinus, Talmudic rabbis provided the most important evidence that *gopher* should be understood as cedar and not pine.

63 On Philo in the sixteenth century, see Joanna Weinberg, "The Quest for Historical Philo in Sixteenth-Century Jewish Historiography," in A. R. Rapoport-Albert and S. Zipperstein, eds., *Jewish History: Essays in Honour of Chimen Abramsky* (London: P. Halban, 1988), 163–87.

64 Ibid., 167, 181 n. 32. Azariah de' Rossi, for example, thought the *Liber Antiquitatum Biblicarum* was genuine. See ibid., 172–4.

65 Guilandinus, *De stirpibus* 8r: "quando Philo Iudaeus, gravissimus auctor in libello cui titulus Biblicae antiquitates, scribit ex cedrinis compactam fuisse: quod ipsum comprobant Hebraeorum eruditissimi, Thargum Talmudistae omnes, R. Nathan, R. Iehosua filius CarchaK, & ceteri, Ghoper Cedrum uno ore omnes exponentes." For the passage in Pseudo-Philo, see Guido Kisch, ed., *Pseudo-Philo's Liber Antiquitatum Biblicum* (Notre Dame, IN: University of Notre Dame, 1949), 115: "et nunc facito tibi arcam de lignis cedrinis." On Rabbi Nathan ben Yeḥiel of Rome, see my discussion in Chapter 3. Rabbi Yehoshua ben Korha was a *tanna* who lived in the mid-second century CE. He is quoted in the Mishnah and in Midrashic literature. See *EJ* 2:452–53. Guilandinus's source for this information was almost certainly Sante Pagnini, *Thesaurus linguae sanctae*. I have used the edition published by Stephanus in Paris, 1548, s.v. גופר, p. 181: "Est (inquit R. D. in li. ra. [Rabbi David Kimḥi in libro radicis]) lignum leve super faciem aquarum. Thargum קדרוס cedri, hoc est cedrinus. Thalmudistae quoque Hebraeorum, quator dicunt esse cedri genera videlicet קדרוס עץ שמן וברוש ארז. In Beresíth rabbáh, R. Nathán exponit lignis דקדרונא cedri. Idem R. Iehosúah filius Carcháh." Regarding the "others" Guilandinus mentions, apart from the unnamed "Thalmudistae" in Pagnini's entry, Guilandinus might have known that Targum Onkelos ad loc. translates *gopher* as קדרום, an alternate spelling for קדרוס, or cedar. Baḥya ibn Paqudah, in turn, cites Targum Onkelos and writes that "gopher is a wood that is called *cedrus*, and it floats on water." See his commentary to Genesis 6:14. Guilandinus may have also been aware of Targum Onkelos by reading the Antwerp Polyglot. See *Biblia Sacra* (Antwerp: Plantin, 1568–72), 8 vols., 1:18–19. See p. 18 for Targum Onkelos and p. 19 for the "chaldaicae paraphrasis translatio," where דאעין דקדרום is rendered as "de lignis cedri."

At times, no source – Jewish, Christian, or pagan – could satisfy Guilandinus or Aldrovandi. In a telling letter to Andreas Patricius, another man affiliated with Padua's botanical garden, Guilandinus analyzed the mysterious plant *kikaion* mentioned in the book of Jonah.[66] In it, Guilandinus is even more vociferous about the inaccuracy of biblical translations. This time Jewish commentators as well as Christian ones earned his disapprobation. The very title of his letter showed his dissatisfaction: "[In which] it is indicated that the Septuagint translators, Aquila, Saint Augustine, Jerome, and Rabbi Ibn Ezra were wrong. It is proved by recent discovery that *kikaion* is *ricinus* [castor oil plant], as opposed to the opinion of all interpreters of the sacred pages of the Jews."[67] Guilandinus was sensible of the fact that he might be accused of excessive boldness in reworking this passage of Jonah. Nevertheless, he emphasized that he was "truly driven to show what the prophet of Nineveh meant when he named the plant *kikai*."[68]

To Guilandinus, fathers of the Western church such as Augustine and Jerome "seemed to fight" over the proper translation of this term, and they wrote "many letters [to one another] on this matter."[69] The Septuagint translated *kikaion* as κολόκυνθα, which had been rendered as *cucurbita* [gourd] in the Vetus Latina. Augustine preferred the old Latin translation *cucurbita*, which Jerome used in his commentary on Jonah.[70] But in Jerome's Vulgate he translated *kikaion* as *hedera* [ivy].[71]

[66] Guilandinus, *De stirpibus*, 11r: Melchior Guilandinus Borussus R. Andreae Patricio Polono S.P.D. Andreas Patricius Polonus (Andrzej Patrycy Nidecki, 1522–87) was a Polish humanist. Patricius published a collection of *Fragmenta* from Cicero: *Fragmentorum M. Tullii Ciceronis Tomi IV. Cum Andr. Patricii adnotationibus* (Venice: apud Iordanum Ziletum, 1561).

[67] Guilandinus, *De stirpibus*, 11r: "Indicatur 72 interpretum, Aquilae, D. Augustini, Hieronymi, & R. Abrahae lapsus, atque KiKaion Ricinum esse praeter omnium sacrae Hebraeorum paginae interpretum opinionem recens invento dogmate comprobatur."

[68] Ibid., 11v: "proinde ego quoque quanquam mihi in eius rei comprehensione (absit arrogantia dicto) non nihil tribuo, tamen ad diffinitionem timide accedo: nec quam ipse serio persuasus sum, tam animose polliceri audeo demonstraturum me tibi ad oculum, qualem Propheta ille Ninivitanus KiKai nomine plantam significaverit."

[69] Ibid., 12r: "nam cum illic exemplaria hebraica habeant KiKaion, nequaquam vel Hederam, vel Cucurbitam vertere oportebat, ut acriter inter se atque pertinaciter digladiari videantur Augustinus et Hieronymus, multis super ea re epistolis conscriptis."

[70] See Paul Antin, ed., *Saint Jérome sur Jonas* (Paris: Sources Chrétiennes, 1956), 108, 113, and 115. See also *PL* 25:1147–50.

[71] Augustine and Jerome exchanged several letters on this topic, which Jerome referred to as the "ridicula cucurbitae quaestio." On this exchange, see J. L. Heller, "Notes on the Meaning of κολοκύντη," *Illinois Classical Studies* 10:1 (1985): 67–116, 81–91.

According to Guilandinus, both were wrong: *kikaion* "ought to be translated as neither gourd nor ivy."[72] *Kikaion* ought to be understood as *ricinum*, or castor oil plant.

The proof for this, as Guilandinus admitted, could be found in Jerome's own description of the plant.[73] "The *kikaion,*" Jerome wrote, "is a kind of shrub, having wide leaves similar to a vine shoot. When transplanted, it soon springs up as a sapling, without the support of any stalk or shaft." Jerome further observed that gourds and ivy do not need external support, since they "support themselves with their stem."[74] Guilandinus knew that Jerome and Augustine were wrong not because he was a better philologist but because he was a botanist. He knew what the plants they described looked like and how they grew. His experience in Padua's botanical garden, coupled with his deep knowledge of Pliny, helped him identify *kikaion* as *ricinus*, or castor-oil tree.

Guilandinus arrived at this identification by broad reading in botanical literature. A plant that exhibits the characteristics of *kikaion* – "rising up into a great shrub, supporting itself on its own stalks, requiring no external support, having leaves like a grape vine or gourd, growing very quickly to a great height, and called *El Keroa* in Syriac" – could be "nothing other than the castor oil plant."[75] As sources for this information, Guilandinus cited various authorities: Ebenbithar, Avicenna, Serapion, Rhazes, and Isahac.[76] To them he added a Jewish commentator, Rabbi Samuel, whom Guilandinus read at secondhand in Sante Pagnini's *Thesaurus linguae sanctae* and who equated *kikaion* with the Arabic *Al Keroam*.[77]

[72] See note 69.

[73] Guilandinus, *De stirpibus*, 13r, "quando Kikaion Ricinum esse, tum Hieronymi verba comprobant."

[74] Ibid., 12v: "Est autem Kikaion genus virgulti lata habens folia in modum pampini, cumque plantatum fuerit, cito consurgit in arbusculam, absque ullis calamorum et hastilium adminiculis, quibus et Cucurbitae et Hederae indigent, suo tronco se sustinens." Jerome, *Epistola* 112. For discussion, see J. L. Heller, "Notes," 84–7.

[75] Guilandinus, *De stirpibus*, 13r: "Etenim arbusti magnitudine consurgere, propriis caulibus inniti, nullis adminiculis aegere, folia ferre Vitis seu Cucurbitae, repente in altitudinem excrescere, et El Keroa a Syris appellari, nulli plantae praeterquam Ricino convenit."

[76] Ibid.: "auctores habeo Ebenbithar, Avicennam, Serapionem, Rasin, Isahac, caeteros."

[77] Ibid.: "adstipulant nostrae sententiae ex Hebraeis interpretibus R. Samuel, citante Pagnino in linguae sanctae Thesauro, Kikaion Arabice AlKeroam vocari perhibens." I have used the Paris, 1548, edition of Pagnini's *Thesaurus linguae sanctae*, p. 1160: "קיק, unde קיקיון, Haederam quidam vertunt … Harabice vocatur אל כרוע inquit R. Semuel." Rabbi Samuel

Guilandinus censured Jewish scholars as often as he praised them. For as remiss as Augustine and Jerome were in translating *kikaion*, at least they attempted to do so. The same could not be said for Abraham Ibn Ezra, whom Guilandinus upbraided immediately after citing Rabbi Samuel. "I do not rashly repudiate the opinion of Rabbi Abraham, who in his commentaries dared to say that by no means may one know what sort of plant the *kikaion* may be."[78] This was a generous misquotation. In the original Hebrew, Ibn Ezra's attitude toward the *kikaion* is even more dismissive. He wrote that "the Spanish sages say that it is a gourd or a poppy. But there is no need to know what it is."[79] For Ibn Ezra, it was not so much that the identity of the plant cannot be known but that there is no good reason to even try to identify it. Guilandinus was appalled.

For the German botanist there simply had to be a way to translate *kikaion*. And he knew that he was bucking a trend. "With great constancy and determination, I defend and protect [my translation], which, as you see, is against the opinion of all interpreters."[80] Guilandinus supported his assertion that *kikaion* should be understood as the castor oil plant by relying on an authority he knew well: Pliny. In *Natural History* Pliny describes a plant called *cici*, whose behavior is similar to that of *kikaion*, whose name had an etymological resemblance to it, and which was "a very common tree in Egypt."[81] Furthermore, Pliny indicated that "some call it [*cici*] *croton*," a Greek term understood as *ricinum* in Latin. For that Greek term, Guilandinus relied on Pliny, too.[82] Although Guilandinus never cites Pliny, it is clear the Roman naturalist was his main source.[83]

is Samuel ben Hophni (d. 1013), Gaon of the rabbinical academy at Sura. On him, see *EJ* 17:770–1.

78 Guilandinus, *De stirpibus*, 13r: "proinde non temere opinionem R. Abrahae reiicio, qui in Commentariis suis affirmare ausus est, cuiusmodi planta sit KiKaion, sciri nulla ratione posse."

79 Ibn Ezra to Jonah 4:6 חכמי ספרד אומרים דלעת או קרה ואין צורך לדעת מהו

80 Guilandinus, *De stirpibus*, 13v: "Ego de Hebraeorum KiKaio contra omnium ut vides interpretum sententiam magna constantia et asseveratione tueor atque defendo."

81 Pliny, *Natural History*, 15:25, "Proximum fit e cici, arbore in Aegypto copiosa (alii crotonem, alii sibi, alii sesamon silvestre eam appellant), ibique, non pridem et in Hispania, repente provenit altitudine oleae, caule ferulaceo, folio vitium, semine uvarum gracilium pallidarumque."

82 Ibid.: "Nostri eam ricinum vocant a similitudine seminis … at in Aegypto, ubi abundat, sine igni et aqua sale adspersum exprimitur, cibis foedum, lucernis exile."

83 Guilandinus, *De stirpibus*, 13r: "Verum enimvero KiKaion, quam Keruam et AlKeroam Arabes nominant, Graeci κρότωνα appelant."

Guilandinus boasted about the support for his theory that he received from the famous anatomist Gabriele Fallopia, the "pillar of the Paduan Academy," who "greatly admired my opinion about *kikaion* … and embraced it with both of his arms."[84] An endorsement for his translation from an illustrious colleague – the "prince of physicians in his time," in the words of a seventeenth-century writer – was important to Guilandinus.[85] And the fact that more than one notable Italian botanist concurred with Guilandinus's assessment lent his argument a patina of legitimacy.

Guilandinus's invocation of Fallopia signals an important aspect of his intellectual project: collaboration. More than a century ago, Charles DeJob argued that the biggest difference between biblical studies in the Middle Ages and the Renaissance could be explained by one word: collaboration.[86] Guilandinus discussed biblical natural history with Paduan theologians in addition to natural philosophers. For example, Girolamo Vielmi's 1575 published lectures on Genesis credit Guilandinus with helping him understand Genesis 1:11 and its mention of "seed-bearing plants."[87] Vielmi refers to Guilandinus as "a most learned man, easily the prince of botanical matters in our time," and relates that they discussed the matter "in casual conversations."[88] The connection between theologians and naturalists is even more explicit in Aldrovandi's case. *Bibliologia*, which contains many discussions of the Hebrew language and biblical *naturalia*, was undertaken at the request of a friend, Camillo Paleotti, the brother of Gabriele, Bologna's bishop. "The first book of

[84] Ibid., "Gabriele profecto ille Fallopius, Patavinae Academiae columen … in nullis non sententiam de KiKaio nostram obvio ore exosculatur, atque ambabas ulnis amplexeratur."

[85] Luigi Lollino, "Melchior Guillandinus stirpium medicarum in Gymnasio Patavino Nomenclator." For full citation, see note 8. Fallopia is described as "medicorum sui aevi princeps." On Fallopia, see *DBI* 44:479–86, where his botanical interests, in addition to his anatomical accomplishments, are discussed.

[86] Charles DeJob, *De l'influence du Concile de Trente sur la littérature et les beaux-arts chez les peuples catholiques: essai d'introduction à l'histoire littéraire du siècle de Louis XIV* (Paris: Ernest Thorin, 1884), 32.

[87] On Vielmi, see Antonino Poppi, *Ricerche sulla teologia e la scienza nella scuola padovana del Cinque e Seicento* (Soveria Mannelli: Rubbettino, 2001), 69ff. I am grateful to Matthew Gaetano for this reference.

[88] Girolamo Vielmi, *De sex diebus conditi orbis liber* (Venice: Giunta, 1575), 335: "Melchior Guilandinus vir doctissimus, et rei herbariae nostra tempestate facile princeps … cum familiaribus colloquiis mecum." I would like to thank Matthew Gaetano for bringing this passage to my attention.

my *Bibliologia*," Aldrovandi recollected in another context to his patron Gabriele, "which deals with the antiquity of letters ... and the use of that very noble paper made in Egypt from papyrus, was written to the illustrious Signore Camillo Paleotti, your brother."[89] As was the case with many of his other writings, *Bibliologia* was dedicated to Gabriele.[90]

Even though Aldrovandi undertook many of his most colorful explorations of the Bible's natural world at the urging of two powerful clergymen in Bologna, he also indicated in side comments that a broader and more extensive group bore responsibility for *Bibliologia*'s genesis. "I am extremely busy and have no leisure time," Aldrovandi lamented, "distracted on the one hand by my private and public studies, and on the other by many friends who constantly write me, and to whom I must respond and explain my opinion about many things that they ask me, in this Natural History."[91] Rather than being the result of a few friends' quest to understand the place of nature in scripture, Aldrovandi's writings on the Bible were the result of widespread interest.

One relationship that had special significance for Aldrovandi's project to decipher the natural language of scripture was his friendship with Benito Arias Montano.[92] Aldrovandi boasted that the Spanish polymath had come to see him and his museum. He remembered when "Arias Montano, that most learned theologian, extremely well versed in ten different languages, and most learned in every kind of science, came to see my museum when he was in Italy."[93] Aldrovandi had many famous visitors

[89] Ms. Aldrovandi 6 (3 vols.), *Lettere e Discorsi*, "Avvertimenti di Ulisse Aldrovandi sopra alcuni capitoli della pittura," 107–17r, 109r–109v: "ho trattato nel primo libro della mia Bibliologia, scritta hora all'Illustre Signore Camillo fratello di V.S. Illustrissima, parlando dell'antichità delle lettere, avanti che si scrivesse et ritrovasse l'uso della carta fatta dal Papiro pianta nobilissima di Egitto." The letter is dated 5 December 1581 (117r).

[90] In his *Bibliologia* Aldrovandi never states this explicitly. See, however, Ms. Aldrovandi 124, vol. 6, dedication.

[91] Aldrovandi, *Bibliologia*, 1:1: "et anchora che io sia molto preocupato che mai non havessi minimo otio, trattenuto parte da mei studii particolari et publici, parte da tanti amici che di continuo mi scrivono, a quali è necessario servirli et dirgli il parer mio di molte cose che mi chiedono in questa historia naturale."

[92] On Arias Montano, see most recently Theodor Dunkelgrün, "The Multiplicity of Scripture: The Confluence of Textual Traditions in the Making of the Antwerp Polyglot Bible (1568–1573)" (PhD diss., University of Chicago, 2012). See also Maria Portuondo, *Secret Science: Spanish Cosmography and the New World* (Chicago: University of Chicago Press, 2009).

[93] Aldrovandi, *Bibliologia*, 1:426: "Ario Montano huomo dottissimo, teologo versatissimo in dieci lingue diverse; che in ogni sorte di scienza e dottrina il quale è sta' a visitare il mio museo, quando è stato in Italia."

come to his museum, but few enjoyed Arias Montano's international reputation. And none was as renowned for their contributions to biblical studies. Comparing Arias Montano's remarks about biblical natural history to Aldrovandi's throws the unusual nature of Aldrovandi's engagement with biblical realia into sharper relief. And studying the way Aldrovandi borrowed from the editor of the Antwerp Polyglot illustrates how widely admired and broadly used Arias Montano's magnum opus was. Finally, observing how Aldrovandi moved beyond Arias Montano's scholarship indicates the limits of theological biblicism for natural philosophers. Though Arias Montano's *Apparatus* to the Antwerp Polyglot could stimulate Aldrovandi's thinking, it could not provide him the answers he sought.

Occasionally Aldrovandi relied on Arias Montano for information about biblical terms. For example, Aldrovandi's extended discussion of *yam suph*, or the Sea of Reeds, was motivated by a comment he openly acknowledged reading in one of Arias Montano's works:

> Benedict Arias Montano, in the third volume of [his] biblical appartus [called] Phaleg, which deals with the dimensions of the earth, says that the Red Sea is called *yam suph* because of the abundance of *gronchi* or papyrus and other similar plants that are used to make writing implements. Suph means *gronco*, or papyrus according to some because it has a stem similar to the *gronco* but a triangular [one], as we have proved elsewhere.[94]

But as we have already seen, Aldrovandi's work went far beyond Arias Montano's; he described the *gronco*, or reed, at great length and specified the difference between the Hebrew term when it meant "reed" and when scripture employed it as a metonym for sea. Aldrovandi acknowledged his source so openly because both he and his readers knew that Arias Montano did not have the final word when it came to matters of natural philosophy. To Aldrovandi, Arias Montano's *Apparatus* provided a stimulant to further investigation.

[94] Ibid., 1:904: "Il Benedetto Aria Montano nel terzo tomo delli Apparati biblici Phaleg dove trata della dimensione della terra, dice che il mare Rosso è chiamato iam suph dalla copìa di gronchi over pappiro et simil piante che sono atte à fare istrumenti da scrivere. Perche suph significa propriamente gronco, overa papiro secondo alcuni, perche fa un fusto simile al gronco ma triangolare come altrove habbiamo provato." See Benito Arias Montano, *Biblia sacra*, vol. 8: *PHALEG, sive de gentium sedibus primis, orbisque terrae situ, liber* (Antwerp: Plantin, 1572), 10.

The same may be said for other passages throughout Aldrovandi's writings. Aldrovandi knew that the Hebrew term עט [*et*] in the Bible means an iron writing implement because it was exclusively paired with the adjective *barzel* – Arias Montano pointed this out in his *Apparatus*.[95] Similarly, Aldrovandi could write about the etymology of *sepher* (book) and emphasize how it originally connoted storytelling, reporting, and narration as opposed to any specific physical property because of a helpful definition of Arias Montano's that Aldrovandi repeated almost verbatim, yet which he did not cite.[96] Finally, Aldrovandi wrote an extended essay on the connections between writing, engraving, and drawing – arts that he considered to be variations of the same central practice, and derivative of the same verbs: *grapho* in Greek and *khakak* in Hebrew.[97] Once again Arias Montano was his most likely source for this idea.[98]

Their divergent discussions of writing in the Bible provide a final example of how Aldrovandi borrowed from but did not duplicate Arias Montano's scholarship. We have already seen how extensive Aldrovandi's discussion of biblical writing and scribal culture is. Arias Montano's *Biblia Regia*, which Aldrovandi owned and thus very likely read,[99] was much briefer and of a different character. In his *Apparatus*,

[95] Aldrovandi, *Bibliologia*, 1:8: "dove il testo latino dice 'stylo ferro et plumbi lamina' il greco testo ha 'ἐν γραφείῳ σιδηρῷ καὶ μολίβδῳ [*sic*: μολίβῳ]' in Hebraico 'בעט-ברצל ועפרת' [*sic*: בעט-ברזל ועפרת] et veramente 'berzel' in hebreo significa proprio ferro, alla qual voce può esser venuto il nome de 'pranzello' che appresso lui ha la potestà delle arme, che si fanno di ferro." Benito Arias Montano, *Biblia sacra*, vol. 7: *Thesauri hebraicae linguae, olim a Sante Pagnino Lucensi conscripti, epitome* (Antwerp: Plantin, 1572): 85, defines the term "עט" as "Stylus aut Calamus: Psal. 45,2 (& Iob 19,24 ubi בעט solum coniungitur cum ברזל ferrum ac si de stylo ferreo; non vero cum plumbo quod postea sequitur)."

[96] Aldrovandi, *Bibliologia*, 1:24: "si legge ספר sepher che significa ben libro ma viene dal verbo ספר saphar che significa raccontare narrare scrivere." Cf. Arias Montano, *Biblia sacra*, vol. 7: *Thesauri hebraicae linguae … epitome*, 80: "ספר Recensere, numerare, narrare, referre, nunciare."

[97] See "Avvertimenti di Ulisse Aldrovandi all Illustrissimo Cardinal Paleotti sopra alcuni capitoli della pittura," in Ms. Aldrovandi 97, *Miscellanea de animalibus et plantis*, 465r–480v, esp. 475r–476r. Paleotti wrote a treatise on painting: *Discorso intorno alle imagini sacre et profane diviso in cinque libri* (Bologna: Alessandro Benacci, 1582). On this work, see Paolo Prodi's introductory remarks to the modern edition in Paolo Prodi, ed., *Discorso intorno alle imagini sacre et profane* (Bologna: A. Forni, 1990).

[98] Arias Montano, *Biblia sacra*, vol. 7: *Thesauri hebraicae linguae … epitome*, 32: "חקק Statuere, scribere, describere, pingere, depingere."

[99] Aldrovandi owned and annotated the *Biblia sacra*. It is mentioned in all three manuscript catalogs of Aldrovandi's library – see BUB Mss. Aldrovandi 27, 107, and 147. Aldrovandi also notes that he made use of Arias Montano's *Apparatus Biblici* in BUB Ms. Aldrovandi

Arias Montano defined the verb "to write" and the noun "writing" in a single entry. That entry summarizes the Spanish polyglot's approach to a practice that was, after all, technological and cultural as opposed to merely linguistic. His entry begins with the observation that "the greatest use for writing is to communicate news of things and actions." He also observed that "writing is a dependable way to pass on news, both to those who are absent and to posterity." When Arias Montano turns to scripture, he provides five biblical quotations, eight from the Old Testament and one from the New Testament, that contain some form of the word "to write" or "writing."[100] But he never uses biblical quotations to contribute to a freestanding history of ancient scribal culture, as Aldrovandi did. The distinction between the two biblical scholars is not evidence of Arias Montano's shortcomings compared to Aldrovandi's achievement; it merely underscores their different scholarly dispositions and illustrates Aldrovandi's propensity to treat the Bible as a text that could enrich natural philosophy.

ALDROVANDI AND OTHER CONTEMPORARY *BIBLIOLOGIAE*

Another way to understand Aldrovandi's tendency to integrate biblical analysis with other sorts of investigations is to compare his *Bibliologia* to other works in that genre. By discussing scribal culture, writing implements, and book history, Aldrovandi was participating in a scholarly trend

48, *Methodus theatri biblici naturalis*. See the list "Authores quibus utor in Theatro Biblico naturali," 1r–1v, 1r.

[100] Benito Arias Montano, *Biblia sacra*, vol. 8, *Liber Ioseph sive de arcano sermone* (Antwerp: Plantin, 1571), chap. 86, "de rebus humano usui inventis," 99: "SCRIBERE, SCRIPTURA: scribendi usus maximus est ad communicandam rerum actionumque notitiam: quando quidem verba ore prolata cum praesentibus tantum communicari possunt, eaque semel emissa non constant, atque auditorum mente saepe excidunt. Scriptura vero eadem multis constansque est; et commissam sibi sententiam fideliter refert, atque ab absentes et ad posteros quoque transmittit, s.s.e. 'Scribe hoc ad monumentum filiis Israel' [Exod. 17] Igitur memoriae conservandae significationem scripturae usus habet. ut, 'Scribes ea super posteis,' etc etc [Deut. 11] 'Ecce scriptum est coram me; non tacebo' [Isa. 65] Testimonii quoque exhibendi et contestandae rei causa res scribuntur, ut 'Scribite vobis canticum istud' [Deut. 31] et Iosue 'scripsit super lapides' [Josh. 8], etc etc 'legem regni scripsit in libro' [I Sam. 10] et 'Scribe visum, et explana sermonem.' [Habac. 2] Rem praeterea maximam, et scitu dignissimam, ac utilissimam scribendi cura alicui imposita significat. ut, 'Audivi vocem de caelo dicentem mihi, Scribe; Beati mortui qui in Domino moriuntur,' etc. [Apocal. 14]. Scribitur aliquid in palmis ad recordationem. ut, 'Ecce in manibus meis scripsi te' [Isai. 49]."

that was well established in his time. At the beginning of the seventeenth century, Justus Lipsius published his *De bibliothecis syntagma*, a study of ancient libraries.[101] Closer to the completion of Aldrovandi's *Bibliologia*, two other Italians wrote works that addressed similar themes: Angelo Rocca, the author of *Bibliotheca Apostolica Vaticana*, and Mutio Pansa, who wrote *Della libraria vaticana*.[102] Neither dealt with the Bible as a source for the history of books and writing, but each was interested in papyrus, Hebrew literature, and the connections between them.

While Rocca's work made little use of Jewish sources and took even less interest in papyrus,[103] Pansa discussed papyrus at length in his *Della libraria vaticana*. Pansa's composition began as a history of the Vatican's collection but grew to embrace a general history of writing. It mentions the Bible more than Rocca's work did but far less than Aldrovandi's. Rocca noted the "heroic acts of the Jews" and observed that Adam's nephews, sons of Seth, created two columns, one of stone and the other of brick, on which they wrote "all arts."[104] These columns, which contained

[101] See Paul Nelles, "The Renaissance Ancient Library Tradition and Christian Antiquity," in R. de Smet, ed., *Humanists and Their Libraries* (Brussels: Peeters, 2002): 159–73; Nelles, "Juste Lipse et Alexandrie: les origines antiquaires de l'histoire des bibliothèques," in Christian Jacob and Marc Baratin, eds., *Le pouvoir des bibliothèques. La mémoire des livres dans la culture occidentale* (Paris: Albin Michel, 1996), 224–42. Lipsius's work was first printed in 1602 and is available in volume 3 of his *Opera Omnia*, 8 vols. (Antwerp: Moretus, 1637). Onofrio Panvinio's *De biblioteca vaticana* was published by Juan Baptista Cardona at Tarragona in 1587. See Nelles, "The Renaissance Ancient Library Tradition," 166; the work was part of Panvinio's *De rebus antiquis*, which remains unpublished. See ibid., 165 and n. 21 for more about Panvinio.

[102] Angelus Rocca, *Bibliotheca Apostolica Vaticana a Sixto V Pont. Max. in splendidiorem, commodioremque locum translata* (Rome: Typographia Apostolica Vaticana, 1591); Mutio Pansa, *Della libraria vaticana ragionamenti divisi in quattro parti* (Rome: Giovanni Martinelli, 1590). For a survey of writings on books and libraries in the early modern period, see Alfredo Serrai, *Storia della bibliografia. V. Trattatistica biblioteconomica*, ed. Margherita Palumbo (Rome: Bulzoni, 1993), 121–92; on Rocca specifically, see 146–55.

[103] For example, in his opening list of "auctorum," or authorities, he mentions "Aben Ezra, Abraam Levita, Gedalia Iachia," all of whom he assigned the honorific "rabini" to. His book does contain an appendix on various uses of writing, including papyrus. Nevertheless, his sources are all works of pagan antiquity; only Josephus, whom he mentions twice, has any connection at all to Jewish literature (see pp. 377 and 380). Still, in neither instance did Josephus directly contribute to Rocca's history of papyrus.

[104] Rocca, *Bibliotheca Apostolica Vaticana*, sig. *3v: "cose Heroiche fra gli Hebrei; tutte l'arti." Rocca's source was almost certainly Josephus, *Jewish Antiquities*, trans. H. S. J. Thackeray (Cambridge, MA: Harvard University Press, 1967), 4.33. For more on these pillars, see Albertus Frederik Johannes Klijn, *Seth in Jewish, Christian and Gnostic Literature* (Leiden: Brill, 1977), 24 n. 82; John Douglas Turner, *Sethian Gnosticism and the Platonic Tradition* (Louvain: Éditions Peeters, 2001), 122.

a digest of Eastern wisdom, made their way to the West through Rome, by the initiative of the "early emperors." Pansa indulged in fairly standard praise for Adam, noting that "he gave a name to all things according to their nature and their properties; no one would ever understand so perfectly the paths of the constellations and the movements of the planets and stars or know so completely the nature of herbs, plants, animals, and all other things in the world as well as he."[105] Such remarks pepper Pietro Andrea Mattioli's more popular work, too.[106]

Pansa's history of papyrus, contained in his first discourse on the "Use of Books and Invention of Letters," presents a conventional account of the natural history of papyrus, and, following Varro, he dates its use to a remarkably late period, Hellenistic Egypt, after the translation of the Septuagint. He claims that after the composition of the Septuagint "a certain kind of paper was found that came from certain small trees called *papiri*, which is a sort of reed similar to cane. It grows in the still waters of the Nile, though Pliny says that they are also in Syria by the Euphrates River."[107] Pansa also insisted that he himself had seen a sample of papyrus and noted that "it was shown to me by the excellent signor Castor Durante, my instructor of blessed memory. While he studied in the Collegio [of Rome], he obtained a sample of it from Padua by the courtesy of Signor Cortuso, very accomplished in the profession of [medicinal] simples."[108] Cortuso was in charge of the botanical garden at

[105] Pansa, *Della libraria*, 2: "Adamo fù creato in somma perfettione da Dio, e di tanto sapere, e di tanta congitione ch'egli impose il nome a tutte le cose secondo la loro proprietà, e natura, e che niuno intendesse mai si bene i giri de cieli, i movimenti de pianeti, e delle stelle, e cognoscesse si perfettamente la natura dell'herbe, delle piante, degli animali, e di tutte l'altre cose del mondo qunato egli."

[106] *Petri Andreae Matthioli medici Caesarei et Ferdinandi Archiducis Austriae Opera quae extant omnia: hoc est, Commentarij in VI. libros Pedacij Dioscoridis Anazarbei de medica materia* (Frankfurt: ex officina typographica Nicolai Bassæi, 1598), sig *2r: "Quod vero rerum omnium scientiam in Adam infuderit ab initio Deus, facile quidem coniicere quisque potest ex Mosaicis monumentis libro primo Geneseos."

[107] Pansa, *Della libraria,* 6: "Fù poi trovata una certa sorte di carta che si faceva da certi piccioli alberi chiamati Papiri, che è una sorte di giunchi simili alle canne, che nascono ne'lagumi del Nilo, se ben Plinio dice, che ve ne sono nella Siria appresso il fiume Euphrate."

[108] Ibid., 7: "Et io affermo haver visto uno di questi Frutici in Roma, mostratomi dall'Eccellente Signor Castor Durante di buona memoria mio precettore, mentre studiava in quel Collegio, havuto da Padoa dal Signor Cortuso, intendentissimo della professione de semplici." Castore Durante's (1529–90) most popular works were *Herbario novo* (Rome: Bartholomeo Bonfadino, & Tito Diani, 1585) and *Il tesoro della sanità* (Pisaro: Bartholomeo Cesani, 1565). See *DBI* 42:105–7, and also Dennis E. Rhodes, *La vita e le opere di Castore*

Padua, where he succeeded Guilandinus, and he had a degree in medicine. Durante was the author of several books of botanical history. While Pansa captures the empirical and botanical spirit of inquiry, he does not think to examine other texts that testify to papyrus's ancient origins. Surprisingly, Pansa failed to connect the fact that Durante's sample of papyrus came from Egypt to the obvious associations between papyrus and Egypt in the early chapters of the book of Exodus. Aldrovandi did integrate Exodus into his study of papyrus. The fact that he did so is testament to his consistent interest in the Bible and his vision of that text's central role not only as a spiritual and divine work but as one that could help scholars write more comprehensive history.

Clearly, Guilandinus and Aldrovandi studied the Bible and did so in unusual ways. To answer lexical questions, such as the meaning of papyrus in the ancient world, and evaluative ones, such as when it was first cultivated and used by humans, Aldrovandi and Guilandinus turned to scripture. They were not concerned with or qualified to comment on the history of biblical texts and translations – issues that deeply engaged contemporary theologians and classicists. In fact, Guilandinus was sharply ridiculed for his alleged incompetence. While he was still alive, shortly after his *Papyrus* was published, the classical scholar and polymath Joseph Scaliger wrote a blistering rejoinder to it that Anthony Grafton has described in detail.[109] According to Scaliger, Guilandinus was simply not fit to comment on philological matters, especially those pertinent to the Bible. For example, Guilandinus made a rash error when he wrote about the Septuagint translators that, "inspired by the holy spirit, they rendered the sacred volumes of the Hebrews from Chaldean into Greek."[110] The Septuagint was translated from Hebrew, not Aramaic, to Greek, and to Scaliger the misstatement was unconscionable. He retorted that the Septuagint translators "who so ineptly translated the sacred

Durante e della sua famiglia (Viterbo: Agnesotti, 1968). Giacomo Antonio Cortuso (1513–1603) was prefect of Padua's botanical garden. He wrote *L'Horto de i semplici di Padoua* (Venice: Girolamo Porro, 1591). On Cortuso, see *DBI* 29:809–11.

109 Grafton, "Rhetoric, Philology, and Egyptomania."

110 Guilandinus, *Papyrus*, 86: "qui sancti spiritus afflatu sacra Hebraeorum volumina de Chaldaico Graeca fecerunt." Azariah de' Rossi proposed that the seventy-two elders translated from an Aramaic version of the Pentateuch. See Joanna Weinberg, "Azariah De' Rossi and Septuagint Traditions," *Italia* 5:1–2 (1985): 7–35, esp. 23–5, 28–32, where she discusses not only de' Rossi's theory but its reception in the sixteenth and seventeenth centuries.

scriptures were inspired by no holy spirit. Furthermore [they translated] from Hebrew, not Aramaic."[111] Isaac Casaubon had an even more scathing remark about Guilandinus's poor linguistic skills. In a dedicatory letter to a collection of Scaliger's minor works, Casaubon quipped about Guilandinus that "in Greek he is completely dependent on his dictionary. This he himself admits, and it is in any case obvious."[112]

There is some truth to what Scaliger and Casaubon alleged: Guilandinus did in fact make mistakes. But it is important to emphasize that Guilandinus was not an editor of texts; he was a natural philosopher. His task was not to establish accurate and readable editions of classical works but rather, in the spirit of Leoniceno, to figure out what Pliny meant. And that intellectual project had practical goals that Scaliger and Casaubon were bound by neither occupation nor inclination to pursue. Those two great Calvinist scholars put the Bible at the center of their historical and antiquarian endeavors: they were involved in interconfessional polemic, which they prosecuted with philological precision. Aldrovandi and Guilandinus did not study the Bible to establish accurate texts, involve themselves in religious conflict, or uphold the truth of any particular confessional perspective. When asked by friends and religious authorities to bring their natural philosophical expertise to bear on the Bible, they obliged. When left to their own devices, they ushered the Bible into an expanding classical canon and used it to supplement their explorations in ancient natural philosophy.

To do so carried risks. Since Aldrovandi and Guilandinus made extensive use of the Bible – and explicitly criticized the Vulgate – they took precautions against attracting unwanted attention from the Inquisition. Gabriele Paleotti acted as Aldrovandi's protector.[113] Either Guilandinus or his publisher thought it prudent to voluntarily submit *Papyrus* to the church authorities for prepublication censorship. Such ecclesiastical

[111] "Profecto nullus afflatus divinus fuit illis, qui tam inepte sacra Biblia traduxerunt. Deinde non ex Chaldaismo, sed ex Hebraismo." Quoted in Grafton, "Rhetoric, Philology, and Egyptomania," 179.

[112] Casaubon, dedicatory letter to Scaliger's *Opuscula varia* (Paris: Drouard, 1610), sig e iiiir: "quippe in Graeca lingua totum se de Lexico suo pependisse, neque ipse diffitetur, et res clamat ipsa." Quoted in Grafton, "Rhetoric, Philology, and Egyptomania," 191 n. 41. Not every evaluation of Guilandinus was so negative; Maffei and Montfaucon, for example, were much more positive.

[113] See my subsequent discussion.

prepublication censorship was stipulated by the Tridentine Index in 1564.[114] As Paul Grendler has argued, from the mid-1560s onward "all authors became careful self-censors."[115] Evidence of Guilandinus's fidelity to this policy may be found in the form of a printed note prefixed to the 1572 edition of *Papyrus,* which explains Guilandinus's actions to readers and assures them the work they are about to read contains nothing offensive to "good morals," the Catholic faith, or its representatives.[116] Given how frequently he quoted the Bible, and how freely he rendered biblical phrases, it is not surprising that Guilandinus or his publisher would have taken this vigilant action.

Aldrovandi drew attention from the Inquisition, too. As a young man, he was arrested in 1549 for suspicion of heresy and was placed under house arrest in Rome for almost a year.[117] He abjured in Bologna's cathedral in September of that year. His specific infraction was fraternization with presumed Protestants. A deposition from 1550 against Francesco Linguardo, a notorious bookseller in Bologna known to have Protestant sympathies, implicates Aldrovandi as a member of his circle.[118] The naturalist's name was cleared, but allegations against his fidelity to the Holy See would resurface throughout his life. He was once again in

[114] The Index was published that year in Venice by Aldus Manutius. See Paul Grendler, *The Roman Inquisition and the Venetian Press, 1540–1605* (Princeton: Princeton University Press, 1977), 148–61.

[115] Ibid., 287.

[116] "Noverint omnes, Papyrum Melchioris Guilandini una cum auctariis exhibitam fuisse antequam typis subiiceretur, tum haereticae pravitatis apud Venetus, et Patavinos inquisitoribus, tum ex Senatus Veneti decreto Bernardino Feliciano, viro cum insigniter docto, tum magnopere humano et Octaviano Magio eidem Senatui a secretis: qui omnes perlectis singillatim libellis omnibus, cum nihil in eis deprehendissent, quod aut fidem catholicam, aut principes viros, aut bonos mores offenderet, atque id syngraphis suis amplissimo Venetorum decemuirali collegio non modo confirmassent sed etiam persuasissent, effectum fuit quod idem collegium decemuirale illos ipsos libellos publicare benigne ac gratiose permiserit, atque in super multam, & poenam ei irrogaverit, qui citra M Antonii Ulmi voluntatem eosdem impresserit, aut alibi impressos importaverit, venales ne habuerit, intra omnes ditiones Venetiae fines." Guilandinus, *Papyrus*, unnumbered page before sig. *2r.

[117] Paula Findlen, *Possessing Nature: Museums, Collecting, and Scientific Culture in Early Modern Italy* (Berkeley: University of California Press, 1994), 162.

[118] Linguardo died before 1566 and was arrested on 26 April 1548. See *DBI* 65:160–1. The deposition charges that Linguardo "ha tenuta da un tempo in qua con molti che sono ne' medesimi errori, come è stato messer Lelio Socino, messer Ulisse aldrovandi, Sebastiano Mainetti, Don Alemano Orlandi gia frate di S. Giacomo, frate Lucio di S. francesco et altri." See ACDF, SO, St. st., L.6.n.,1b, fols. 57r–58v; reproduced in Baldini and Spruit, *Catholic Church and Modern Science* 1:738–41, 739.

trouble with the Inquisition in the 1570s.[119] This time the charges were similar. On 14 July 1571 Antonio Balducci, the inquisitor of Bologna, wrote to Scipione Rebiba, cardinal of Pisa, and insisted that "since 1548 Aldrovandi had [participated] in a circle where there were Lutheran readings."[120] Five months earlier Balducci had written to Rebiba and denounced Aldrovandi with stinging language: he called him a "most perfidious heretic."[121]

But Aldrovandi did not lack defenders. An anonymous, undated, and unpublished testimony of Aldrovandi's activities and his value to the larger community of clergymen was sent to the pope. It lucidly articulates Aldrovandi's reputation for sacred studies. "In his histories," the authors write,

> he has inserted all natural and inanimate things of which Holy Scripture makes mention, such as gems, plants, and animals; truly this conforms to what Saint Augustine says.... There can be no doubt that this incredible effort is much desired by scholars, philosophers, physicians, and theologians. How much utility might these histories bring to the whole world; they could strengthen the faith of many Christians, as they have for some illustrious and most revered cardinals who have seen his Museum, such as Paleotti, Gaetano, Sforza, Valieri, Borromeo, Ascolano, Sfondato, Sega, and many others. Being a reasonable demand, I hope that Your Holiness will grant him your universal blessing.[122]

In a similar vein, his powerful friend and patron Gabriele Paleotti wrote to the Roman Inquisition to assure it that he had read Aldrovandi's work

[119] See Ugo Baldini, "Cardano e Aldrovandi nelle lettere del Sant'Uffizio romano all'Inquisitore di Bologna (1571–1573)," *Bruniana e Campanelliana* 6 (2000): 145–63.

[120] ACDF, SO, St. st., EE.1b, fol. 831r; reproduced in Baldini and Spruit, *Catholic Church and Modern Science*, 1:737. "Ulisse del 1548 in circa dove fu letta una lectione alla lutherana."

[121] Balducci to Rebiba, 10 February 1571. ACDF, SO, St. st., EE.1b, fols. 810v–811r; reproduced in Baldini and Spruit, *Catholic Church and Modern Science*, 734–5.

[122] "Aldrovandi Ulisse Memoriale agli assunti dello Studio," Bologna, Archivio Isolani, F. 30 (30/1–2–3). "Et in queste sue istorie inserisse tutte le cose naturali, delle quali si fa mentione nella Sacra Scrittura, o siano cose inanimate, come gioie, overo piante, o animali, dichiarandole conforme a S. Agostino nel libro secondo della Dottrina Christiana trigesimo nono. La qual fatica non è dubbio che è molto desiderata da tutti i studiosi, philosophi, medici e theologi. E quanta utilità possino apportare queste istorie à tutt'il mondo, ne possono far fede molti Signori e particolarmente alcuni Illustrissimi et Reverendissimi Cardinali, c'hanno veduto il suo Museo, come Paleoto, Gaetano, Sforza, Valieri, Bonromeo, Ascolano, Sfondrato, Sega et molti altri. Et per essere giusta domanda spera che V.B. per beneficio universale gli la concederà." Unnumbered pages addressed to Beatissimè Pater.

on biblical natural philosophy, *Theatrum biblicum naturale*, and that it contained nothing offensive:

> Doctor Aldrovandi, a public professor in the *studium* of Bologna, has produced after much time and great labor a most copious and useful natural history which addresses, among other things, the trees, plants, birds, and minerals that Sacred Scripture mentions in conformity with what Saint Augustine says in book 2, chapter 39, of *De doctrina cristiana*.[123]

Paleotti went on to explain that though Aldrovandi wished to have his work printed, and that he was urged to do so by others, he could not accomplish this without the approval of the Holy Office. To that end he humbly submitted that the recipients of his letter would do him the honor of allowing Aldrovandi's work to be printed since it would be for the great benefit of the public.[124] Paleotti's letter, like the advance presentation of Guilandinus's work to inquisitors, was a farsighted attempt to secure advance approval from church authorities.

In sixteenth-century Italy, laymen who wrote about the Bible, even its natural imagery and terminology, could raise suspicions. Apart from Aldrovandi's brief period of house arrest in Rome as a young man – long before he wrote about the Bible – neither he nor Guilandinus was ever convicted of any crime against the Catholic Church or punished for any theologically offensive utterance. But these two naturalists, who steered clear of confessional polemics and focused on scientific and antiquarian matters, still piqued curiosity and possessed the power to generate controversy. They lived in a world in which one needed to

[123] Bologna, Archivio Isolani, F. 30/30 (3): Agli Illustrissimi et Reverendissimi Cardinali della Congregatione sopra l'Indice Per Il Dottore Ulisse Aldrovandi Bolognese raccomandato dal Signor Cardinale Paleotti (with the annotation: "si trattò di questo memoriale nella Sacra Congregatione dell'Indice la quale concesse la gratia dimandata Maii 1596"): "Il dottore Ulisse Aldrovandi publico professore nello studio di Bologna, dopo haver con gran lunghezza di tempo et con molta fatica posto insieme una historia naturale copiosissima et utilissima, nella quale oltre l'altre cose si tratta degl'arbori, delle piante, degli ucelli, dei minerali che fa mentione la Sacra Scrittura, con dichiararli conforme a S. Agostino lib. 2 de doctrina christiana, c. 39 hora che ha posto mano alla stampa essortato a ciò et aiutato anco da' Signori principali et di giuditio, non può passar oltre, poichè nell'Indice nuovo si ordina, che alli ministri a' quali tocca il rivedere et sottoscrivere li libri che si stampano, si devano dar l'opere le quali doveranno rivedere rescritte." Another version of this letter was published by Baldini and Spruit, *Catholic Church and Modern Science*, 741–3.

[124] Bologna, Archivio Isolani, F. 30/30 (3).

seek ecclesiastical approval to print a book on any topic concerning religion or morals.

CONCLUSION

Ulisse Aldrovandi integrated the Bible into his study of ancient booklore much more thoroughly than his contemporaries did. His scientific training, interest in Hebrew, and diligent examination of the Bible enabled him to put that sacred text to new and creative uses. Among them was his tendency to use the Bible as a historical rather than a theological source. And a roiling debate concerning Pliny's *Natural History* gave him and his colleague Melchior Guilandinus an opportunity to combine biblical studies and natural philosophy to an unprecedented degree. Rather than folding their scientific learning into their biblical commentaries, as many of their contemporaries did, Aldrovandi and Guilandinus folded their biblical learning into their scientific commentaries. The result was a new approach to the Bible that considered scripture as more than an inerrant source for religious doctrine: it became a mine for valuable scientific and historical material as well.

3

"The Grandeur of the Science of God"

David de' Pomi and the Stones of the High Priest's Breastplate

David de' Pomi, a Jewish physician and lexicographer who lived in late sixteenth-century Venice, believed in the medical efficacy of biblical stones. Placing his trust in the powers of *tarshish*, one of the stones featured in the high priest's breastplate,[1] he confessed that he "had no greater hope in times of plague" than that stone,

> for I wear it fastened in a ring on my finger, and, peering down at it in suspicious places, it provides me such a measure of comfort that I am bewildered by it. Indeed, I notice at once how, by means of perspiration, the poisonous vapors evaporate and evacuate from my body, and I rest content as does he who is liberated from a fierce fever. Infinite times I have accidentally touched infected persons, and, knowing they were infected, have immediately felt the infestation of that infection in me. I then look at the diacinto, and in no time at all I have passed into a greatly improved state. I have known the power of this stone and the truth about how it often changes into different colors when the quality of the air shifts.[2]

1 See Exodus 28:20 and 39:13.

2 David de' Pomi, *Tsemaḥ David Dittionario novo Hebraico, molto copioso, dechiarato in tre lingue* (Venice: Giovanni de Gara, 1587), 86:2: "Io n'ho fatta nel tempo del contagio ogni maggior'esperienza, perciò che portandolo ligato in un'anello nel dito, mirandolo ne' luogi di sospetto, mi dava conforto tale, che ne rimanevo stupefatto, anzi mi avedevo che subito per sudore sboravano et uscivano dal mio corpo vapori velenosi, rimanendo contento a guisa di quel che resta liberato dal'ardentissima febre, et infinite volte m'è occorso toccare casualmente l'infettati e conoscere la loro infettione dalla gran mutatione quale in me stesso subito sentivo, e guardato poi il Diacinto senz'intervallo di tempo in meglior stato mi tras-mutavo. Conoscesi la bontà di detta pietra e la vera dal mutar'ella spesso colore secondo la varietà del aere." "Diacinto" is de' Pomi's Italian translation for *tarshish*. His entry for *tarshish* refers the reader to his description of the *diacinto* stone (see 232:2), which he explains in full under the heading (86:2) יקנטין, the Aramaic term for hyacinth. See יקנטין,

This personal reflection comes from *Tsemaḥ David* (The sprout of David), de' Pomi's lexicographical work published in Venice in 1587 by Zuan di Gara.[3] De' Pomi translates *tarshish* as *diacinto*. *Diacinto*, or *hyacinthus* in Latin, was known to possess curative properties. But few translators, lexicographers, or biblical commentators paired the scientific reputation of hyacinth with the Bible's mysterious stone *tarshish*.[4] This chapter explores how and why de' Pomi did this. Since the author of *Tsemaḥ David* does not reveal his sources for information about *tarshish* or *diacinto*, the pages that follow do. My intention is to delineate the options de' Pomi had, assess which he chose, and reflect on what those choices indicate about his intellectual proclivities and the broader project of probing the Bible's natural world, which his work represents.[5] I argue that de' Pomi translated *tarshish* as *diacinto* in order to attach data from Renaissance mineralogy to a biblical term that would underscore *tarshish*'s medical efficacy. He did so by using empirical evidence of *diacinto*'s curative powers, as well as oral and written Greek traditions. De' Pomi's writings on *tarshish* underscore the prominence of Greek learning in Italian Jewish intellectual life of the sixteenth century, the persistence of oral traditions in a notoriously bookish age, and the importance of empirical evidence in biblical analysis.

Like many other sixteenth-century lexicographers, collectors, and medical doctors in Europe, David de' Pomi took an avid interest in the

Aramaic for hyacinth, at 86:2. The first number refers to the page, the second to the column. David de' Pomi himself endorses this pagination: see "avertimento," sig. B1r.

3 On Zuan di Gara, see Abraham Habermann, *Ha-madpis Zu'an di Garah u-reshimat sifre bet defuso, 324–370 (1564–1610)* (Lod: Mekhon Haberman, 1982). Di Gara published several other dictionaries of note, including Marco Marini's *Arca Noë*.

4 In one edition of David Kimḥi's *Sefer HaShorashim*, translated by Sebastian Münster as *Dictionarium Hebraicum ex rabbinorum commentariis collectum* (Basel: Froben, 1535), *tarshish* is equated with hyacinth. See sig. bb3–bb4: "item תרשיש lapis pretiosus qui in rationali summi sacerdotis ... quem quidam chrysolitum vocant ... alii dicunt quod habeat formam תכלת hyacinthi." Two other mid-sixteenth-century editions of this work, however, equate *tarshish* with *chrysolithus*. The Basel 1539 edition has "lapis pretiosus.... Quem quidam chrysolitum vocant ... Chaldaeus interpretatur Aphricam." The Basel 1564 edition has "lapis preciosus.... Quem quidam chrysolitum vocant." Since we do not know which edition de' Pomi read we cannot determine the source of his rendering of *tarshish* as hyacinth.

5 A great many other entries in *Tsemaḥ David* address the antiquarian and scientific life of the biblical world. Of them, a fair number are lengthy: *qorban* (sacrificial offering, 174:3), *re'em* (unicorn, 181:3), and *sambation* (a mythical river, 150:2), for example. Each could be profitably explored as examples of de' Pomi's integration of natural philosophy with biblical studies.

antiquarian and medical aspects of biblical gemstones. His responsibilities as a physician motivated him to seek out effective remedies against all sorts of maladies. As Richard Palmer observed, Italian doctors of the Renaissance were trained to believe that ancient cures were the best ones.[6] The recurrent plagues that afflicted northern Italy during the course of de' Pomi's career created a sharp demand for new, ever more effective prophylactics against the "bad air" of plagues.[7] Furthermore, his immersion in the cosmopolitan world of sixteenth-century Venice afforded him numerous opportunities to see modern-day derivatives of these stones and speak to the merchants who sold them, the sailors who brought them back, the pharmacists who prescribed them, and the fortunate owners who had the resources and connections to purchase them. For example, he acquired his *diacinto* stone, and much information about its provenance in the East Indies, from a man he described as a "great Muslim merchant."[8] In other writings besides his dictionary de' Pomi boasted of his prowess in curing people during times of plague. On 1 July 1589, de' Pomi wrote to Pope Sixtus V to request permission to treat Christian patients. He informed the supreme pontiff that "it will likewise be attested that during the plague which broke out here I performed immense services to the state in visiting and caring for the afflicted without any reward."[9] Testimonies to de' Pomi's skill came from other pens as well. Earlier in 1589, Archbishop Matteucci, the papal nuncio in Venice, wrote to Sixtus V noting that de' Pomi "has the

6 Richard Palmer, "Medical Botany in Northern Italy in the Renaissance," *Journal of the Royal Society of Medicine* 78 (February 1985): 149–57.

7 Katharine Park has shown how in medieval Florence frequent contagion provoked a crisis of confidence in traditional medicine, prompting healers to combat the plague by other means. See her *Doctors and Medicine in Early Medieval Florence* (Princeton: Princeton University Press, 1995). De' Pomi's Jewish colleague Abraham Yagel emphasized that biblical incense could counter the effects of plague and urged his readers to carry around a piece of sponge cake modeled on the oil bread mentioned in Exodus 29:23 as a prophylactic against the plague. See his *Moshia Ḥosim* (Venice: Zuan di Gara, 1587), 17b–18a and 21b, respectively. On the notion that Yagel moved beyond traditional Galenic medicine to cures based in his own religious tradition, see David B. Ruderman, *Kabbalah, Magic and Science: The Cultural Universe of a Sixteenth-Century Jewish Physician* (Cambridge, MA: Harvard University Press, 1988): 33.

8 De' Pomi, *Tsemaḥ David*, 232:3.

9 See Archivio Segreto del Vaticano, Dispacci del nunzio a Venezia all Segreteria di Stato, filza 28, f. 282, published in David Chambers and Brian Pullan, eds., *Venice: A Documentary History, 1450–1630* (London: Blackwell, 1992), 341.

reputation of being, although a Jew, a good man" and that he "effected some remarkable cures at the time of the plague."[10]

Late Renaissance natural philosophers wrote at length about precious stones, and David de' Pomi was no exception. The most prominent group of entries that treat mineralogical topics in *Tsemaḥ David* includes those defining and describing the stones of the high priest's breastplate.[11] Within that group, de' Pomi's entry on *tarshish*, the tenth stone listed in Exodus 28, is the most fruitful for examination. De' Pomi flagged the value of this entry, in which he defined *tarshish* as *diacinto*, on the title page of his book.[12] Because it is easily the most elaborate of the twelve entries on the breastplate's stones, and because it departs most radically from the lexicographical tradition de' Pomi inherited, it tells us much about de' Pomi's approach to the natural philosophy of the ancient Jewish world. In order to ascertain why de' Pomi departed so radically from received lexicography, we must take a wide look at all the sources available to him to comprehend why he chose to identify the stones as he did and expand a single entry into an edifying personal anecdote, a scientific treatise in miniature, and a philological discourse.

David de' Pomi was born in 1525 at Spoleto, a city that, as he himself put it, had been ravaged by the Italian wars.[13] He received his early education at home from his father, Rabbi Isaac, and subsequently lived in Todi where he studied "at the feet of the chief of the physicians," Yehiel Alatino.[14] In 1545 de' Pomi matriculated at the University of Perugia,

[10] Dated 4 February 1589. Archivio Segreto del Vaticano, Dispacci del nunzio a Venezia all Segreteria di Stato, filza 26, f. 477, published in Chambers and Pullan, *Venice*, 340.

[11] See Exodus 28:17ff.

[12] Title page, Hebrew section: ועל כח הנפלא שיש בדיאצינטו

[13] The best source of information on de' Pomi's life is the Hebrew autobiography included in *Tsemaḥ David*. See *Tsemaḥ David*, sig. 5ar–5av. *EJ* 16:366–7, also has a useful entry on de' Pomi. See also Ariel Toaff, *Gli ebrei a Perugia* (Perugia: Deputazione di storia patria per l'Umbria, 1975), 146–9; Ladislao Münster, "L'*Enarratio brevis de senum affectibus* [bref commentaire aux maladies des vieillards] de David de' Pomi, le plus grand médecin israélite au XVIe siècle," *Revue d'Histoire de la Médicine Hebraique* 20 (July 1954): 7–16, 125–36; Cecil Roth, *Jews in the Renaissance* (Philadelphia: Jewish Publication Society, 1959), 223–5; Harry Friedenwald, "Apologetic Work of Jewish Physicians," *Jewish Quarterly Review*, n.s., 32 (1941–2): 228–30, 407–8.

[14] On Yeḥiel (Vitale) Alatino, who served as physician to Pope Julius III (1550–5), see Oscar Scalvanti, "Lauree in medicina di studenti israeliti a Perugia nel secolo XVI," *Annali della facoltà di Giurisprudenza di Perugia*, 3rd ser., 8 (1910): 91–129; for briefer mentions of Alatino, see Moses Shulvass, *The Jews in the World of the Renaissance*, trans. Elvin L. Kose

where he followed a traditional medical curriculum. Six years later he received his doctorate in medicine and philosophy.[15] He was not the only Jew to earn a medical degree at Perugia during this time; at least two others did as well.[16] After practicing as a physician in a variety of towns in northern Italy, de' Pomi spent the last twenty-four years of his life, from 1569 to 1593, as a doctor in Venice. In that city he received permission several times to treat Christian patients.[17] In addition to *Tsemaḥ David*, his best-known work, de' Pomi published a defense of Jewish physicians, a treatise on the conditions of old age, a translation of Ecclesiastes with an essay on suffering, and a short work on plagues.[18] De' Pomi also wrote at least two undated and unpublished texts: a historical treatise in

(Leiden: Brill, 1973), 208, and Roth, *Jews in the Renaissance*, 223. See also Toaff, *Gli ebrei a Perugia*, 147–8 and bibliography there.

15 For detail on the typical medical curriculum of the mid-sixteenth century, see Paul Grendler, *The Universities of the Italian Renaissance* (Baltimore: Johns Hopkins University Press, 2002), 319–28, and notes there. For more on de' Pomi's doctorate, including the diploma's text, see Ariel Toaff, *The Jews in Umbria* (Leiden: Brill, 1993), 3:1282–5 (doc. no. 2525), 27 November 1551. De' Pomi's degree is also published in Scalvanti, "Lauree in medicina," 34–7.

16 Salomone di Benigno Turani di Orvieto took his degree in 1552. Angelo di Laudadio de Blanis took his in 1547. For more on them, see Scalvanti, "Lauree in medicina," 31–3 and 38–9, respectively.

17 De' Pomi's 1589 license to practice medicine is published in David Chambers and Brian Pullan, eds., *Venice: A Documentary History, 1450–1630* (London: Blackwell, 1992): 340–1.

18 *De medico hebraeo enarratio apologica* (Venice, 1588); *Enarratio brevis de senum affectibus praecavendis atque curandis* (Venice, 1588); *Discorso intorno a l'humana miseria e sopr'al modo di fuggirla* (Venice, 1572); and *Brevi discorsi et efficacissimi ricordi per liberare ogni città oppressa dal mal contagioso* (Venice, 1577). De' Pomi contributed scholia to *Dioclis epistola ad Antigonum asiae regem, pro tuenda valetudine conscripta, ac scholiis non spernendis exposita* (Venice, 1588). Julius Fürst claims that de' Pomi published an *Index novus in singulis Hippocratis libris* (Venice, n.d.) in his *Bibliotheca Judaica* (Leipzig: W. Engelmann, 1849–63), 3:111–13. Another list of de' Pomi's publications may be found in Münster, "L'*Enarratio brevis de senum affectibus* de David de' Pomi," 162–3 n. 3. Münster dates the *Index novus* to 1591. I have never seen either the *Dioclis epistola* or the *Index novus*, nor have I found a record, let alone description of them, in any library catalog. The text on pages 10 to 28 of de' Pomi's *Enarratio Brevis De Senum affectibus praecavendis atque curandis* consists of a Latin translation of a work by Diocles of Carystus (fourth century BCE) entitled *Pro tuenda valetudine*. Münster believes de' Pomi translated this from the original Greek into Latin, though he adduces no proof to support his assertion. A Latin translation of *Pro tuenda valetudine* had been published some twelve years before by Mizaldus. For more on Diocles of Carystus, see Philip J. van der Eijk, *Diocles of Carystus: A Collection of the Fragments with Translation and Commentary*, 2 vols. (Boston: Brill, 2000). For the Greek text of the letter itself with facing translation, see ibid., 1:310–21; for van der Eijk's commentary, see 2:352–60.

Italian on the fall of Cyprus in 1571 to the Turkish Sultan Selim II and a messianic work in Hebrew on exile and redemption.[19]

David de' Pomi wrote in three languages, published several books in his lifetime, and supplied Christian as well as Jewish scholars with information about the Hebrew language and the cultural world of the Bible and postbiblical texts.[20] More importantly, because he wrote about medicine, the Bible, and the natural world of scripture, de' Pomi's work is an ideal resource for mapping the intersection of biblical studies and natural philosophy in late Renaissance Italy. In spite of the advantages that attend a close study of de' Pomi, scholarship on the Spoletan doctor has not been extensive. While physicians and philologists have studied de' Pomi in recent years, few historians have. Unfortunately, studies of de' Pomi undertaken by medical doctors tend to be fairly impressionistic.[21] Although modern doctors such as these bring a certain knowledge of medical details to their scrutiny of de' Pomi, their studies tend to lack awareness of the social and cultural contexts that inform his work. Another approach modern scholars of de' Pomi have taken is philological.[22] As

[19] The historical treatise is *Discorso maraviglioso sopra la guerra promossa da Selim Imperator di Turchi*. The best description of this work is in the *Christie's* catalog of the A. L. Shane Collection of Judaica and Hebraica, auctioned on 24 June 1998, p. 155. There is an extant copy in Bologna, Biblioteca dell'Archiginnasio, Ms. A 428. Guido Bartolucci notes this manuscript in his article "Venezia nel pensiero politico ebraico rinascimentale: un testo ritrovato di David de' Pomis," *Rinascimento* 44 (2005): 225–47, 227 n. 6. The messianic work is in Budapest, Library of the Hungarian Academy of Sciences, Ms. Kaufmann 556, pp. 43–97; see also Jewish National and University Library microfilm F 15191. It is entitled חבור על גלות וגאולה. Abraham David briefly describes this manuscript in *Kirjat Sefer* 58 (Hebrew) (1983): 198. חבור על גלות וגאולה is also mentioned in M. Weisz, *Katalog der Hebräischen Handschriften und Bücher in der Bibliothek des Dr. David Kaufmann* (Frankfurt: Kauffmann, 1906).

[20] Ulisse Aldrovandi owned and annotated *Tsemaḥ David*. See Biblioteca Universitaria di Bologna, Ms. Aldrovandi 147 for a list of Aldrovandi's books. Aldrovandi's copy of *Tsemaḥ David* has the shelf mark A.VI.D.IV.2.

[21] James L. Fuchs, "Jewish Medical Compendia and Jewish-Christian Relations in Early Modern Europe," *World Congress of Jewish Studies* 10, B2 (1990): 83–90; Angelo Mecchia, "Cenni di geriatria in un'opera del medico umbro Davide de' Pomi (1525–1600)," *Pagine di storia della medicina* 10 (1996): 58–62; Ladislao Münster, "L'*Enarratio brevis de senum affectibus* ('Bref commentaire aux maladies des vieillards') de David de' Pomi, le grand médicin israélite en Italie au XVIe siècle," in Gad Freudenthal and Samuel Kottek, eds., *Mélanges d'histoire de la médicine hébraïque; études choisies de la "Revue d'histoire de la médicine hébraïque" (1948–1985)* (Leiden: Brill, 2003): 161–81. Originally in *Revue d'histoire de la médicine hébraïque* 20 (1954).

[22] Massimo Pazzini, "Registrazione e definitione del lemma nel dizionario di Rabbi David de Pomis," *Liber Annuus* 43 (1993): 261–76.

detailed and thorough as studies such as these may be, they tells us little about the themes in de' Pomi's work or its significance to early modern or Jewish history.

Historians have not completely neglected de' Pomi. Cecil Roth, for example, adopts a hagiographic tone when writing about the Spoletan physician and insists that de' Pomi made certain medical discoveries well in advance of his Christian colleagues: there is an apologetic element to Roth's writing about de' Pomi.[23] Roth questions the scientific "accuracy" of de' Pomi's discourse on the use of a ram's horn in medical recipes.[24] Remarks such as these indicate that Roth glorified Jewish cultural achievement and minimized what he saw as its superstitious or pseudoscientific qualities. In order to assess the scientific and cultural contributions of de' Pomi, we must situate his work in the context of his time and refrain from evaluating the "accuracy" of his observations – a modern concern that tells us more about those studying de' Pomi than de' Pomi himself.

DAVID DE' POMI AND GREEK EDUCATION

Of the many tools de' Pomi used to define and describe classical and post-classical Hebrew words, the Greek language was one of the most important. He knew Greek and frequently mentions Greek words and phrases in his published works. His knowledge of Greek enabled him to seek out alternative editions of the Bible such as the Septuagint. Greek terms proved to be sturdy pegs upon which de' Pomi could hang scientific and antiquarian knowledge. In turn, that knowledge enriched the religious tradition of which he was enamored. Interest in Greek, attentiveness to material culture, and an emphasis on experimentation are all hallmarks of sixteenth-century medical humanism.[25] Educated during medical humanism's heyday, David de' Pomi not only absorbed its teachings but, more importantly, applied them to his examination of the Bible.

[23] See Cecil Roth, *The Jews in the Renaissance* (Philadelphia: Jewish Publication Society of America, 1959), 223.

[24] Ibid., 233.

[25] Vivian Nutton, "The Rise of Medical Humanism," in Ian Maclean, ed., *Logic, Signs, and the Order of Nature in the Renaissance* (Cambridge: Cambridge University Press, 2002); A. Wear, R. K. French, and I. M. Lonie, eds., *Medical Renaissance of the Sixteenth Century* (Cambridge: Cambridge University Press, 1985).

The Spoletan physician learned Greek while he was a medical student at the University of Perugia. Like all universities on the Italian Peninsula that awarded medical degrees, Perugia placed a heavy emphasis on *lettere umane*, which were taught every day, once in the morning at hour 17 (eleven o'clock) and again in the afternoon at hour 22 (four o'clock).[26] University records from the middle of the sixteenth century cite the importance of Greek in helping to "understand the etymology of words and the structure of Latin sentences."[27] In the late 1540s, when de' Pomi was a student, Cristoforo Sassi held the chair of *lettere umane* and was a competent Hellenist. Sassi held that position for more than forty years – evidence of his courses' popularity with students[28] – and was a pupil of the renowned classicists Francesco Maturanzio and Riccardo Bartolini.[29] In 1550, the year before de' Pomi took his degree, the university hired Antonio Galeota da Urbino, a man who favored Greek letters over Latin ones in his teaching and research.[30] De' Pomi learned Greek at a university that valued its instruction.

De' Pomi's passion for Greek did not wane after he completed his studies; his mature work, including *Tsemaḥ David*, amply displays his interest in Greek history and literature. As A. C. Dionisotti pointed out, modern scholars should be cautious about assuming a premodern writer knew Greek just because he quoted a word or two; one could find stray Greek words in a variety of Latin dictionaries in the Middle Ages and Renaissance.[31] But the frequency of de' Pomi's use of Greek obviates this concern. In *Tsemaḥ David* a number of entries mention Greek. The work's Latin preface explains that "quite a few external terms," meaning

[26] G. Ermini, *Storia della università di Perugia* (Bologna: N. Zanichelli, 1947), 208. The morning session focused on poetry, the evening one on rhetoric and oratory. For more on university schedules, see Grendler, *The Universities of the Italian Renaissance,* 147.

[27] Cited in Ermini, *Storia della università di Perugia*, 537.

[28] Paul Grendler argues in *The Universities of the Italian Renaissance* (Baltimore: Johns Hopkins University Press, 2002) that it was crucially important for professors to attract students to their lectures in light of threats from Jesuit *studii* and private instruction.

[29] Ermini, *Storia della università di Perugia*, 543–4.

[30] Ermini notes that Galeota was "ricordato spesso con lode come poeta e grecista" (ibid., 545).

[31] A. C. Dionisotti, "Greek Grammars and Dictionaries in Carolingian Europe," in Michael W. Herren, ed., *The Sacred Nectar of the Greeks: The Study of Greek in the West in the Early Middle Ages* (London: Kings College London Medieval Studies, 1988): 1–56, 2.

those that are not Hebrew, "may be found in many commentaries."[32] The most common of these were Persian, Arabic, and Greek. But of those three de' Pomi lavishes the most attention on Greek. For example, his remarks on *gematria*, or exegesis based on the numerical value of Hebrew words, distinguish between the rabbinic sense of the term and what ancient Greeks meant by it.[33] *Tanais*, de' Pomi explains, was the Roman term for a place that Greeks referred to as *Thanai*.[34] The rabbis often used the word *listeis*, or "assassin," de' Pomi informs us, "along with many other Greek terms."[35] Describing the *matatron*, or angel that ministers to God, de' Pomi points out that *matator* is Greek for "guard."[36] According to de' Pomi, the word *siman*, or sign, is "more Greek than anything else."[37] This sampling of Greek terms in *Tsemaḥ David* indicates de' Pomi's abiding interest in the language and its traces in rabbinic literature. Later in this chapter we will see how Greek served him in his quest to identify and understand *tarshish*. But before we are able to examine the important role Greek played in de' Pomi's

[32] *Tsemaḥ David*, sig. A3v: "caeterae vero externae voces praeter Chaldaicas, quibus pro legis interpretatione interpretes usi fuere, perpaucae existunt in commentariis vero quamplures reperiuntur; Persianae videlicet, Arabes, Graecae (ut modo dictum est) nec non aliae."

[33] Ibid., 31:4: on the original Greek meaning de' Pomi observes לכן צריכים אנו לידע חכמת המדוד והוא נקראת גיאומט"ריאה בלשון יון

[34] Ibid., 72:4: "nome di provincia così chiamata (al mio parere) per il fiume ch'ivi corre, da latini tanais, e da greci è detto tanai."

[35] Ibid., 110:2 In his Hebrew entry, but in neither the Latin nor the Italian that follows, de' Pomi credits Levita as a source for this insight: אמר ר' אליה בלשון יון קורין לגזלן ליסטיס וכן בדברי רז"ל ליסטים מזוין "Questa voce ליסטים *listes* è greca e significa assassino, e se ne sono serviti li Rabini spesse volte, come de molte altre voci greche." The Greek word is properly spelled λῃστής. If de' Pomi had encountered the word in Hebrew script he would not have known whether the first י stood for ι, as he supposed, or η, which is correct. The word means "robber." A proper transliteration would be *leistes*. Abraham Portaleone justified the study of Greek on the grounds that ancient rabbis spoke it. See *SG*, 4r.

[36] *Tsemaḥ David*, 116:2–3. De' Pomi makes this observation in both his Hebrew entry (ובלשון יון מטטור שמעתי שמורה כמו שומר) and his Latin one: "graece, ut aiunt, מטטור custodem significat." Conspicuously, *Metatron* was a technical term in Kabbalah. See Daniel Abrams, "The Boundaries of Divine Ontology: The Inclusion of Metatron in the Godhead," *Harvard Theological Review* 87:3 (1994): 291–321; Moshe Idel, "Enoch Is Metatron," *Immanuel* 24–5 (1990): 220–40; Lawrence Kaplan, "Enoch and Metatron Revisited: A Critical Analysis of Moshe Idel's Method of Reconstruction," *Kabbalah* 6 (2001): 73–119. I am grateful to Yaacob Dweck for these references.

[37] *Tsemaḥ David*, 152:4. Curiously, only the Hebrew and Italian portions of this entry make this point; the Latin is silent. Hebrew: (והוא לשון יוני ממש קורין לאות סימן); Italian: "Questa voce סימן è più tosto greca che di altra sorte de lingua e significa segno; si truova nulla dimanco nella Sagra Scrittura che v'è composto verbo, come dir segnare."

writings, we must explore the acknowledged traditions *Tsemaḥ David* inherited and responded to: natural philosophy, Hebrew lexicography, and Renaissance mineralogy.

NATURAL PHILOSOPHY IN *TSEMAḤ DAVID*

The stated aim of *Tsemaḥ David* was to clarify confusing language in scripture. In his Latin preface to the work, de' Pomi noted that Hebrew terms possess various meanings and that "ambiguous words may be regularly found among Hebrew [writers]."[38] One who studies de' Pomi's dictionary, as a Hebrew passage on the title page advertised, "will scarcely need any other commentary to understand and discern the interpretation of literary matters and [their] plain sense."[39] Similarly, the Latin section of *Tsemaḥ David*'s title page emphasized that diligent readers could use the dictionary to interpret the Holy Scriptures "with ease."[40] But de' Pomi's work had broader applications apart from elucidating the true meaning of scripture. It also introduced readers to postclassical Hebrew writings. And the sorts of writings de' Pomi had in mind were not only "declarations and discourses on the divine and Mosaic law" but also those "about many of the liberal arts."[41] His dictionary helped readers "clearly understand the force of the meaning of every term written by diverse Hebrew authors about various fields of learning."[42] Words like *tarshish* had substantial afterlives in late antique and medieval Hebrew writings. De' Pomi's tendency to apply scientific learning to the Bible and biblical learning to modern science is a particular feature of *Tsemaḥ David*.

As did many physicians of the late Renaissance, David de' Pomi infused his work with colorful digressions on a variety of natural philosophic topics. Essays such as the one on the ram's horn that Roth mocked were

[38] Ibid., Prefatio, sig. A3v: "verborum quin etiam aequivocatio non raró apud hebraeos reperitur."

[39] Ibid., title page, Hebrew section:באופן שכל מי שיקראהו לא יצטרך כמעט לפירוש אחר להבין ולהשכיל פשר דבר ופשט ישר

[40] Ibid., Latin section: "ut quisque conceptum suum haebraice eleganter exprimere scripturasque singulas sacras interpretari perfacile valeat."

[41] Ibid., Italian preface: "alli signori lettori": "discorsi sopra la Divina e Mosaica legge, e sopra molte delle arti liberali."

[42] Ibid., "parendo loro esser'utile a chiunque disidera brevemente intendere la forza della significatione di ciascuna voce scritta da diversi Autori hebrei intorno a varie scienze."

not exceptions to de' Pomi's scientific acumen. Though they may have clashed with Roth's modern sensibilities, they are nonetheless representative of de' Pomi's overall approach to natural philosophy. De' Pomi's specific interest in natural philosophy is manifest in both the Hebrew and Latin sections of *Tsemaḥ David*'s title page. The Hebrew portion of the title page claims that the dictionary reveals "secrets and mysteries of nature, particularly in discussing precious stones and pearls."[43] Furthermore, the Hebrew text broadcasts that the dictionary conveys the "true capacity and wondrous power that the *diacinto* possesses against the plague as well as other matters that are hidden from the masses."[44] The Hebrew front matter not only calls attention to the conspicuous role of natural philosophy in the work but also spotlights the efficacy of the very stone this chapter examines.

The Latin section of the title page is even more explicit about *Tsemaḥ David*'s originality and its scientific bent. De' Pomi claims that his lexicon is "exceedingly detailed, such as has never existed before," and boasts that the work deals with "pearls, unicorns, amber, hyacinth, and other new precious stones, somewhat removed from general knowledge, which will be deemed mysterious to most people." Like the Hebrew portion of the title page, the Latin section highlights the central scientific preoccupation of *Tsemaḥ David*. It does so, however, with greater specificity.[45]

De' Pomi's focus on stones, gems, and other marvels of biblical natural science was not unique in late sixteenth-century Italy. Other scholars, including at least one lexicographer, took a similar interest in the scientific realia of the biblical world. For example, David de' Pomi acknowledged Marco Marini in the Latin preface to *Tsemaḥ David*, writing that "one can easily supplement anything lacking" in his dictionary with the work of the "distinguished Reverend and Abbot, the most learned master Marcus Marini, who, having no equal among Latin scholars, illuminated

[43] Ibid., title Page, Hebrew section: ונגלו בו ג"כ סודות מה ורזי הטבע ובפרט בספור אבנים טובות ומרגליות The title page also announces plenty of material about אמברה וקרן ראם

[44] Ibid.: ועל בחינת האמתי ועל כח הנפלא שיש בדיאצינטו נגד השנוי ... ודברים אחרים נסתרים לרבים

[45] Ibid., title page, Latin section: "Lexicon novum haebraicum locupletissimum quantum nunquam antea … cum quadam Margaritarum, Unicornis, Ambrae, Hyacinti nec non caeterorum lapidum praeciosorum nova et minime obscura universali cognitione, quae tamquam arcana a quam plurimis existimabitur."

the Hebrew language."[46] Marini's *Arca Noë*, completed in April 1581 but not published until 1593, advertises its concern with scientific terminology in Hebrew. In his preface "to the reader who loves Hebrew" (*ad* φιλεβράιον *lectorem*), Marini insists that the language is rich in scientific value. He writes, "If we desire learning, we shall find no other language richer in learning, for I marvel that, in a way, it embraces all scientific, divine, and human learning."[47] Marini's readers evidently agreed and flagged *Arca Noë*'s scientific value. In a laudatory epistle written in Hebrew by Israel Zifroni of Guastalla[48] and included in the front matter of Marini's dictionary, the Jewish printer and savant points out how valuable the dictionary is, especially since it contains information about the "*shoham* stones, *avnei miluim*" and also the "*urim ve tumim*," the prophetic stones used by the high priest to predict the future.[49] Zifroni also insists that "everything that the author truly vocalized with his hand is correct for the discerning one and accurate for those who find understanding; your eyes will see and you will rejoice."[50] In directing his readers to Marini's work, de' Pomi identified an intellectual comrade in late

[46] "Qui si mancus in re aliqua extiterit, alii perfacile supplere poterunt, Reverendus praesertim Abbas ac Doctissimus Dominus Marcus Marini, qui non parum apud latinos haebraicam linguam illustravit." Ibid., sig. A3v. Marco Marini played a central role in editing the Basel Talmud of 1578–80. On his role in that project, see Joseph Prijs, *Die Basler hebraïschen Drucke 1492–1866* (Olten: Urs Graf-Verlag, 1964), 176, 179. Our best source for information on Marini's life is Giovanni Mingarelli's *Marci Marini Vita*, included in *Marci Marini Brixiani canonici regularis congregationis Rhenanae sanctissimi salvatoris annotationes literales in Psalmos nova versione ab ipsomet illustratos* (Bologna: apud Thomam Colli ex Typographia Sancti Thomae Aquinatis, 1748), x–xxii. Mingarelli notes that Leon Modena, Samuel Archivolti, Israel Zifroni, and de' Pomi himself all lauded Marini: "Hebraeorum vero illa aetate in Italia doctissimi, Leo Mutinensis, David Pomarius, Samuel Archivoltus, atque Israel Zifronius, cum ipsum, tum ipsius scripta laudibus maximis celebrarunt. Et merito quidem." Ibid., xxii.

[47] Marini, *Arca Noë Thesaurus linguae sanctae novus* (Venice: Giovanni di Gara, 1593), sig. *3r: "Nam si doctrinam quaerimus, nullam hac lingua doctrinis copiosiorem inveniemus, cum omnes tum divinae, tum humanae etiam scientiae doctrinas miro quodam modo complectatur." See Chapter 1 for Aldrovandi's similar take on the scientific value of Hebrew.

[48] On Zifroni, see A. M. Habermann, "The Printer Israel ha-Zifroni and His Son Elishma, and the List of Books Which Were Printed by Them" (Hebrew), in his *Studies in the History of Hebrew Printers and Books* (Jerusalem: R. Mas, 1978), 215–92; and Marvin Heller, "Ambrosius Froben, Israel Zifroni and Hebrew Printing in Freiburg im Breisgau," *Gutenberg-Jahrbuch* 80 (2005): 137–48.

[49] Marini, *Arca Noë*, sig. **5v.

[50] Ibid., sig. **5v: כל הדברים אשר נקד המחבר מידו ממש כלם נכוחים למבין וישרים למוצאי דעת ועיניכם תראינו ושמחתם

sixteenth-century Italy, one whose authority other Jews such as Zifroni would endorse several years later. De' Pomi's work, though unique, was not conceived or carried out in intellectual isolation.

DAVID DE' POMI AND RENAISSANCE LEXICOGRAPHY

De' Pomi's fellow naturalists were not his only intellectual peers. A broader class of learned men entreated him to polish and publish his scattered notes. Just as Aldrovandi was impelled to investigate the Bible's natural world by Gabriele Paleotti, de' Pomi was persuaded to do the same by certain Venetian nobles. In an Italian preface to his work, de' Pomi explains its genesis, recounting that he had "compiled in my infancy, and in my youth a dictionary in Hebrew, Latin, and Italian for my own use." Some friends had seen it and urged him to publish it, since

> being in my study, my composition (completed many years ago and then laid aside) was seen by some noble and learned men. They persuaded me in the most effective way, and even eventually implored me (since they had the authority to order me) to see that this work be published.... Judging that their demand was no less just than honest, I allowed myself to be persuaded to mollify them in this, their ardent desire.[51]

De' Pomi tells his readers that his nameless admirers "added that my labor was greater by a significant measure than those written by others."[52] De' Pomi does mention Lorenzo Massa, secretary of the Venetian senate and, in de' Pomi's view, a man "not unlearned in Hebrew."[53] Not

51 *Tsemaḥ David*, sig. A3v: "Havendo io, nella mia fanciullezza e nella giovenil età, composto per mio uso e dechiarato in hebreo, in latino et in volgare un Dittionario.... Et essendo nel mio studiolo stata veduta questa mia compositione (fatta certo già di molti anni e posta da banda) da alcuni Nobili e Dotti, mi hanno con ogni meglior modo persuaso, anzi con grandissima instanza pregato (ancor che havessero autorità di commandarmi) a permetter'io che tal opra vada in luce ... giudicando la lor dimanda esser non meno giusta, che honesta, mi sono lasciato persuadere a compiacergli in questo lor'ardente disio."

52 Ibid., "soggiongendo, che la mia fatica è stata di gran lunga magiore di quella che vien da alcuni compresa."

53 Massa was the nephew of the well-known physician Nicolò Massa. See Richard Palmer, "Nicolò Massa, His Family, and His Fortune," *Medical History* 25 (1981): 385–410, esp. 387 n. 14. Nicolò supported his nephew's education at Padua; Lorenzo studied arts there in 1552–3 and subsequently studied medicine in Northern Europe. Some letters from Lorenzo are included in Nicolò's *Epistolarum medicinalium tomus alter* (Venice: ex officina Stellae Jordani Zilleti, 1558), which was no doubt meant to smooth Lorenzo's entry in the

coincidentally, Massa had helped de' Pomi publish some of his Latin writings. Just as natural philosophy was a social enterprise strengthened by the bonds of friendship, so was lexicography.

Dictionaries were a major preoccupation of Renaissance intellectual life.[54] By the sixteenth century, Hebrew lexicography had a storied past. In Jewish culture, systematically defining biblical words was a project that had begun in the Gaonic period (seventh to eleventh centuries). Gerrit Bos has shown how Jews in medieval Western Europe translated some of the Bible's natural terminology into Latin and Romance vernaculars as well.[55] And Israel Ta Shema has written about medieval lexicographers, such as Nathan ben Yeḥiel of Rome, the eleventh-century polymath who wrote the Middle Ages' most comprehensive Hebrew dictionary.[56] The presence of Greek words in Ben Yeḥiel's dictionary

Venetian civil service, since Massa dedicates it to the doge. The younger Massa's career took wing: in 1561 he was in Rome as secretary of the Venetian embassy, and by 1573 he was secretary of the doge. See Palmer, "Nicolò Massa, His Family, and His Fortune," 399. As far as de' Pomi's claim about Massa's Hebraic proficiency, Massa's nineteenth-century biographer Emmanuele Antonio Cicogna stated that he was "peritissimo poi nelle lettere greche e latine non solo, ma eziandio nelle ebraiche ne conosceva gl'intimi sensi per modo che alcuni fra' principali giudaici dottori che chiaman rabbini, diecevano essere più nota la lor lingua al Massa, che ad essi medesimi, e a quelli che nelle più solenni loro scuole la insegnavano." See Cicogna, *Delle inscrizioni veneziane*, 6 vols. (Venice: Giuseppe Orlandelli, 1824–53), 5:19–20.

54 John P. Considine, *Dictionaries in Early Modern Europe: Lexicography and the Making of Heritage* (Cambridge: Cambridge University Press, 2008).

55 Gerrit Bos, "The Creation and Innovation of Medieval Hebrew Medical Terminology: Shem Tov ben Isaac, 'Sefer ha-Shimmush,'" in Anna Akasoy and Wim Raven, eds., *Islamic Thought in the Middle Ages: Studies in Text, Transmission and Translation, in Honour of Hans Daiber* (Leiden: Brill, 2008), 195–218; Bos, "A Late Medieval Hebrew-French Glossary of Biblical Animal Names," *Romance Philology* 63 (2009): 71–94; Bos, "The Literature of Hebrew Medical Synonyms: Romance and Latin Terms and Their Identification," *Aleph: Historical Studies in Science and Judaism* 5 (2005): 169–211; Bos, "Shem Tov ben Isaac, Glossary of Botanical Terms, Nos. 1–18," *JQR* 92:1–2 (July–October 2001): 21–40.

56 See Israel Ta-Shema, "The Italian Setting of Rabbi Nathan ben Yehiel of Rome's 'Arukh'" (Hebrew), in *Keneset Mehkarim, Iyyunim bisifrut harabanit biyemei habenayim,* vol. 3: *Italy and Byzantium* (Jerusalem: Bialik, 2004), 3–8; and the philologically detailed studies of Shifra Sznol, "Medieval and Jewish Greek Lexicography: The Arukh of Nathan ben Jehiel," *Erytheia* 30 (2009): 107–28; Luisa Ferretti Cuomo, "Dalle glosse giudeo-italiane dell' 'Arukh': accessori," in Francesco Aspesi et al., eds., *Il mio cuore è a oriente: studi di linguistica storica, filologia e cultura ebraica dedicati a Maria Luisa Mayer Modena* (Milan: Cisalpino, 2008): 435–56; see also Raimundo Griñó, "El Meturgeman de Elías Levita y el 'Arukh' de Natán ben Yehiel como fuentes de la lexicografía targúmica," *Biblica* 60:1 (1979): 110–17; Shraga Abramson, "The 'Arukh' of Rabbi Nathan ben Yehiel of Rome" (Hebrew), *Sinai* 95:1–2 (1984): 27–42.

may have made it even more appealing to de' Pomi.[57] Other philologists such as David Kimḥi and Abraham Ibn Ezra flourished several centuries before de' Pomi.[58]

In Latinate culture, by contrast, the sixteenth century was a transformative period. Perhaps the most important Renaissance dictionary was Ambrogio Calepino's appropriately named *Cornucopiae,* published in 1502 in Reggio. As a student of early modern dictionaries observed, "during the whole period of the Renaissance scarcely an important dictionary was published which did not reflect directly or indirectly the influence of the Calepine."[59] This work, written in Latin, incorporated seven languages into its entries. In the years after Calepino's death, the dictionary was enlarged considerably, and by 1590 four new languages were added, including Polish and Hungarian.[60] Yet Calepino's dictionary was more than a simple mechanism for defining words. One unique feature is its polyglot nature; another is its tendency to move beyond simple definitions and treat the many associations of each word. In fact, DeWitt Starnes pointed out that Calepino's work functions as much as an encyclopedia as a dictionary; the same could be said for de' Pomi's.[61] A major source of this tendency for Calepino, and for lexicographers who followed in his train, was Franciscus Grapaldus's *Lexicon de partibus aedium*. In that work, Grapaldus's discussion of the term *apotheca*, for example, moves from a discussion of wine shops to wine cellars to different types of wines and ultimately to the vessels that contain them.[62] Abraham Portaleone was similarly interested in the vessels and storage facilities that were a key part of pharmacological culture in late Renaissance

[57] See the unsigned essay "Toldot rabbenu Nathan, ish romi, ba'al heArukh veQorot sifro," in *Bikurei HaIttim* (Vienna, 1829), 8–9, 28–29.

[58] On these scholars and on medieval Hebrew studies more generally, see Nicholas de Lange, ed., *Hebrew Scholarship and the Medieval World* (Cambridge: Cambridge University Press, 2001); William Horbury, ed., *Hebrew Study from Ezra to Ben-Yehuda* (Edinburgh: T&T Clark, 1999). See also Steven Harvey, ed., *The Medieval Hebrew Encyclopedias of Science and Philosophy* (Dordrecht: Kluwer Academic Publishers, 2000).

[59] DeWitt T. Starnes, *Renaissance Dictionaries: English-Latin and Latin-English* (Austin: University of Texas Press, 1954): 52.

[60] I have used Andrea Calepino, *Dictionarium linguarum septem* (Basel: Henric-Petrina, 1575).

[61] Starnes, *Renaissance Dictionaries*, 52.

[62] Jonathon Green, *Chasing the Sun: Dictionary Makers and the Dictionaries They Made* (New York: Henry Holt, 1996): 50–1.

Mantua.[63] De' Pomi shares the same digressive and associative style that characterizes other Renaissance dictionaries and encyclopedias, in which their authors could display their broad learning.

John Considine has identified another cluster of sixteenth-century dictionaries that explicitly served cultural historians and antiquarian scholars. Three of the French Hellenist Guillaume Budé's early works display this approach to classical antiquity. His *Annotationes* (1508) on the first twenty-four books of the *Pandectae*, an early text of Roman law, applied his knowledge of everyday life in the ancient world to a study of its laws. *De asse et partibus eius libri quinque* (1514) examined ancient numismatics and glossed many ancient texts that mentioned money. He poured his considerable knowledge of ancient legal practices into another work, his *Commentarii linguae graecae* of 1529.[64] In an analogous way de' Pomi infused his lexicographical work with his deep knowledge of natural philosophy. In the late Renaissance, dictionaries served many purposes besides providing definitions of words. They frequently functioned as outlets for authors to display their erudition.

The study of Hebrew underwent a renaissance in the sixteenth century, just as Latin and Greek did, and engaged Jews and Christians alike. Well-known Christian Hebraists like Sebastian Münster and Johannes Buxtorf compiled Hebrew dictionaries. Elia Levita composed a Hebrew dictionary in which he discussed Aramaic forms of Hebrew words.[65] Sante Pagnini wrote a Hebrew dictionary as well.[66] *Tsemaḥ David* belongs to this renascent genre of sixteenth-century dictionaries as well as to the established tradition of Hebrew lexicography from the Middle Ages. Like Calepino and other Renaissance lexicographers, de' Pomi conceived of his work as an amplification of other texts. The Hebrew portion of *Tsemaḥ David*'s title page announces that the text expatiates upon every word in Nathan ben Yeḥiel's *Arukh*, the *Meturgeman* and *Tishbi* of Elia Levita,[67] and many "other words besides those, exceedingly numerous."[68] Rather than expand on those works, de' Pomi's dictionary

[63] See Chapter 5.
[64] Considine, *Dictionaries in Early Modern Europe*, 31–3.
[65] See Gérard E. Weil, *Elie Lévita humaniste et massorète (1469–1549)* (Leiden: Brill, 1963).
[66] Sante Pagnini, *Thesaurus linguae sanctae* (Paris: Stephanus, 1548).
[67] On these works and their place in *Tsemaḥ David*, see the discussion below.
[68] *Tsemaḥ David*, title page, Hebrew section: ומלות אחרות זולתן אין מספר

supersedes them. Nathan ben Yeḥiel, David Kimḥi, and Elia Levita rarely expatiate upon topics in their definitions; de' Pomi frequently does. His entry on *qorban* (sacrificial offering), for example, runs to two printed columns in Hebrew, five in Latin, and two in Italian.[69] The breadth and detail of the Latin entry for *qorban* reveals that de' Pomi wished his Christian readers to know much more about sacrificial offerings than they could by merely reading the Bible. This antiquarian essay on animal sacrifices condenses Mishnaic and Talmudic scholarship on this topic and presents it, complete with the original terminology, for his readers' instruction.

HYACINTH AND *TSEMAḤ DAVID*

Many entries in *Tsemaḥ David* are expansive and anecdotal. De' Pomi's definitions of precious stones are no exception. And it is no accident that de' Pomi reserves the longest and most fulsome treatment of any biblical stone for *tarshish*, which he equated with hyacinth. In the sixteenth century hyacinth was commonly used as a prophylactic against the plague. But precisely how de' Pomi equated these two terms and the products they represented is a more complicated matter. De' Pomi's Latin entry for *tarshish*, like his Hebrew one, provides a skeletal outline of the issue. Indeed, Latin and Hebrew entries are often nearly identical in *Tsemaḥ David*, perhaps because its author wished Jews to improve their Latin by reading the language alongside a Hebrew translation; conversely, Christian scholars well versed in Latin could deepen their knowledge of Hebrew by comparing it to the Latin that followed. In contrast, the Italian portion of de' Pomi's entry is where he expands on themes introduced in the Hebrew and Latin, and where he presents the appropriate medical data. Indeed, de' Pomi almost always reserves his most extensive remarks for the vernacular portions of his entries. By using the vernacular rather than Latin to fully develop his ideas, de' Pomi followed in the footsteps of several sixteenth-century writers.[70]

[69] Ibid., 174:3–178:3.

[70] Chiara Crisciani has convincingly argued that the vernacular was an increasingly serious medium for writing in the Renaissance. See her "Histories, Stories, Exempla, and Anecdotes: Michele Savonarola from Latin to Vernacular," in Gianna Pomata and Nancy Siraisi, eds., *Historia: Empiricism and Erudition in Early Modern Europe* (Cambridge, MA: MIT Press,

To get a sense of how de' Pomi frames the discussion of *tarshish*, it is worth quoting the Latin entry in full:

> The word refers to an island of Africa, and means hyacinth, a precious stone, which, according to the account of a certain great merchant who traveled around India for many years, is said to be born from a [kind of] pregnancy, and to come from a specific region of that island. When the rains fall at a specific time (and this we may confirm as true, since when the rains do not fall, these stones are never found), pearls spring up from five species of mollusk, which are called *ostricha* in the vernacular. When the rains fall at the proper time, the crustaceans absorb droplets, which, in time, become pearls.[71]

While de' Pomi claims that the *tarshish* stone comes from an eponymous island in Africa and is a type of pearl that emerges from crustaceans only after periods of prolonged rain, the Latin tells us nothing of the value of the stone or of its medical properties; de' Pomi's Italian entry develops these themes.

After stating that *tarshish* may be understood as *iacinto*, the Italian word for hyacinth, de' Pomi gives oral testimony regarding the provenance of the stone. The Spoletan physician cites one of his rabbinic colleagues and an anonymous Turkish merchant,[72] who testifies to the

2005), 297–324. See also Brian Richardson, *Print Culture in Renaissance Italy: The Editor and the Vernacular Text, 1470–1600* (Cambridge: Cambridge University Press, 1994). On vernacular Bible translations in Italian Jewish culture, see Giuseppe Sermoneta, *Un volgarizzamento giudeo-italiano del Cantico dei Cantici* (Florence: G. C. Sansoni, 1974), 21–31; Sermoneta, "Considerazioni frammentarie sul giudeo-italiano," *Italia: Studi e ricerche sulla cultura e sulla letteratura degli ebrei d'Italia* 1 (1976): 1–29; 2 (1978): 62–106.

[71] *Tsemaḥ David*, 232:3: "Haec vox תרשיש significat insulam Aphricae et hyacinthum lapidem praetiosum, qui (ex relatu cuiusdam magni mercatoris per Indiam per multos continuos annos vagantis) oritur ex praegnitie (ut aiunt) cuiusdam terrae illius regionis, dum in certo tempore aquae pluviales descendunt. Et indicio est hoc veritatem possidere, quoniam, pluvia illo in tempore non descendente, lapides illi nullo pacto inveniri [*sic*: inveniuntur]. Sic ortum habere margaritas dixit in conchilium specie illa, quae ostrichae [*sic*: ostricha] vulgo dicitur; aperiuntur etenim dum pluit in praefisso tempore et recipiunt guttas illius aquae, qua congelata, in margaritas vertitur [*sic*: vertuntur]." With regard to "praegnitie," de' Pomi uses an alternative spelling for "praegnatione." I have seen few other instances of this spelling in medieval Latin. See, for example, Pierre Berchoir (d. 1320), *Dictionarii seu Repertorii Moralis Petri Berchorii Pictaviensis ordinis divi benedicti Pars Prima* (Venice: apud Haeredem Hieronymi Scoti, 1574), 496: "certe sic, praegnities enim lactationem praecedit."

[72] It is worth noting that the Italian reads "un gran mercante turcho," but the Hebrew is less specific about the nationality of the man, stating only "an important Ishmaelite": ישמעלי אחד חשוב

truth of what de' Pomi conveyed in the Latin and Hebrew portions of the entry. He recounts that

> Rabbi Isaac of Avila, one of my most faithful compatriots, told me that a great Turkish merchant, worthy of implicit trust, informed him that he had been to the East Indies many times and had indeed spent a very long time there. As a matter of curiosity he had sought out and investigated with great diligence the origins of precious stones. He found places [amenable] to the appearance [of precious stones] where the rainwater descends from the mountains at a specific time. Since he had not come at the proper season, the jewels did not appear.[73]

De' Pomi interrupts the Turkish merchant's account to summarize the relevance of the episode; then he proceeds to discuss the medical properties of the stone. "It is not surprising, therefore, that many of these stones possess great virtue against the plague, especially the *diacinto*, which I have experimented with in times of infestation in this great city. Because of a heavenly influx in certain constellations, plague arises, since God wills it to be so."[74] De' Pomi's entry ends by directing the reader to an

[73] *Tsemaḥ David*, 232:3: "me disse Rabi Isaac d'Avila mio fedelissimo compadre, che un gran mercante turcho, degno d'ogni credenza, gli disse esser diverse volte stato nelle Indie Orientali, et ivi fermatoseci per longissimo tempo e, come curioso, haver con ogni maggior diligenza cercata et investigata la origine delle gioie et haver'al fermo trovato nascere per ingravidarsi alcuni di quei monti di l'acqua della pioggia venuta a certo tempo determinato, per ciochè, non venendo in quella prefissa stagione, le gioie non nascono." I have not been able to identify Rabbi Isaac of Avila. A Portuguese Jew of the same name did turn up in Amsterdam in the middle of the seventeenth century. See Yosef Kaplan, "Wayward New Christians and Stubborn New Jews: The Shaping of a Jewish Identity," *Jewish History* 8:1–2 (1994): 27–41, 31.

[74] The entry on *tarshish* runs from 232:1 to 233:1. "Non è meraviglia donque, se molte di esse posseggono gran virtù, particolarmente il diacinto, contra la peste come ho io isperimentato nel tempo del contagio che venne in questa magnifica citta, perciochè nascono per influsso celeste in alcune costellationi, secondo che piace al Signor Iddio." On the general connection between astrology and medicine, see Nancy Siraisi, *Medieval and Early Renaissance Medicine: An Introduction to Knowledge and Practice* (Chicago: University of Chicago Press, 1990), 67. Also see H. Darrel Rutkin, "Astrology," in Katharine Park and Lorraine Daston, eds., *Cambridge History of Science*, vol. 3: *Early Modern Science* (Cambridge: Cambridge University Press, 2008), 541–61, esp. 544–6; Lauren Kassell, "'The Food of Angels': Simon Forman's Alchemical Medicine," in William R. Newman and Anthony Grafton, eds., *Secrets of Nature: Astrology and Alchemy in Early Modern Europe* (Cambridge, MA: MIT Press, 2001), 345–84; Anthony Grafton and Nancy Siraisi, "Between the Election and My Hopes: Girolamo Cardano and Medical Astrology," in ibid., 69–131. On the notion that plagues had astrological causes, see, for example, David Ruderman, *Kabbalah, Magic, and Science: The Cultural Universe of a Sixteenth-Century Jewish Physician* (Cambridge, MA: Harvard University Press, 1988), 33.

excursus about hyacinth in the Aramaic section of *Tsemaḥ David*.[75] The lengthy Italian entry in this section simply serves to describe how pearls emerge from crustaceans on a certain Indian island owing to the influence of seasonal rains. Before de' Pomi could accurately expand upon the medical properties of the *tarshish* stone, he first had to equate it to hyacinth and give a full account of its origin. Having done so, the stage was set for a medical explanation of the benefits of the hyacinth stone. These preliminary remarks also signal the conspicuous interest in precious stones both within the Jewish community and outside of it.

De' Pomi's Hebrew entry states that the "true" hyacinth stone is exceedingly rare and found only in small numbers; it is "extremely dear to one who knows its power and ability, which is great."[76] In the Hebrew entry, but not in the Italian or Latin, de' Pomi dismisses quacks and unlettered merchants. As David Gentilcore has shown, many university-trained physicians calumniated against such medical practitioners.[77] De' Pomi cautions his readers that "the unlearned, artisans, and stone merchants call the *diacinto* a stone of golden color, but it is not like that at all."[78] The real color of the *diacinto*, de' Pomi maintains, is red. After remarking that the "true" stone comes only from Ethiopia and India, de' Pomi addresses the medical relevance of the gem. The Hebrew entry points out that the ancient rabbis knew that the stone could help prevent the spread of the plague; the Italian entry says nothing about rabbis, but does remark that the "ancient and learned authors" praised its value against the plague.[79] Clearly, de' Pomi's praise for and belief in the medical efficacy of *tarshish* far exceeds his faith in any of the other stones of the breastplate. His claims about its immediate, even magical effect against contagious disease testify to the value of the stone in his eyes. The rest of the entry explains how to go about examining these stones to distinguish true from false – a theme that twenty years later Abraham

[75] *Tsemaḥ David*, 232:3: "E perche s'è ragionato della virtù del diacinto nelle dittioni יקנטין non dirò altro di esso al presente."

[76] Ibid., 86:3: ויש לדעת שהאבן הלז האמיתי לא נמצא אלא במספר מעט ... והוא יקר מאד למי שיודע כחו ופעולתו כי רבה היא

[77] David Gentilcore, *Healers and Healing in Early Modern Italy* (Manchester: Manchester University Press, 1998); Gentilcore, *Medical Charlatanism in Early Modern Italy* (Oxford: Oxford University Press, 2006).

[78] *Tsemaḥ David*, 86:3: ועמי הארץ וגם רבים מאומני ומתגרי האבנים טובו' קוראים דיאצינטו אבן א' זהבי בצבעו ואין ממנו בשום אופן

[79] Ibid.

Portaleone would develop with even greater energy.[80] Finally, de' Pomi excuses himself for the lengthy digression, stating that, "even though with this narrative I may have departed from the order of the dictionary, I hope that readers will not deem me worthy of censure, considering that it was for their benefit, and not mine, that I wrote these things."[81]

The first acknowledged source for David de' Pomi's comments on precious stones is medieval Jewish lexicography. As he himself noted on the title page of *Tsemaḥ David*, the work was designed as an amplification of three major works: the *Arukh*, by the eleventh-century Roman lexicographer Nathan ben Yeḥiel; and the *Meturgeman* and *Tishbi* of Elia Levita, the fifteenth-century Jewish grammarian and lexicographer who tutored Sebastian Münster in Hebrew.[82] Given that all three of these works are explicitly dedicated to explaining postclassical Hebrew, none of them would have been of much help to de' Pomi in his effort to define the scientific language of scripture.

The one medieval Jewish lexicographer from whom de' Pomi drew considerably is David Kimḥi, the late twelfth-century exegete and grammarian. Although de' Pomi does not mention Kimḥi on the title page of his work, the front matter of *Tsemaḥ David* signals Kimḥi's importance to de' Pomi's work three times. *Tsemaḥ David*'s Latin preface states that the twenty-four books of the Bible contain the "pura hebraica lingua." On these rich linguistic depositories, Kimḥi, "that illustrious man" (*insignis ille vir*), based his grammar. Furthermore, Kimḥi was the first, according to de' Pomi, to divide his dictionary into biblical words and nonbiblical words: a taxonomic principle that guides *Tsemaḥ David*.[83] In the Hebrew preface to his work, de' Pomi mentions Kimḥi again, suggesting that Kimḥi was de' Pomi's first point of reference for the meaning of words after Nathan ben Yeḥiel's *Arukh*. Only after exhausting the *Arukh* and Kimḥi's works did de' Pomi turn to Levita's linguistic compositions. "I compiled this composition from all of these [sources]," de' Pomi writes.[84]

[80] See Abraham Portaleone, *SG*, 58v–59r.

[81] *Tsemaḥ David*, 87:2: "ancor che con questa narrativa io sia uscito da l'ordine del dittionario, tuttavia spero che li signori lettori non mi faranno per questo meritevole di censura, considerando che non per mio, ma per lor'utile ciò sia stato da me detto."

[82] See Weil, *Elie Lévita*.

[83] Sig. A3r.

[84] Sig. A5r.

Kimḥi's work was extremely important for de' Pomi as he struggled to define the precious stones of the high priest's breastplate. Of the three stones that de' Pomi discourses upon most prolifically, he takes his definitions of two of them directly from Kimḥi, most likely via the edition with Levita's Latin glosses. Indeed, if we systematically compare the identifications of the twelve stones carried out by Kimḥi and de' Pomi, we see that half the definitions are exactly the same.[85] In short, de' Pomi was seriously indebted to Kimḥi and Levita for the Latinate scientific vocabulary that corresponded to the precious stones. Yet de' Pomi found little of intrinsic interest when it came to the scientific content of Kimḥi's definitions. De' Pomi, a medical doctor, craved more substantial material on the medical properties of the stones. Identifications, in the form of names, may have come directly from Levita's edition of Kimḥi. Descriptions, however, and medical excurses, came from other, less predictable, sources.

Examining Kimḥi's comments on three stones in particular underscores de' Pomi's originality. For *pitdah*, Kimḥi notes that it is "a stone from among the precious stones. They say that it is green, and Rabbi Yona writes that it is called זמרד in Arabic."[86] In the margin next to this gloss, we find the words "Lapis praeciosus, smaragdus."[87] Kimḥi's remarks on *yahalom*, the next stone that de' Pomi discourses upon at length, are scarcely more developed. Kimḥi quotes Abraham Ibn Ezra, who maintains that a Spanish sage noted that it is called אל מא״ס in Arabic. On the chemical composition of the stone, Kimḥi writes, "it breaks all stones and bores holes through them." In the margin next to these remarks we read "Iaspis."[88] For *tarshish*, Kimḥi offers even less specificity. He writes, "a precious stone that looks like תכלת. We have already discussed it in the entry for רשש." In

[85] De' Pomi draws on Kimḥi's definitions of *odem, pitdah, sapir, yahalom, shevo,* and *shoham.*

[86] Kimḥi is referring to Rabbi Jonah ibn Janah, an eleventh-century Spanish grammarian. His *Kitāb al-Tanqīh* (Book of Minute Research) was translated by Judah ibn Tibbon as *Sefer HaDikduk*. It contains a dictionary of biblical Hebrew entitled Kitāb al-Usūl, which ibn Tibbon translated as *Sefer HaShorashim* (Book of Roots). These works were widely available in the Middle Ages and exerted considerable influence on many thinkers, including David Kimḥi. See *EJ* 9:680–3.

[87] David Kimḥi, *Sefer HaShorashim Thesaurus linguae sanctae sive dictionarium hebreum* (Venice: Giustiniani, 1547), col. 352.

[88] Ibid., col. 115.

the margin next to this entry, Kimḥi writes "Chrysolithus."[89] Such is the level of depth and content in Kimḥi's glosses.

Yet there was more to the world of medieval Hebrew writings on precious stones than just lexicographical works. Though he never acknowledges them, David de' Pomi may have drawn from a significant and growing body of lapidaries that circulated in manuscript throughout the later Middle Ages and early modern period. By de' Pomi's time there were several Hebrew manuscripts concerning precious stones.[90] Some of these lapidaries were arranged according to the alphabetical order of non-Hebrew mineralogical terms, others according to the names of the twelve tribes of Israel, and still others according to the Hebrew terms for the stones mentioned in the book of Exodus. The affinities between some of these works and de' Pomi's entry on *tarshish* are strong. One text extols the placement of precious stones in rings as a way of keeping a curative nearby. Others identify *tarshish* as *iacinto* but say nothing about the salubrious properties of the stone. Still others assess precious stones besides *tarshish* in nearly identical ways to how de' Pomi describes *iacinto*'s medicinal value. But in the many medieval and Renaissance lapidaries that were distributed under various authors' names, only a few addressed the medicinal properties of either *tarshish* or *iacinto* in a way that corresponds to de' Pomi's entry, and these were written, without exception, by Italian or Greek physicians in the later Middle Ages and Renaissance. Renaissance Jewish physicians in Greek-speaking areas turned to Greek renderings of the Bible. Italian Jewish physicians did so, too.

Rings are frequently mentioned in medieval Hebrew lapidaries, as are observations about the efficacy of stones against the plague. A discussion of the *bezoar* stone in a Hebrew lapidary attributed to Aristotle and copied in 1382 in an Italian script describes the secrets of that stone

[89] Kimḥi, *Sefer HaShorashim*, col. 543. In the entry רשש there is barely any more of interest, except that that entry indicates that תרשיש is a name of a place, too.

[90] See the texts collected in *Sefer segulot ha-avanim tovot* (Jerusalem: Yerid Ha-Sefarim, 2004). The works in this volume date from the thirteenth to the nineteenth century. In its breadth and diversity, the collection is an excellent one with which to contextualize de' Pomi's lexicographical work. Sadly, the book lacks a critical apparatus, introductory remarks, or justification for the inclusion or exclusion of various texts. Still, it is the best printed resource for understanding medieval Hebrew lapidaries. I wish to thank Gad Freudenthal for making this text known to me.

in a manner reminiscent of de' Pomi's discussion of *iacinto*.[91] The text makes two points that connect to de' Pomi's work: "its characteristic is that it is effective against all plant and animal poisons, and from the bite of rodents and their stings";[92] and it explicitly mentions that this stone may be worn as a ring: "Whoever places a ring [made] of it on his finger will be respected by all who look upon him."[93]

An anonymous late medieval text from the end of the fourteenth century goes so far as to identify *tarshish* with *iacinto*. Apart from some reflections on the stone's color and its homiletic significance for being paired with the tribe of Asher, the most significant part of this entry is the simple statement: "*Tarshish* is *iacint*[*o*]."[94] This text may have helped de' Pomi equate *tarshish* and hyacinth, but it did not offer any explanation for why the biblical stone should be understood as *iacinto*.

A third text provides even more clues. In the early years of the sixteenth century, a Cretan Jewish doctor named Moses ben Eliahu Galina, who was also known as "the master of the secret," wrote a work called

[91] The text, entitled *Secrets of Stones and Pearls*, was published in a 1908 work by Moshe Gaster entitled *Secret of Secrets*. The manuscript of *Secrets of Stones and Pearls* is in the British Library, Ms. Oriental 2396. For a description of it, see G. Margoliouth, *Catalogue of Hebrew and Samaritan MSS in the British Museum*, vol. 3 (London: British Museum, 1965), 158–60. See also Moritz Steinschneider, *Die hebraeische Uebersetzungen des Mittelalters und die Juden als Dolmetscher* (Berlin: Kommissionsverlag des Bibliographischen Bureaus, 1893), 245. The text in question is in fact not an independent manuscript but rather a section of *Secrets of Stones and Pearls* called (at 123r): המאמר השמיני בחוכמות מיוחדות וסודות נימוסיות מהצלמים והטוב הנפשות וסגולות האבנים היקרות והצמחים והחיונות ומלות נפלאות מסודות הרפואה ומה שדומה הארסים ואינו צריך לרופא ובלעדי זה ממה שיועל כמו שזכרנו On 134v it is called שער בחכמות מיוחדות יסודות נימוסיות וזיכר סגולות אבני מרגליות See *Sefer segulot ha-avanim*, 76. *Bezoar* refers to concrements found in different organs of mammals, birds, reptiles, sea creatures, and plants. The most prized of these came from the gallstones of Persian goats. For more on that stone, see Deborah Harkness, *The Jewel House: Elizabethan London and the Scientific Revolution* (New Haven: Yale University Press, 2007), 33. See also Peter Borschbert, "The Euro-Asian Trade in Bezoar Stones (approx. 1500 to 1700)," in Michael North, ed., *Artistic and Cultural Exchanges between Europe and Asia, 1400–1900* (Aldershot: Ashgate, 2010), 29–43, 30.

[92] *Book of Secrets of Precious Stones*, 76: סגולתו שהוא מועיל מן הארסים כולם החיונים והצמחים ומנשיכת השרצים ועקיצתם [true pagination British Library Ms.: 135r].

[93] Ibid., 76: ומי שישים ממנו טבעת בידו יכבדו אותו כל האנשים וכל מי שיביט עליו [true pagination British Library Ms.: 135r].

[94] Ibid., 82: "תרשיש היא יכנ"ט" The work is entitled *These Are the Specifics of the Stones of the Breastplate* אלה הפרטים של אבני החשן The manuscript is from Oxford, Bodleian Ms. 647. The name of the copyist is Shmuel, and we have no other information regarding either the author of the work or its scribe. The work was copied in 1388, and pages 29b–30a of the Oxford manuscript contain this text.

Divrei Ḥakhamim.[95] It was not published until 1730 but circulated in manuscript form in the sixteenth century. Galina did see the publication of another of his works during his lifetime, a treatise on chiromancy and phrenology entitled *Toldot Adam*, published in Venice in 1517. Galina's entry on *iacinto* is similar to de' Pomi's definition in emphasizing *iacinto*'s curative properties. Galina does not identify the biblical stone *tarshish* with *iacinto*, but his treatment of *iacinto* strongly resembles that of de' Pomi. Galina defines three types of *iacinto* stone (as does de' Pomi) and observes that "the third type of this stone protects man so that he is not struck by the arrows of lightning that descend upon him in fury from the heavens. Additionally, he who wears it will not die from the plague because the ring purifies the air around him. And it removes from him the poison that is collected within it [the air]."[96] Galina and de' Pomi shared two important things in common: they were both physicians, and they both relied upon Greek traditions in their explication of the Bible. The fact that Galina, a Jewish physician from a Greek-speaking milieu, described the hyacinth stone in terms redolent of those de' Pomi used indicates the role that Greek learning may have played in identifying *tarshish* with *iacinto*.[97]

Another even more probable source for de' Pomi's equation of *tarshish* with *hyakinthos* was oral tradition. It is not surprising that northern Italian Jews would have absorbed Greek teachings concerning the precious stones of the Bible. As many as fourteen thousand Greeks lived in Italy between 1566 and 1596.[98] Greek Jews were prominent in

95 See Israel Ta-Shema, "The Book 'Ta'alumot ḥokhma' of Rabbi Elihu Galeno" (Hebrew), in *Keneset Meḥkarim: Iyyunim bisifrut harabanit biyimei habenayim*, vol. 3: *Italy and Byzantium* (Jerusalem: Bialik, 2004), 331–5. See 332 n. 5, for the appellation "בעל הסוד." See also Gerrit Bos, "Hayyim Vital's *Kabbalah Ma'asit we-Alkhimiyah* (Practical Kabbalah and Alchemy), a Seventeenth-Century 'Book of Secrets,'" *Journal of Jewish Thought and Philosophy* 4 (1994): 55–112; 61 n. 66.

96 *Book of Secrets of Precious Stones*, 131: האבן הזאת מהמין השלישי תשמור האדם שלא יכו בו חצי הברקים שירדו בזעף מן השמים. וגם לא ימות במגפה מי שנושאו עליו מפני שמזכך האויר שהוא סביבותיו ומסיר ממנו הארס הגנוז בו

97 David Jacoby has described the affinities between Greek and Hebrew learning among Jewish physicians in late medieval Crete in his "Jewish Physicians and Surgeons in Crete under Venetian Control" (Hebrew), in Reuven Bonfil, Menahem Ben-Sasson, and Joseph Hacker, eds., *Tarbut ve-hevrah be-toldot Yisrael bi-yeme-ha-benayim* (Jerusalem: Zalman Shazar, 1989): 431–44; see esp. 436–7.

98 In general, see Giorgio Fedalto, *Ricerche storiche sulla posizione giuridica ed ecclesiastica dei Greci a Venezia nei secoli XV e XVI* (Florence: L. S. Olschki, 1967). For this statistic, see

Venice and throughout the Veneto.[99] Significantly, many Italian doctors served as Venetian envoys and resident physicians in places with Greek-speaking Jewish communities, such as Constantinople and Crete.[100] And unattributed Greek etymologies in *Tsemaḥ David* suggest that de' Pomi may have heard oral communications from Greek speakers regarding the role of Greek in Hebrew literature. At the beginning of the twentieth century, the romance philologist David Blondheim showed how persistent oral traditions of the names of biblical stones were in the Jewish communities of medieval Europe; those oral transmissions gave rise to disparate renderings of these terms.[101] Long ago Joseph Perles proved that vernacular translations of the names of the stones were regularly taught to Jews in school.[102] Blondheim published manuscript fragments in Romance languages, written in Hebrew characters, that gave vernacular equivalents for the stones' names. Many of those translations show the influence of Greek. Indeed, a late fourteenth-century Greek translation of the Bible known as the *Graecus Venetus*, undertaken by a Jew who converted to Christianity, equates *tarshish* with *hyakinthos*.[103]

Closer to de' Pomi's own time, his colleague and coreligionist Abraham Portaleone not only gave his own rendition of the twelve stones in Italian but supplied that of his teacher, Moses Provenzali. Provenzali never published his translation, and Portaleone remarks that he "received

Heleni Porfyriou, "La diaspora greca in italia dopo la caduta di Constantinopoli: Ancona, Napoli, Livorno e Genova," in Maria Francesca Tiepolo and Eurigio Tonetti, eds., *I greci a Venezia* (Venice: Istituto Veneto di Scienze, Lettere, ed Arti, 2002), 151–84.

[99] See Benjamin Arbel, "Jews in International Trade: The Emergence of the Levantines and Ponentines," in R. C. Davis and B. Ravid, eds., *The Jews of Early Modern Venice* (Baltimore: Johns Hopkins University Press, 2001), 73–96.

[100] Jacoby, "Jewish Physicians and Surgeons in Crete under Venetian Control." See also Zvi Ankori, *Encounter in History: Jews and Christian Greeks in Their Relation through the Ages* (Hebrew) (Tel Aviv: Center for the History and Culture of the Jewry of Salonica and Greece, 1984), esp. 157–98 on Greek as a shared language between Jews and Christians in the former Byzantine Empire.

[101] David Blondheim, *Les parlers judéo-romans et la* Vetus Latina*: étude sur les rapports entre les traductions bibliques en langue romane des juifs au moyen âge et les anciennes versions* (Paris: É. Champion, 1925), 73 n. 1. See also Joseph Perles, *Beiträge zur Geschichte der hebräischen und aramäischen Studien* (Munich: Theodor Ackermann, 1884), 123.

[102] Perles, *Beiträge*, 124. See also M. Güdemann, *Geschichte des Erziehungswesens und der Cultur der Juden in Italien während des Mittelalters*, 2 vols. (Vienna: Alfred Hölder, 1884), 2:206.

[103] See Oscar Gebhardt, ed., *Graecus Venetus. Pentateuch Proverbiorum Ruth Cantici Ecclesiastae Threnorum Danielis versio graeca* (Leipzig: F. A. Brockhaus, 1875), Exodus 28:10.

the solution to the identity of the precious stones from the academy of the great, exalted master, the awe-inspiring man of God, our honorable teacher and rabbi, Rabbi Moses Provenzali of blessed memory."[104] While Portaleone ultimately did not agree with Provenzali, Provenzali's tradition regarding *tarshish* was to equate it with *iacinto*. David de' Pomi did not study with Provenzali, nor did he have the chance to read Portaleone's encyclopedia; it was not published until several years after his death. But Provenzali's translation, identical to de' Pomi's, demonstrates Italian Jews' tendency to use Hellenic traditions to elucidate the Bible's natural science.[105]

As significant as the Hebrew lapidaries and oral traditions were, the most important sources for scientific information on the precious stones for a sixteenth-century Italian physician like de' Pomi did not come from Jewish texts written in Hebrew but from Christian ones written in Latin. While Hebrew lapidaries and oral teachings may have helped him translate *tarshish* as hyacinth, they could not provide much information about the properties of that stone. By the High Middle Ages, Western European scholars could draw from a rich well of materials on the supposedly natural properties of precious stones.[106] One of the most prolific writers on this topic was Albertus Magnus (d. 1280). Renaissance figures, including de' Pomi, quote his work, and still more allude to or borrow from his writings.[107]

Albertus Magnus's *De mineralibus* was an important though unacknowledged source for de' Pomi. Indeed, de' Pomi's use of the Tarshish stone closely follows Albertus Magnus's own description of the physical uses particular to hyacinth. Describing hyacinthus, Albertus Magnus

[104] SG, 45r: ומבית מדרשו של הגאון המופלא איש האלהים נורא כמהר"ר משה פרוונצאלי ז"ל קבלתי פתרון האבנים טובות

[105] On a related point, see Joanna Weinberg's argument about Mantuan Jews' interest in the Letter of Aristeas in her "Azariah de' Rossi and Septuagint Traditions," *Italia* 5 (1985): 7–35, esp. 9–17.

[106] Moritz Steinschneider, "Lapidarien, ein kulturgeschichtliches Versuch," in George Alexander Kohut, ed., *Semitic Studies in Memory of Rev. Dr. Alexander Kohut* (Berlin: S. Calvary, 1897), 42–72.

[107] See, for example, Nancy Siraisi's comments about Albertus Magnus's books in Antonio Benivieni's library in her *The Clock and the Mirror: Girolamo Cardano and Renaissance Medicine* (Princeton: Princeton University Press, 1997), 154. There were a number of editions of *De mineralibus* that would have been available to de' Pomi by the middle of the sixteenth century.

writes that, "physically, its use is that when suspended from the neck or worn on the finger it keeps a traveler safe and makes him welcome to those who entertain him. It also protects him in regions infected with the plague."[108] As we have seen, de' Pomi champions an identical use for this stone, in terms of both the manner in which it ought to be worn and the tutelary uses to which it may be put. Even though de' Pomi does not mention Albertus Magnus as a direct source for this practice, the close resemblance between the two texts is striking and provides evidence that de' Pomi was reading, or at the very least knew about, Albertus Magnus's work.

Another unacknowledged medieval source de' Pomi drew from is Serapion, a Christian physician.[109] David de' Pomi's contemporary and colleague Abraham Portaleone refers to Serapion's work numerous times, and though de' Pomi does not, we may assume he knew about Serapion, given how fundamental his works were to sixteenth-century medical culture. De' Pomi learned much about hyacinth from Serapion's work: the color and appearance of the best sort of *tarshish* gem, and several of its salutary properties. In particular, Serapion maintains that there are three kinds of hyacinth stone but that "the red variety is better than the others. When a fire is lit near it, it glows increasingly red."[110] Beyond this simple description of its physical appearance, de' Pomi also may have taken some medical details from Serapion. The medieval Arab physician asserted that "the power of Hyacinth is such that whoever carried it with himself, as either a little figurine or some other type thereof, and enters into a place or a province in which many people have fallen, or into a plague-stricken region, no harm will befall him and he will remain safe from danger; no lightning will ever strike him. This property

[108] *De mineralibus,* book 2: *De lapidibus pretiosis*, tractatus 2: *De lapidibus nominatis et eorum virtutibus*, cap. 8: *De incipientibus ab I litera*, p. 232: "in ligaturis autem physicis est usus eius, quod collo suspensus vel digito gestatus, tutum reddit peregrinum et gratum hospitibus, et est contra pestiferas regiones." Quoted in Girolamo Cardano, *De Subtilitate*, ed. Elio Nenci (Milan: FrancoAngeli, 2004), 598 n. 19.

[109] He was known as Johannes Serapion or Serapion the Younger in the Christian West, to distinguish him from his ninth-century predecessor who wrote in Syriac. On Serapion, see George Sarton, *Introduction to the History of Science,* 3 vols. in 5 (Baltimore: William & Wilkins, 1927–48), II, i: 229.

[110] Quoted in Cardano, *De Subtilitate*, 598, n. 18: "et rubeus est melior aliis, quia quando incenditur ignis super eum, rubescit multum."

of hyacinth is well known and much praised among men."[111] De' Pomi seems to have taken as much from Serapion as from Albertus Magnus, and each scholar provided valuable information on the medical value of the hyacinth stone.

The most likely way de' Pomi learned about these medieval figures was by reading Renaissance medical writers. Perhaps the first text David de' Pomi would have turned to for information about the medical properties of stones was Marsilio Ficino's *De vita libri tres*. In fact, this book was one of the most popular medical works of the late fifteenth and early sixteenth centuries.[112] Virtually any university-educated physician would have been familiar with its contents. At various points in his work, Ficino discusses the magical and medical properties of precious stones, explaining that these properties are inherently magical and quasi divine: "Since properties of this kind and their effects could not come into being by elemental power, it follows that they proceed from the life and spirit of the cosmos, particularly through those very rays of the stars; and that therefore through them the spirit is affected as much and as soon as possible and exposed very much to celestial influences."[113] Ficino believed that the cosmos was animate and that divinely infused *spiritus* from the heavens affected things on earth. To Ficino, precious stones were repositories for *spiritus* – an idea that would have been appealing to de' Pomi. Moving on to discuss some particular stones, Ficino observes that "it is for just this reason that emerald, jacinth, sapphire, topaz, ruby, unicorn's horn, but especially the stone which the Arabs call bezoar, are endowed with occult properties of the Graces."[114] Because of their divine nature, supernatural origin, and medical efficacy, many of these objects, or their Hebrew equivalents, receive lengthy and detailed entries in de' Pomi's dictionary. In yet another parallel to de' Pomi's prophylactic use

[111] Ibid.: "est autem virtus hyacinthi, quod qui portaverit eum secum, aut sigillaverit aliquid cum aliqua specie ipsorum, et portaverit sigillationem super se, et intraverit in regionem aliquam, vel provinciam, in qua cadunt fulgura multa, seu in terram pestiferam, nullatenus nocebit ei, et fit tutus ab eis, quoniam non cadet fulgur super eum. Et haec quidem virtus est multum divulgata et honorata inter homines."

[112] On the popularity of *de vita*, see Marsilio Ficino, *Three Books on Life*, ed. and trans. Carol V. Kaske and John R. Clark (Binghamton, NY: Medieval and Renaissance Texts and Studies, 1989), introd.

[113] Ibid., book 3, chap. 12:300–1.

[114] Ibid. See also Thorndike, *A History of Magic and Experimental Science* (New York: Macmillan, 1929), 2:909–10, citing Pietro d'Abano and 4:224–5, citing Antonio Guaineri.

of hyacinth, Ficino remarks about these gems that "not only if they are taken internally, but even if they touch the flesh, and, warmed thereby, put forth their power, they introduce celestial force into the spirits by which the spirits preserve themselves from plague and poison."[115] This observation legitimizes the practice of wearing a gem, as it substantiates the salutary power of gems that merely come into contact with the skin and need not assimilate directly into the body. Ficino acknowledges Serapion as his major source for this information. He notes that "Serapion writes that he who wears a jacinth, or a signet made from one, is safe from lightning; and that this power of it is very widely known."[116] In terms of both its particular emphasis on the properties of the hyacinth stone and its general ascription of divinity to the healing powers of stones, Ficino's *De vita libri tres* was a likely source for de' Pomi.

Closer to his own time, de' Pomi might well have drawn from the work of Girolamo Cardano, who wrote extensively about precious stones in the seventh book of his encyclopedia of natural history, *De subtilitate libri XXI*.[117] It is especially noteworthy that so many of the stones Cardano studied were understood by contemporary Europeans as being the modern-day equivalents of biblical gems. Near the beginning of his extended essay on precious stones, Cardano writes that "most excellent among gems are green *smaragdus*, red *carbunculus*, sparkling *adamas*, milky pearl, dark-blue sapphire, golen *chrysolithus*, and various types of opal ... hyacinth may be added to these."[118] Nearly all of these stones were taken by biblical commentators, lexicographers, and natural scientists to represent either the stones in the high priest's breastplate or those in Revelation. Cardano upholds the medical efficacy of stones, stating that "not only are they alive, but they also alleviate sicknesses, old age, even death."[119] Moving from general observations

[115] Ficino, *Three Books on Life*, 300–1.

[116] Ibid. The Serapion quotation comes from *Liber aggregatus in medicinis simplicibus* (Venice, 1503), chap. 398, pp. 156.4–157.1–2, as cited in Ficino, *Three Books on Life*, 440 n. 7.

[117] On Cardano as a physician, see Siraisi, *The Clock and the Mirror*.

[118] Cardano, *De Subtilitate*, 595: "Praecipuae inter gemmas, smaragdus viridis, carbunculus rubens, adamas candidus, margarita lactea, sapphirus caeruleus, chrysolithus aureus, opalus varius. Precia eo ordine nunc apud nos se habent, nisi quod opalus smaragdum sequitur. His hyacinthus addatur."

[119] Ibid., 595: "neque solum vivunt, sed morbos, et senectutem, et post etiam mortem patiuntur."

about gems to specific remarks on their individual properties, Cardano discusses hyacinth at length and calls upon the testimony of familiar medieval authorities. He writes that "men of worthy authority attribute to Hyacinth much praise. Among them is Serapio, whom in [my] commentary on *Ars medica* I taught was [the same person as] John of Damascus, and who argues that [hyacinth] will render safe from lightning those who wear it – it will indeed protect them.[120] And just as a wax seal whose engravings are imprinted upon it, so will [hyacinth] make its mark on those who wear it."[121] Following these remarks, Cardano repeats the familiar wisdom that hyacinth keeps its wearers safe from lightning and the plague. Even though Cardano is more concerned with how the stone protects people from lightning and thunder, devoting several pages to an examination of precisely how the stone does this, he also states that the stone is capable of affording protection from pestilence. Finally, as marker of the two men's similar inclinations, Cardano himself wore a hyacinth stone on a ring, just as de' Pomi did. Cardano admitted that "I am accustomed to wearing quite a large stone, and it seems not to act as a soporific. My own stone is not crimson, which is the best sort, but golden, and far from the best. The crimson [stone] is the best."[122] The similarities between Cardano's work on hyacinth and de' Pomi's definition of *tarshish* are evident, and they indicate that de' Pomi may have borrowed much from him.

Another contemporary scientific source de' Pomi drew on for information about the biblical stone *tarshish* may have been François de la Rue's *De gemmis … explicatio*. De la Rue, or Rueus as he was known

[120] See "Ars curandi parva, quae est absolutissima medendi methodus," in Cardano's *Opera Omnia* (1663), 7:143–98.

[121] Cardano, *De subtilitate*, 597–8: "Hyacintho tribuunt non paucas laudes viri autoritate digni; inter quos Serapio, quem nos Ioannem Damascenum in Commento super Artem Medicam esse docuimus; quod a fulgure tutos reddat gestantes atque adeo tutos, ut vel cera quae illius caelaturae subiecta fuerit, etiam illud gestata arceat."

[122] Ibid., 599: "Ego praegrandem soleo gestare, videturque aliquid, non tamen multum conferre ad somnum; verum non puniceus hic meus est, atque ex illo optimo genere, sed aureus, multumque ab optimo desciscens. Optimus enim puniceus est, qui raro lentis superat magnitudinem." Cardano told the story of how he lost his ring on two other occasions. See *De vita propria liber*, chap. 30, in *Opera Omnia* 1:21. For an English translation, see *The Book of My Life*, trans. Jean Stoner (New York: New York Review Books, 2002), 101–2. See also his collection of *Paralipomena*, book 3, chap. 6, "de portento quod mihi apparuit," in *Opera Omnia* 10:459–60.

throughout the Latin world, originally published his work in Paris in 1547. *De gemmis* is organized not around the account of the high priest's breastplate in Exodus 28, but around John the Apostle's vision of the thirteen stones descending from the Jerusalem sky in the penultimate chapter of Revelation.[123] Clearly, de la Rue's scholarly point of departure, as well as his main area of interest, is the mineralogy of the New Testament rather than that of the Old Testament. Even so, many of the stones mentioned in Revelation are identical to those in Exodus or, more importantly, were conflated by Renaissance readers. Not surprisingly, de la Rue's entry on hyacinth bears some vivid similarities to de' Pomi's. After describing the appearance of the stone at some length, de la Rue suggests that, "moreover, when one looks at its features, it thickens and restores stubborn coldness from bodies, brings on sleep, guards powers (of the heart especially), and it is believed to keep away the plague from those who wear it, bringing its hidden properties to light."[124] As we have seen, de' Pomi also believed in hyacinth's ability to ward off the plague. Beyond this, de la Rue mentions other medical attributes of hyacinth, including its promotion of mental alacrity and its defense against the evil portents of thunder.[125] Lastly, de la Rue states that hyacinth is most effective as a medicament when it is "hung around the neck as an amulet close to the heart, so that it touches the skin."[126] In spite of the key similarities in de' Pomi's and de la Rue's treatment of the hyacinth stone, one must bear in mind that de la Rue's discussion of hyacinth was grounded in a study of New Testament, as opposed to Old Testament, stones. Nevertheless, de la Rue may have been a source

[123] François de la Rue, *De gemmis aliquot, iis praesertim quarum d. Ioannis Apostolus in sua Apocalypsi meminit*, bound with Levinus Lemnius, *Similitudinum ac parabolarum quae in Bibliis ex herbis atque arboribus desumuntur, dilucida explicatio* (Frankfurt: ex officina Paltheniana, 1596), 204.

[124] Ibid., 219: "porro quod ad facultates spectat, pertinaci frigiditate corpora densare atque reficere, somnum conciliare, virtutes (cordis praesertim) tueri, a populatim saeviente peste, cum manifesta sua qualitate, tum recondita quadam proprietate gestantem adserere, creditur."

[125] Ibid. In the Middle Ages, Marbode of Rennes (1035–1123) wrote about similar uses for the hyacinth stone in his *De lapidibus*, which was first printed in 1511. In a chapter of *De lapidibus* entitled *De iacinto*, Marbode of Rennes writes, "sed quodcunque genus collo suspendere possis, / Vel digito portes terras securus adibis, / Nec tibi pestiferae regionis causa nocebit." See John M. Riddle, *Marbode of Rennes' (1035–1123)* De lapidibus (Wiesbaden: Steiner, 1977), 52.

[126] François de la Rue, *De gemmis aliquot,* 219: "Ideoque pro amuleto collo suspenditur e regione cordis, ut cutem contingat."

for de' Pomi. Renaissance physicians believed deeply in the power of the hyacinth stone. Medical men as different as François de la Rue, Girolamo Cardano, and David de' Pomi all wore it in nearly identical fashion.[127]

Some of de' Pomi's Christian contemporaries had a distinct approach to the stones of the Bible, one that emphasized their theological significance more than their medical properties. Andrea Bacci's work on this subject, published at Rome in the same year as de' Pomi's dictionary, exemplifies this trend and provides a helpful point of comparison and contrast.[128] Even though Bacci emphasized doctrinal issues at the expense of scientific ones, his main interest, even in a book on an ostensibly theological subject, was natural philosophy. Near the beginning of *Le XII Pietre Pretiose*, Bacci noted that "it has always been the opinion of the great [natural] philosophers, and has been confirmed by the holy doctors of the church, that in all of nature works of greater wonder than gems and precious stones are not to be seen." For Bacci the church fathers merely confirmed what science had already taught him. But his book enriched patristic teachings with medieval and modern science. *Tsemaḥ David* displays the same complementary relationship between religious and scientific authority. Given the similarities between Bacci's and de' Pomi's work, and also the simultaneous publication of their books, a closer look at Bacci's *Le XII Pietre Pretiose* helps clarify the dynamic between science and faith in *Tsemaḥ David*.

Andrea Bacci was an exact contemporary of de' Pomi, and their research interests were similar. Born in 1524 in Sant'Elipidio a Mare, in Piceno, Bacci never earned a medical degree but, owing to papal intervention, was granted a chair in 1567 in botany at the University of Rome (La Sapienza). He remained in this position all his life and in 1587 was named chief physician to Pope Sixtus V.[129] That same year, Bacci wrote his

[127] A few other examples include Lodovico Dolce, *Trattato delle gemme che produce la natura* (Venice: G. Battista and G. Bernardo Sessa, 1565); Raniero Gnoli and Attilia Sironi, eds., *Istoria delle pietre* (undated Ms. from 1570s) (Turin: Umberto Allemandi, 1996); Camillo Leonardo (or Leonardi), *Speculum lapidum* (Venice: per Melchiorem Sessam et Petrum de Rauanis sociis, 1516); and Scipione Vasolo's 1577 *Le miracolose virtù delle pietre pretiose per salute del vivere humano*, published by A. Mottana in *Rendiconti Lincei* 16:1 (2005): 19–73.

[128] Andrea Bacci, *Le XII Pietre Pretiose, le quali per ordine di dio nella santa legge, adornavano i vestimenti del sommo Sacerdote* (Rome: Giovanni Martinelli), 1587.

[129] This biographical sketch comes from M. Crespi's entry in *DBI* 5:29–30. For more on Bacci, see Nancy Siraisi, "Rome: Medicine, Histories, Antiquities, and Public Health," in

short work on the precious stones of the Bible, dedicated to Alessandro Peretti, the cardinal of Montalto. It is striking that Bacci's piece and de' Pomi's dictionary were published the same year and noteworthy that Bacci's and de' Pomi's title pages emphasize a focus on precious stones and their occult secrets – even the very same stones.[130] Bacci was widely recognized for his mineralogical work. In a dedicatory poem to one of Bacci's later books, a natural history of wine in the ancient world, the Neapolitan theologian Giovanni Francisco Lombardo recalled Bacci's celebration of stones in Exodus and praised him for "adorning nature with his learned talents."[131]

Bacci's work on precious stones is in many ways similar to de' Pomi's. The Roman botanist confirms de' Pomi's belief that merely looking at precious stones gives strength to the observer. Bacci cites a passage from book 3 of Josephus's *Antiquities* explaining that, in biblical times, Jews would bring these stones with them into battle. According to Josephus, the glow of the stones would strengthen the Israelites' resolve and weaken that of their enemies.[132] Bacci also proposes that those who wear stones as ornaments or as fixtures in rings have wonderful access to occult powers.[133] These brief passages from Bacci's preface correspond to de'

her *History, Medicine, and the Traditions of Renaissance Learning* (Ann Arbor: University of Michigan Press, 2007), 168–93, 318–26; Siraisi, "Historia, Natural History, Roman Antiquity, and Some Roman Physicians," in Pomata and Siraisi, *Historia,* 325–54, esp. 348 n. 14 for additional literature.

[130] See title page of *Tsemaḥ David*, Latin section: "cum quadam Margaritarum, Unicornis, Ambrae, Hycinti, nec non caeterorum lapidum praeciosorum nova, et minime obscura universali cognitione, quae tamquam arcana a quam plurimis existimabitur." Bacci's title page announces discourses on "il diamante, le margarite, e l'oro ... con un sommario dell'altre pietre pretiose."

[131] Andrea Bacci, *De naturali vinorum historia* (Rome: ex typographia Nicolai Mutii, 1596), sig. a4r: "Quas gemmas celebrat sacra Exodus, inde recenset, / adiectis quas Rex possidet Aethiopum. / Occultas rerum caussas penetratque metalla, / naturae ut pateant plurima facta palam. / Describit radio cunctarum exordia rerum, / dira venena docet, praebet et antidota. / Quis non *Andreion* vocet hunc, Iasoline, virum, quem / tot Natura ornat dotibus ingenii?"

[132] Bacci, *Le XII Pietre Pretiose,* 2: "Onde Iosepho nel 3 dell'Antichità fa testimonianza essere stato antico costume de gli Hebrei di comparire nelle guerre loro co'l confalone Sacerdotale di queste xii gemme, perchè, prima che l'essercito si movesse, si vedeva uscirne tanto splendore, che abbagliati i nimici, i suoi, all'incontro, pigliavano animo della vittoria et di haver Dio in aiuto loro." See Josephus, *Antiquities* 8:9.

[133] Bacci, *Le XII Pietre Pretiose*, 3: "queste veramente si hanno a proporre per le principali virtù delle Pietre pretiose, le quali a vederle o portarle addosso, o ne gli anelli, o in altri ornamenti si dicono operare mirabilmente per proprietate occulta."

Pomi's similar claims and testify to the wide diffusion of these ideas. They suggest that de' Pomi was not alone among sixteenth-century Italian physicians in believing that the precious stones of the Bible had miraculous and medically benevolent powers.

But Bacci's work departs from de' Pomi's in two important ways: both his translation of names for biblical stones and his analysis of their secret properties are quite different. In the case of *tarshish*, Bacci follows the Vulgate and translates it as *chrisolito*. The divergence between de' Pomi and Bacci is not surprising. The identification of this stone was a troublesome matter for sixteenth-century Italians: Sante Pagnini, Marco Marini, Andrea Bacci, David de' Pomi, and Abraham Portaleone all came to different conclusions regarding its proper identity. Some natural philosophers, such as Abraham Yagel, even proposed two translations for the Hebrew term.[134] This multiplicity of opinions regarding the stones' true identity, especially in Jewish communities, led Augustinus Steuchus to muse in his *Veteris testamenti recognitio* of 1529 that Jews were "more casual than all other people in contriving knowledge of these matters."[135] Bacci's entry on *chrisolito,* for example, is short and says little about the medicinal properties of the stone. After listing possible alternative names for the stone, he notes, in step with de' Pomi, that the best version of the stone comes from Ethiopia, while lesser versions originate in Arabia. At the very end of the entry, he observes that the stones "guard against evil spells most effectively when they are worn on the left arm."[136] Apart from this mention of the health benefits of *chrisolito*, Bacci says nothing else about the stone's ability to protect people from the plague.

[134] Abraham Yagel, בית יער הלבנון (The House of the Forest of Lebanon), Oxford, Bodleian Ms. Reggio 10, chap. 69, הטור הרביעי תרשיש שוהם וישפה (The fourth row: *tarshish, shoham, and yaspeh*), where on 161v and 162r he translates *tarshish* in two different ways: היאצינטו (hyacinth), which he may have got from de' Pomi, and הקריסוליטו (chrysolithus), respectively. For more on Yagel and his encyclopedia of natural philosophy, see Ruderman, *Kabbalah, Magic and Science*.

[135] Augustinus Steuchus, *Veteris testamenti recognitio* (Lyon: Gryphius, 1531 [1529]), 464: "cum in his lapidibus interpretandis Hieronymus semper Septuaginta sequatur, et eorum in ea re approbarit aeditionem, non mihi visum est affere in medium, quae de his lapidibus ab Hebraeis dicuntur: cum et ipsi vehementer a Septuaginta et Hieronymo discrepent, et levior apud eos de hisce rebus inveniatur cognitio, quam omnes alias gentes."

[136] Bacci, *Le XII Pietre Pretiose*, 15: "Conservano dalle fascinationi, massime portati nel braccio sinistro."

Bacci analyzes the more quotidian health benefits of other stones in the high priest's breastplate. In fact, precious stones had a secure place in Galenic medicine as remedies for a variety of afflictions.[137] Bacci notes, for example, that *topatio* (Hebrew: *pitdah*) is effective against "sadness and other afflictions of the soul" and that it "mitigates against anger and fury."[138] *Smeraldo*, similarly, when "worn around the neck, cures the Hemitritean fever, the worst sort."[139] He is also interested in etymologies, clearly specious to the modern reader,[140] and in Jewish commentators' views of certain stones – even if only to dispute them. For example, discussing *sapphiro*, Bacci remarks "although some Jewish interpreters describe it as being of similar color to crystal, and others to *purpura nigra*, which is the color of violets, these commentators are mistaken; it is common knowledge that sapphire is the color of the air in the clearest sky."[141]

The ultimate difference between these two natural philosophers is that while de' Pomi focuses on the scientific and curative properties of stones, Bacci is concerned above all with the spiritual significance and doctrinal relevance of the stones' identity. Labeling himself a "Christian philosopher" in his work on unicorns, Bacci's allegiance was to the dominant figures in Christian thought.[142] Accordingly, when he assessed the significance of the names of biblical stones, Bacci faithfully follows

[137] See Galen's account of the medicinal uses of stones in his *De simplicium medicamentorum temperamentis ac facultatibus libri XI*, book 9, chap. 2, in C. G. Kühn, ed., *Opera*, 12:192–208. Hyacinth is prescribed, along with jaspis, indico, and other stones, as a cure for a variety of ailments. See ibid., 207. See also Galen's list of items that can be substituted as medicaments for various gemstones in *De succedaneis liber*, in ibid., 19:734–45. In this later work, which may be pseudo-Galenic but was transmitted with Galen's works, *beryllus* may be substituted "pro lapide hyacintho," indicating that hyacinth was a popular enough remedy not only for Galen to mention it but for him to list a substitute for it. Ibid., 735.

[138] Bacci, *Le XII Pietre Pretiose*, 8: "vale contra la mestitia, et altre passioni dell'animo et buttata per esperienza nell'acqua bollente, fa cessare maravigliosamente il bollore, onde alcuni hanno preso occasione di dire che mitiga la colera, et l'ira."

[139] Ibid., 9: "Tenuto al collo sana la febre Hemitriteo, pessima febre."

[140] For example, he claims that *sardius* is so called because it comes from Sardinia (Sardo). Ibid., 7.

[141] Ibid., 11: "et benche alcuni interpreti Hebrei lo descrivano di colore simile al cristallo, et altri alla purpura nigra, che è il color delle viole, questi però s'ingannano, perche di commun parere il sapphiro è del color dell'aria nel cielo chiarissimo." I have not been able to locate Bacci's source of information regarding these "Jewish commentators."

[142] See Andrea Bacci, *L'Alicorno* (Florence: Giorgio Marescotti, 1573), 53: "essendo io Filosofo Christiano e curioso di sapere, e di scrivere la verità sopra a tutti i miei desiderii, mi ritratterrò molto volentieri."

Saint Jerome and Epiphanius, the fourth-century bishop of Cyprus who wrote an influential work on precious stones in Revelation. For example, regarding the *diaspro*, Bacci explains that it is mentioned in Exodus "in order to prefigure the heavenly Jerusalem in the Apocalypse with the fundamentals and marvels of the *diaspro*, since the strength of the *diaspro* and the grandeur of the science of God overpower and overcome all false doctrine."[143] For de' Pomi, the ultimate strength of biblical stones lay in their curative powers, not their theological ones. Bacci shared a belief with de' Pomi that attending to the natural products of the biblical world could positively change present-day circumstances.

As were the church fathers Jerome and Epiphanius, to whom Bacci paid eloquent deference, Bacci was chiefly concerned with the symbolic features of the high priest's stones. In fact, the Roman botanist undertook his work because those theologians deemed the precious stones worthy of investigation.[144] As such, it is not surprising that Bacci's identifications of the stones match those of the Vulgate precisely; taking his lead from Epiphanius, he had no reason to deviate from church tradition. In spite of Bacci's and de' Pomi's many similar tendencies and overlapping professional interests, their different means of employment affected their approach toward the scientific content of scripture. Bacci lived in Rome and, in addition to his teaching responsibilities at La Sapienza, was working as the chief physician to Pope Sixtus V when he published his book on precious stones. His personal circumstances led him to follow the fathers of the church and refrain from speculation on the medical and magical applications of biblical products. Still, to understand the role patristic writings played in Italian naturalists' efforts to understand the precious stones of the Bible, we must consider the availability of those writings in de' Pomi's and Bacci's time, as well as their significance.

Bacci was not alone in introducing his work as a continuation of patristic writings; many other Italian naturalists grounded their investigations of science and scripture in a discussion of one or more fathers

[143] Bacci, *Le XII Pietre Pretiose*, 12: "Onde nell'Apocalisse vien figurata la celeste Hierusalem c'habbia i fondamenti, et le muraglia di diaspro, significando secondo S. Hieronimo, che la forze del diaspro e la grandezza della scienza di Dio espugna et supera ogni falsa dottrina."

[144] Ibid., sig. +2r–v: "la quale tratta delle Dodici pietre pretiose, che, secondo la interpretatione di S. Gieronimo e di S. Epifanio Arcivescovo antico di Cipri, si legge, che per ordine di Dio nella Sacra Scrittura, se ne dovesse ornare il manto del Sommo Sacerdote."

of the church.[145] De' Pomi may have turned to their writings as well. We know that learned Jews in sixteenth-century Italy such as Azariah de' Rossi read patristic writings, especially in the new Latin translations of Greek patristic works coming out in the sixteenth century.[146] And Christian scholars also directed an increasing amount of attention to the church fathers as the century wore on.[147]

Neither Epiphanius nor Jerome, the two church fathers Bacci openly acknowledges as direct influences, identifies *tarshish* as hyacinth or describes the medical benefits of that stone. Epiphanius, in his short work on the precious stones of the Bible, which was available in several editions by the middle of the sixteenth century,[148] was concerned above all else with describing their appearance and predicting their efficacy in aiding "pious meditations."[149] Because Epiphanius focused his attention on the spiritual properties of the stones, and because his renderings of their names remained in the mainstream of Catholic tradition owing to their identical match with the language of the Vulgate, Epiphanius was a trusted source for scholars like Bacci.

Jerome, a slightly younger contemporary of Epiphanius, had not defined *tarshish* as hyacinth but praised it as a "most precious stone" and speculated that it might be a variant of *ligurius*, the stone he designates as *leshem*. In a letter on the priest's garments, Jerome wondered why hyacinth, "a most precious stone, is not included among them, unless perhaps it is another name for *ligurius*."[150] And, in general, Jerome displayed very little interest in the medical properties of stones.

[145] See Chapter 1 where I discuss how Aldrovandi cast his work on nature and the Bible as a response to Augustine's *De doctrina christiana*.

[146] Azariah de' Rossi, *The Light of the Eyes*, trans. and ed. Joanna Weinberg (New Haven: Yale University Press, 2001), introd., xxxviii–xxxix.

[147] See Eric Cochrane, *Italy, 1530–1630* (London: Longman, 1988), 189; Pio Paschini, "Un cardinale editore: Marcello Cervini," in his *Cinquecento Romano e Riforma Cattolica* (Rome: Facultas Theologica Pontificii Athenaei Lateranensis, 1958), 185–217.

[148] Conrad Gesner, *De omni rerum fossilium genere* (Zurich: Gesner, 1565), in which one finds *De gemmis XII Rationalis*, attributed to Epiphanius. Quoted in Petrus Franciscus Fogginius, ed., *S. Epiphanii ... De XII Gemmis Rationalis summi sacerdotis Hebraeorum liber* (Rome: Typis Zempellianis, 1743). For a modern edition, see Migne, *Patrologiae cursus completus ... series graeca*, (Paris: J.-P. Migne, 1857–99), 43:310.

[149] *De duodecim gemmis quae erant in veste Aaronis liber*, in Migne, *Patrologia Graeca*, 43:294–304, 294: "colores sive formas, locos, et quae faciunt inde ad pietatem meditationes."

[150] Epistola LXIV ad Fabiolam, "*De veste sacerdotali*," in *PL* 22:607–22, 616: "Satisque miror cur hyacinthus pretiosissimus lapis in horum numero non ponatur, nisi forte ipse est alio nomine 'ligurius.'"

As they were for Epiphanius, homiletics were his primary interest. Jerome did mention Symmachus, the late second-century translator of the Bible into Greek, and he was aware of gaps between Symmachus's rendering of the names of the stones and his own. He noted, for example, that Symmachus did not translate *bareqet* as *smaragdus* but prefers *ceraunius*.[151] In another place, Jerome directly took up the issue of whether *tarshish* is best understood as *chrysolithus* or hyacinth and suggested that the very word *tarshish* expressed the blueness of the sea. According to Jerome, the stone took its name from this color.[152] The fact that he did so is evidence that, from late antiquity to the sixteenth century, the proper identification of this stone was a matter of controversy.

But without question the church father who took the most sustained interest in hyacinth was Symmachus, of whom sixteenth-century scholars were well aware. Symmachus rendered the Hebrew term *tarshish* as *hyakinthos* in virtually all instances for which we have record of his work. Symmachus's Greek translation of the Bible dates from the late second century. Scholars have long debated Symmachus's translations as well as his religious identity. Eusebius and Jerome believed that he was an Ebionite, or Jewish heretic. Epiphanius maintained that he was a Samaritan who converted to Judaism.[153] In the nineteenth century, Abraham Geiger concluded that certain Midrashic renderings in Symmachus's translations proved his status as an Ebionite.[154] Most modern scholars have agreed.[155]

Whatever his religious identity, Symmachus was the only ancient translator of the Bible into Greek who rendered *tarshish* as *hyakinthos*.[156]

[151] Ibid., 615.

[152] Epistola XXXVII ad Marcellam, in *PL* 22:462: "Quaeras si Tharsis lapis chrysolithus sit, aut hyacinthus, ut diversi interpretes volunt, ad cuius coloris similitudinem Dei species scribatur, quare Jonas propheta Tharsis ire velle dicatur (*Jonae* 1) et Salomon et Josaphat in Regnorum libris naves habuerint, quae de Tharsis solitae sint exercere commercia (2 *Reg.* 10). Ad quod facilis est responsio ομώνυμον esse vocabulum, quod et Indiae regio ita appelletur et ipsum mare, quia caeruleum sit et saepe solis radiis percussum colorem supra dictorum lapidum trahat, a colore nomen acceperit."

[153] Alison Salvesen, *Symmachus in the Pentateuch* (Manchester: Journal of Semitic Studies Monographs 15, 1991).

[154] Abraham Geiger, "Symmachus der Übersetzer der Bibel," *Jüdische Zeitschrift für Wissenschaft und Leben* 1 (1862): 39–64.

[155] Salvesen, *Symmachus in the Pentateuch*, 297.

[156] Frederick Field, ed., *Origenis Hexaplorum quae supersunt sive veterum interpretum graecorum in totum Vetus Testamentum fragmenta*, 2 vols. (Hildesheim: Georg Olms

Even in biblical passages where *tarshish* is employed as an adjective rather than as a noun, Symmachus renders it as some variant of hyacinth.[157] Scholars as varied as Augustinus Steuchus, the exegete, and Antonio Carafa, the primary editor of the Sixtine Greek Bible, knew of Symmachus's Bible translation and occasionally accepted his interpretation. The Jewish convert to Christianity Sixtus Senensis wrote an entry on Symmachus in his *Bibliotheca Sancta*.[158] Although I have not yet found any printed text from de' Pomi's lifetime that notes Symmachus's translation of *tarshish* as *hyakinthos*, we do know of manuscripts that contain Symmachus's glosses. Natalio Fernandez Marcos has reported that between 1565 and 1575 the library of a certain Konstantinos Barenos contained a complete translation of the Psalms by Symmachus and other bits of the Old Testament.[159] And Steuchus and Carafa are merely two examples of de' Pomi's contemporaries who were aware of Symmachus's work. Ulisse Aldrovandi approvingly quotes one of Symmachus's glosses, and even prefers one of Symmachus's renderings of a precious stone in Ezekiel to that of Jerome.[160] Aldrovandi's patron Gabriele Paleotti mentions Symmachus as well in a badly damaged letter in Bologna's Archivio Isolani.[161] Augustinus Steuchus observed that the "true septuagint was most holy among the Jews ... but it did not satisfy Symmachus or Theodotion, who established other interpretations."[162] Steuchus knew that Symmachus's renderings of the Hebrew Bible presented an alternative to the Septuagint. He also stated that he had access to various Greek Bible commentaries in the library of

Verlagsbuchhandlung, 1964 [1865]), 1:131, Exodus 28:20: תרשיש, *chrysolithus*; Origen: χρυσόλιθος; Symmachus: ὑάκινθος.

157 Ibid., 2:770, Ezek 1:16: כעין תרשיש: Vulgate: quasi aspectus chrysolithi. Origen: ὡς εἶδος θαρσείς. Aquila: ὡς ὀφθαλμός χρυσολίθου. Symmachus: ὡς ὅρασις ὑακίνθου. Jerome: "*Tharsis*, quam nos in *mare* vertimus: Aquila *hyacinthum* posuit, qui lapis caeli habet similtudinem." See ibid., n. 42.

158 Sextus Sinensis, *Bibliotheca Sancta*, 2 vols. (Venice: Gryphius, 1566), 1:471.

159 Natalio Fernández Marcos, *Introducción a las versiones griegas de la Biblia* (Madrid: Consejo Superior de Investigaciones Cientificas, 1979), 110.

160 BUB Ms. Aldrovandi 91, *De lucentibus*, "Excellentissimo ac valde Reverendissimo Alfonso Paleoto Canonico S. Petri Cathedralis Ecclesiae dignissimo," 372r–377r, 372r: "Et novem istae gemmae Ezechielis ex quatuor ordinibus tres occupabant: nam in primo ordine erant sardius, topatius, smaragdus. Symmachus dissentit in Smaragdo Corauneum pro eo transferens."

161 Bologna, Archivio Isolani, F. 60/134, CN 88, p. 401.

162 Steuchus, *Veteris testamenti ... recognitio*, sig. a2v.

the Venetian cardinal Domenico Grimani: "Greek fathers, who were most vigilant in matters of sacred scripture, are commonly cited, for we have a great number [of them] in the divine library of the most learned man, the most excellent in all virtues, Domenico Grimani."[163] While it cannot be proved that de' Pomi himself had access to Grimani's collection – de' Pomi was a small child when Grimani died, and parts of his collection were dispersed soon after his death[164] – we know from Moritz Steinschneider's research that Grimani had cordial relations with Jews and even hired Abraham de Balmes as his Hebrew teacher. De Balmes dedicated a 1523 Latin composition to Grimani.[165] Finally, we know that de' Pomi's Jewish compatriot Azariah de' Rossi was familiar with Symmachus's works – even if only at secondhand. In his *Meor Enayim* (Light of the eyes), de' Rossi wrote that "the books which were translated by the seventy elders did not retain their true meaning in the Greek language. And so Aquila, Symmachus, and Theodotion made other translations which were different from it." In contrast to Aquila and Theodotion, de' Rossi suggested, Symmachus "gave more consideration to the meaning of the text."[166]

And there is one final way de' Pomi might have come across Symmachus's rendering. A corpus of eleventh-century Greek glosses to the sixth-century Codex Ambrosianus testifies to the persistence of Symmachus's translations throughout the Middle Ages. In these texts, a Jewish glossator broke from the standard rendering of *tarshish* as

[163] Ibid., 9–10.

[164] The best source for information about Grimani's library, especially his Greek manuscripts, is in Aubrey Diller, Leendert G. Westerink, and Henry D. Saffrey, eds., *Bibliotheca graeca manuscripta cardinalis Dominici Grimani (1461–1523)* (Venice: edizione della laguna, 2003). Upon Grimani's death in 1523, he bequeathed part of his library to his nephew Marino Grimani and the rest to the Augustinian monastery Sant'Antonio di Castello. Eventually the latter was absorbed into the library of San Marco. In 1597, for example, when the Holy Office under the direction of Cardinal Agostino Valier surveyed the contents of religious libraries in Venice, 112 of the original 392 Greek manuscripts were still available in the monastery's collection, which was nominally open to the public. See Marino Zorzi's *presentazione* to this work, pp. v–xi.

[165] Moritz Steinschneider, "Une dédicace d'Abraham de Balmes au Cardinal Dom. Grimani," *REJ* 5 (1882): 112. Most recently on de Balmes, see Ennio de Bellis, "Cenni sulla dottrina della *demonstratio* nel pensiero di 'Avraham de Balmes," in Fabrizio Lelli, ed., *Gli ebrei nel Salento: secoli IX–XVI* (Galatina: Congedo Editore, 2013), 285–99 and works cited there.

[166] Azariah de' Rossi, *Light of the Eyes*, 172. De' Rossi likely learned this from Jerome, *Praefatio in librum chronicorum Eusebii*. See *PL* 27:35–6.

chrysolithus and translated the Hebrew stone as *hyakinthos*.[167] As de' Pomi sought to import a corpus of scientific knowledge into the camp of scriptural studies, Symmachus's translations may have provided a valued link.

Though de' Pomi roamed far and wide to find information about the stones of the high priest's breastplate, there were sources within his own cultural tradition that may have inspired him as much as Albertus Magnus or Girolamo Cardano did to wear the *diacinto* stone as a prophylactic against the plague. A Talmudic legend in the tractate *Bava Batra* relates that "a precious stone hung from the neck of Abraham, our father. Whoever looked upon it was instantly cured."[168] Although de' Pomi nowhere mentions this passage, early modern Jews, in spite of the ban against printing the Talmud in Italy after 1554, knew it well.[169] De' Pomi, as an educated Jew, was almost certainly aware of this passage. It attests to a belief, enshrined in one of Judaism's canonical texts, in the curative properties of precious stones. De' Pomi may have drawn from the Talmud to buttress his belief, buoyed by scientific learning, in the curative properties of stones. Though it may have legitimized his own practice of hanging a stone around his neck, the Talmudic legend about Abraham did not specify what stone it was.[170] As we have seen, de' Pomi had to look far beyond classical Jewish traditions and medieval Hebrew lexicography to equate hyacinth with *tarshish* and augment his faith in the latter with the science of the former. De' Pomi and his Jewish colleagues such as Abraham Portaleone balanced contemporary learning with received tradition. Such a commitment was a constant challenge, a stimulus to further study, and an exercise that strengthened their faith.

[167] The best study of this text is the unpublished *tesi di laurea* of Mariachiara Fincati, *Il restauro medievale dell'Esateuco ambrosiano A 147 inf.* (Milan: Università Cattolica del Sacro Cuore, 2008). See also her "Per la storia dell'Esateuco ambrosiano A 147 inf.," *Aevum* 83 (2009): 299–339.

[168] BT Bava Batra 16v: אבן טובה היתה תלויה בצוארו של א"א שכל אחד הרואה אותה מיד נתרפא

[169] See Isaiah Sonne, "Journeys through the Place Where Reality and the Book – History and Bibliography – Are Adjacent" (Hebrew), in *Alexander Marx Jubillee Volume* (New York: Jewish Theological Seminary, 1950), 209–35. See also Amnon Raz Krakotzkin, *The Censor, the Editor and the Text: The Catholic Church and the Shaping of the Jewish Canon in the Sixteenth Century* (Philadelphia: University of Pennsylvania Press, 2007).

[170] A very similar use for the Bezoar stone is attested in British Library, Ms. Oriental 2396. The author of that manuscript writes (135r): ואם יתלו ממנו בצואר הנער שלא נרפא ולא אירע לו מאורע יציל אותו מהמאורעים "If they hang it [Bezoar] upon the neck of a young person who was not cured, and if no incident befell him, it will rescue him from any further incidents."

CONCLUSION

For David de' Pomi, Greek traditions and empirical evidence connected premodern science to scripture, allowing him to import a body of scientific knowledge into scriptural studies. While he professed his allegiance to medieval Hebrew lexicography, he supplemented that tradition with other sources. For his work on the precious stones of the Bible, at least, de' Pomi favored medieval and early modern Latin lapidaries as well as a corpus of medieval Hebrew writings on precious stones. Oral traditions may have informed de' Pomi's views, too. Venice was crowded with Jews from all over the Mediterranean world, and as writers in both the sixteenth and twentieth centuries emphasized, rendering the names of biblical stones into the vernacular was a common practice – and one that each community performed differently.

De' Pomi's sensitivity to and interest in Greek terminology for the Bible's recondite vocabulary is representative of broader trends in Italian Jewish culture of the late Renaissance.[171] Joanna Weinberg has clearly shown how important the Septuagint was in Jewish culture in the middle of the sixteenth century and has argued that Azariah de' Rossi was familiar with the Greek Bible in spite of the fact that he did not know Greek very well.[172] Abraham Portaleone and his teacher Moses Provenzali used Italianized Greek words to gloss scripture.[173] The physician and antiquarian Girolamo Mercuriale invoked a line from Horace

[171] See Moses A. Shulvass, "The Knowledge of Antiquity among the Italian Jews of the Renaissance," *Proceedings of the American Academy of Jewish Research* 18 (1948–9): 291–300. See also Joanna Weinberg, "Azaria de' Rossi and Septuagint Traditions," *Italia* (1985): 7–35.

[172] It is worth noting that in spite of his considerable learning de' Rossi lacked a university degree and was therefore deprived of the best opportunity to study Greek. De' Rossi himself lamented that he did not know Greek as well as he wished: ואני הצעיר לא ידעתי ספר ולשון יוני כאבת נפשי *Me'or Enayim* (Mantua, 1573–5), 2. In spite of this deficiency, he discusses the rabbis' use of Greek in several places (Weinberg trans., 577–8, 596) and is also aware of differences between literary and spoken Greek, which he refers to as לשון מיוחד להעלות על ספר and ידבר בו איש אל רעהו respectively. See Weinberg trans. 687 and Cassel edition (Vilna: Y. R. Rom, 1866), 462.

[173] Portaleone cultivated his Greek studies in other settings, too. In several letters in his collected medical *consilia*, Portaleone investigates Greek expressions, even when he wrote to other Jews. See, for example, his 1569 *consilium* to Abraham Provenzali, in *Abrahami Portaleonis medici mantuani hebrei responsorum et consultationum medicinalium liber*, Paris, Bibliothèque nationale, Ms. Latin 13004, 293r–v.

when he urged students to study Greek "day and night" in his popular work on medical studies.[174] His language may have reminded biblically literate Jews of similar wording in a scriptural exhortation to study day and night.[175]

In sixteenth-century Italy the examination of precious stones from the Bible was an intellectual endeavor that stood at the intersection of medicine, antiquarianism, and biblical studies. For de' Pomi, and for other Italian physicians as well, medical science and biblical studies had a reciprocal relationship. De' Pomi's scientific training helped him understand scripture by introducing him to Latin books and traditions that, properly understood, could reveal the Bible's hidden meaning. And his education at Perugia instilled a lifelong interest in Greek that stimulated de' Pomi's curiosity about Greek renderings of the Bible as indicative of the text's true meaning. But de' Pomi's fascination with biblical gemstones was not merely bookish; it was nurtured by the commercial setting he lived in. His professional experience as a physician put him into regular contact with several Venetian merchants who dealt in precious stones. In de' Pomi's mind, some of those stones, including *hyacinthus*, became physical instantiations of biblical words. However, university education and medical culture did not merely offer their services to biblical commentary; they were enriched by biblical traditions, too. De' Pomi believed that a biblical product whose arcane properties were exposed by modern science could be the best cure for disease. And in a time of devastating plagues such as the one that struck Venice in 1571–2, medical practitioners of all sorts enthusiastically sought new remedies. When Andrea Bacci invoked the "science of God" and its "grandeur" in his discussion of the high priest's stones, he articulated a belief that the natural philosophy of the biblical world could solve contemporary problems. He easily could have been speaking for his Jewish colleague from Spoleto.

[174] See Richard J. Durling, "Girolamo Mercuriale's *De modo studendi*," *Osiris*, 2nd ser., 6 (1990): 181–95, 188: "Ceterum Graeci ii sunt de quibus id Horatium dicere cogor 'Nocturna versate manu, versate diurna.'"

[175] Joshua 1:8: והגית בו יומם ולילה

4

Jewish-Christian Relations in Sixteenth-Century Italy

Abraham Portaleone's Correspondence with His Gentile Colleagues

In the 1580s and 1590s, Abraham Portaleone, a Jewish physician of Mantua, corresponded with several of his Catholic colleagues. The very fact that Portaleone corresponded with Catholic physicians such as Giovanni Battista Cavallara and Alessandro Magno presents new evidence of sustained social and intellectual contact between Jews and Christians in early modern Italy. Their letters also augment our knowledge of key topics in late Renaissance natural philosophy, such as alimentation and embryology. Most importantly, Portaleone's correspondence with Cavallara and Magno suggests that the boundaries separating religious scholarship from scientific research were porous and that religious differences promoted rather than impeded the free flow of information and ideas across those boundaries.

In sixteenth-century Italy, the medical profession promoted interconfessional dialogue. Jewish and Christian medical students attended the same universities, treated patients of different faiths,[1] and, in some cities such as Mantua, were members of the same colleges of physicians. They also wrote each other letters, which contain passages that signal

[1] Throughout the sixteenth century Jews needed a license to treat Christian patients. Fewer licenses were granted after 1555 during the papacy of Paul IV. In his bull "Contra medicos hebraeos" (1581), Pope Gregory XIII strengthened the restrictions Paul IV had imposed. See Harry Friedenwald, "Jewish Physicians in Italy: Their Relation to the Papal and Italian States," in his *The Jews and Medicine*, 2 vols. (Baltimore: Johns Hopkins University Press, 1944), 2:551–612, esp. 582–9. Friedenwald includes a facsimile reproduction of Gregory XIII's bull between pages 550 and 551 and provides an English translation on pages 584–6.

A portion of this chapter previously appeared as "Abraham Portaleone and Alessandro Magno: Jewish and Christian Correspondents on a Monstrous Birth," *European Journal of Jewish Studies* 5:1 (2011): 53–66.

familiar and enduring relationships. To the historian of Jewish-Christian relations in the premodern period, these exchanges indicate two important things. First, they suggest that some Jews and Christians formed and sustained intellectual alliances that were not predicated on, or poisoned by, interfaith polemic. Second, they reveal how medicine catalyzed this form of social intercourse more than any other profession. Of all the professional settings in the early modern world where educated men of different religions interacted, medicine facilitated the closest collaboration between Jews and Christians. And of all the places in early modern Europe where medical men of different faiths enjoyed social intercourse, northern Italy and especially the city of Mantua serve as prominent examples.

Religious polemic is entirely absent from the letters Portaleone exchanged with his Christian correspondents; antiquarian and natural scientific exchanges dominate.[2] Still, religious scholarship was not absent from these exchanges. Issues of faith instigated them and steered epistolary conversations in new philosophical and philological directions. For example, considerations of permitted and prohibited foods during the Passover holiday stimulated Portaleone's thinking about ancient bread and shaped his response to Cavallara. Similarly, concerns about ritual practices such as baptism, circumcision, and postpartum maternal purification sparked Portaleone's exchange with Magno about neonatal viability and embryonic development. Though none of the correspondents – Portaleone, Magno, or Cavallara – enunciated those concerns, they are a key component of these letters.

Using religious texts in scientific deliberations, Portaleone and his correspondents developed new applications for the former and stretched the epistemological boundaries of the latter. Religious scholarship not only flourished in the context of ritual, doctrine, and exegesis but took root in the field of natural philosophy, too. And sixteenth-century natural

[2] The correspondence of the Italian physician Girolamo Mercuriale with the Protestant physician Theodor Zwinger provides an intriguing parallel. In an extensive epistolary relationship that Nancy Siraisi has studied in detail, the two medical men avoided religious topics entirely. See Nancy G. Siraisi, "Mercuriale's Letters to Zwinger and Humanist Medicine," in Alessandro Arcangeli and Vivian Nutton, eds., *Girolamo Mercuriale: medicina e cultura nell'Europa del Cinquecento. Atti del convegno 'Girolamo Mercuriale e lo spazio scientifico e culturale del Cinquecento' (Forlì, 8–11 novembre 2006)* (Florence: L. S. Olschki, 2008), 77–95.

science needed new sources with which to answer a flurry of difficult questions. The discoveries of new lands unknown to ancient geographers and naturalists revealed new species of flora and fauna that had to be identified and understood. The spread of apparently unprecedented diseases unfamiliar to classical physicians created a demand for novel cures. And the metastasizing interest in ancient quotidiana that affected doctors as much as it did lawyers, clergymen, and classicists spurred researchers to find untapped resources with which they could satisfy their curiosity.[3] Among them were classical Jewish texts, especially the Talmud.

PORTALEONE'S MEDICAL LETTERS AND JEWISH-CHRISTIAN RELATIONS IN RENAISSANCE ITALY

Contemporary scholarship acknowledges that Jewish and Christian physicians attended the same universities, belonged to the same colleges of physicians, and even worked together in the early modern period.[4] However, there is scarcely any published evidence of correspondence. Portaleone's medical letters provide plenty of such evidence. Abraham Portaleone maintained epistolary relationships with many Christian physicians, who were among the late sixteenth century's most prolific and respected medical doctors. Evidence of those relationships may be found in Portaleone's *Book of Medical Responses and Consultations*.[5] That volume was "collected and compiled" in 1607 by Portaleone's son David, also a physician.[6] It consists of 626 numbered folios and contains

[3] On lawyers and their interest in all aspects of life in the ancient world, see Donald Kelley, *Foundations of Modern Historical Scholarship: Language, Law and History in the French Renaissance* (New York: Columbia University Press, 1970), esp. 48.

[4] On the first point especially, see David B. Ruderman, *Jewish Thought and Scientific Discovery in Early Modern Europe* (New Haven: Yale University Press, 1995), 100–15 and the bibliography cited there.

[5] *Excellentissimi D. Abrahami Portaleonis medici mantuani hebraei responsorum et consultationum medicinalium liber, per me David eius filium collectae et conscriptae cum indice locupletissimo anno MDCVII*, Paris, Bibliothèque nationale, Ms. Latin 13004. Henceforth *Responsorum et consultationum medicinalium liber.*

[6] For more on David and his medical practice, including the dispensations he received from Clement VIII and Gregory XV to treat Christian patients, see Shlomo Simonsohn, *History of the Jews in the Duchy of Mantua* (Jerusalem: Kiryath Sepher, 1977), 646. Daniel Carpi provides more information about David b. Abraham Portaleone, including a transcription of his doctoral diploma, which was signed by Galileo Galilei, in "Jewish Graduates

an extensive six-folio index. Given its meticulous penmanship, substantial index, and clear layout, this text was most likely a fair copy intended for printed publication. Indeed, collections of medical case studies were frequently printed in the sixteenth century and were extremely popular among contemporary physicians.[7] One such collection, by Portaleone's Italian colleague and correspondent Girolamo Mercuriale, appeared in print under an almost identical title.[8] But Portaleone's medical letters were never printed. At the bottom of the title page, a small printed note pasted there states that the manuscript was bequeathed to the monastery at St-Germain des Prés by the Duke of Coislin in 1732. By 1774 it had been absorbed into the Bibliothèque du Roi's collection,[9] where it remains today.

This chapter presents and analyzes correspondence between Portaleone and two Catholic physicians: Alessandro Magno and Giovanni Battista Cavallara. In addition to these letters, Portaleone's *Responsorum et consultationum medicinalium liber* includes epistles to and from Girolamo Fabrizi da Aquapendente, Scipio Cassola, Marcello Donati, Girolamo Mercuriale, and thirty-five others.[10] The very fact that Portaleone corresponded with so many notable gentile physicians is itself worthy of note. Scrutiny of Portaleone's medical letters sharpens our knowledge of Jewish-Christian relations in Renaissance Italy.

of the University of Padua During the 16th century" (Hebrew), in *Be-tarbut ha-Renesans u-ven ḥomot ha-geto: meḥkarim be-toldot ha-Yehudim be-Italyah ba-me'ot ha-14–17* (Tel Aviv: University Publishing Project, 1989), 96–130, 101, 117. Some of David ben Abraham Portaleone's own *consilia* are preserved in a manuscript, now in Budapest, Library of the Hungarian Academy of Sciences, entitled *Consulti medici di Guglielmo Portaleone Mantovano e d'altri Italiani dal MDLXXII al MDCLXV*. David Kaufmann describes the manuscript in "Jewish Ethical Wills: Texts and Additions," *JQR*, o.s., 4:2 (1892): 333–41.

7 Danielle Jacquart, "Theory, Everyday Practice, and Three Fifteenth-Century Physicians," in Michael R. McVaugh and Nancy G. Siraisi, eds., *Renaissance Medical Learning: Evolution of a Tradition* (Philadelphia: History of Science Society, 1991): 140–60.

8 Girolamo Mercuriale, *Responsorum et consultationum medicinalium tomus primus, nunc primum a Michaele Columbo collectus et in lucem editus* (Venice: apud Iolitos, 1587). They were also published a year later as *Liber responsorum et consultationum medicinalium nunc primum a Michaele Columbo collectus et in lucem editus* (Basel: Conradum Valdkirch, 1588). For discussion, see Siraisi, "Mercuriale's Letters to Zwinger and Humanist Medicine."

9 See Léopold Delisle, *Inventaire des manuscrits latin conservés à la Bibliothèque nationale sous les numéros 8823–18613, et faisant suite à la séries dont le catalogue a été publié en 1774* (Paris: A. Durand et Pedone-Lauriel, 1863–71), 84.

10 For a list, see the index to *Responsorum et consultationum medicinalium liber*, which I have transcribed and included as Appendix I.

Historians who write about Jews living in Italy during the Renaissance typically advance one of two possible lines of argument. Robert Bonfil, for example, claims that Jews defined themselves in opposition to Christian culture, which threatened the cohesion and continuity of Judaism and Jewish life.[11] Bonfil insists that once Jews were forced to live in northern Italian ghettos, they embraced Christian culture more than they had when they were integrated among their Christian neighbors.[12] Cecil Roth, on the other hand, paints a brighter picture of Jewish-Christian relations in Renaissance Italy, which the recent work of Stephanie Siegmund confirms, although with modifications.[13]

Intellectual historians acknowledge that Jewish and Christian scholars worked together and learned from each other in fifteenth- and sixteenth-century Europe. For example, the German Jewish grammarian Elias Levita (1468–1549) taught Cardinal Egidio da Viterbo Hebrew in exchange for instruction in Greek.[14] But there has been little debate about who benefited most from those working relationships: historiographical orthodoxy claims that Jewish-Christian intellectual exchanges usually favored Christians. Frank Manuel, for example, has insisted that Christians approached Jewish texts with the sole aim of furthering their own theological ends.[15] Similarly, David Ruderman has documented

[11] Robert Bonfil, "Aspects of the Social and Spiritual Life of the Jews in the Venetian Territories at the Beginning of the Sixteenth Century" (Hebrew), *Zion* 41 (1976): 68–96.

[12] Robert Bonfil, "Change in the Cultural Patterns of a Jewish Society in Crisis: Italian Jewry at the Close of the Sixteenth Century," *Jewish History* 3:2 (September 1988): 11–30; reprinted in David B. Ruderman, ed., *Essential Papers on Jewish Culture in Renaissance and Baroque Italy* (New York: New York University Press, 1992), 401–25, esp. 411–13. For a response to Bonfil's thesis, see David Ruderman, "The Italian Renaissance and Jewish Thought," in Albert Rabil Jr., ed., *Renaissance Humanism: Foundations, Forms, and Legacy*, vol. 1: *Humanism in Italy* (Philadelphia: University of Pennsylvania Press, 1988), 382–433, esp. 412–17.

[13] Cecil Roth, *The Jews in the Renaissance* (Philadelphia: Jewish Publication Society, 1959); Stephanie Siegmund, *The Medici State and the Ghetto of Florence* (Stanford: Stanford University Press, 2006).

[14] See Gérard E. Weil, *Elie Lévita humaniste et massorète (1469–1549)* (Leiden: Brill, 1963), 221–34. Also see Christoph Daxelmüller, "Zwischen Kabbala und Martin Luther – Elija Levita Bachur, ein Jude zwischen den Religionen," in Ludger Grenzmann et al., eds., *Wechselseitige Wahrnehmung der Religionen im Spätmittelalter und in der frühen Neuzeit* 1 (2009): 231–50; Deena Aranoff, "Elijah Levita: A Jewish Hebraist," *Jewish History* 23 (2009): 17–40; Shimon Iakerson, "An Autograph Manuscript by Elijah Levita in St Petersburg," *Studia Rosenthaliana* 38 (2005–6): 178–85.

[15] Frank E. Manuel, *The Broken Staff: Judaism through Christian Eyes* (Cambridge, MA: Havard University Press, 1992), 62.

how Elijah Delmedigo studied with Pico della Mirandola from 1480 to 1485, when Delmedigo translated Averroistic texts for his Christian pupil. Those translations helped Pico formulate his syncretist philosophy, the full expression of which may be found in his *Theses* of 1486.[16]

It was not only Christians who benefited from Jewish instruction and Hebrew texts; Jewish culture was also shaped by its encounter with and absorption of Christian intellectual traditions. As Robert Bonfil writes, a cursory look at Renaissance Hebrew books "dispels all doubt that their authors were conscious of sharing ideas, mentalities and even cultural content with the Christian society in which they lived."[17] Through various media – face-to-face interactions, published debates, and epistolary exchanges – the intellectual dialogue between Jews and Christians in Renaissance Italy was extensive and embraced a variety of topics outside the ken of interfaith polemic. As one recent historian put it, in Renaissance Italy Jews and Christians related to one another in ways that were "sociable, respectful, and amicable."[18]

In early modern Italy, medicine was one field in which Jews and Christians frequently encountered one another and where they were often on cordial terms. An effective way to deepen our knowledge of those encounters is by studying the letters Jewish and Christian physicians exchanged. Portaleone's *consultationes* and *responsa* allow us to do that, and the specific content of those letters merits deeper exploration. Before we examine the topics Portaleone and his interlocutors discussed, it is essential to describe the genre to which those letters belonged.

Rare in medieval Europe, medical *consilia* containing narratives about individual patients began to appear at the beginning of the fourteenth

[16] David Ruderman, "The Italian Renaissance and Jewish Thought," in Albert Rabil Jr., ed., *Renaissance Humanism: Foundations, Forms, and Legacy*, vol. 1: *Humanism in Italy* (Philadelphia: University of Pennsylvania Press, 1988), 382–433, 387; *Johannis Pici Mirandulae conclusiones* DCCCC (Rome: Eucharius Silber, 1486). For a modern edition, see Bohdan Kieszkowski, ed., *Conclusiones sive theses DCCCC Romae anno 1486 publice disputandae, sed non admissae* (Geneva: Droz, 1973). For a translation, see Stephen Alan Farmer, ed. and trans., *Syncretism in the West: Pico's 900 Theses (1486): The Evolution of Traditional, Religious, and Philosophical Systems* (Tempe, AZ: Medieval and Renaissance Texts and Studies, 1998).

[17] Robert Bonfil, "Aliens Within: The Jews and Antijudaism," in Thomas Brady, Heiko Oberman, and James Tracey, eds., *Handbook of European History, 1400–1600: Late Middle Ages, Renaissance, and Reformation*, vol. 1: *Structures and Assertions* (Leiden: Brill, 1994), 263–97, 290.

[18] Siegmund, *The Medici State and the Ghetto of Florence*, 292.

century.[19] During the fifteenth and sixteenth centuries *consilia* evolved into more historical, anecdotal, and epistolary forms. Several factors hastened this evolution. First, court culture became much more vibrant. At this time, more physicians were called to serve rulers at court – and write for broader audiences. Abraham Portaleone was one of those physicians. Second, humanist trends that emerged in Italian culture in the Renaissance influenced the medical profession and elevated the importance of and social value placed on good writing, especially in Latin. Third, the civic environment of Renaissance Italy encouraged physicians to share their writings with other sorts of professionals besides doctors.[20] Portaleone's letters, for example, mention his consultations with merchants, spice grinders, and scholars.

In the generation immediately preceding Portaleone's, *consilia* became vehicles for extended treatments of various subjects. Commercially, the genre of medical letters achieved unprecedented popularity after 1556–7, when Giunti published a successful compendium of five different writers of medical letters.[21] In literary terms, Nancy Siraisi has shown how in Renaissance Europe medical case studies evolved into a genre that offered physicians the opportunity to pen "short essays on a variety of freely chosen topics."[22] That evolution, in turn, was accelerated by fifteenth-century developments in classical studies: as Anthony Grafton

[19] See C. Crisciani, "L'individuale nella medicina tra medioevo e umanesimo: i consilia," in R. Cardini and M. Regoliosi, eds., *Umanesimo e medicina: il problema dell' "individuale"* (Rome: Bulzoni, 1996), 1–32; C. Crisciani and Jole Agrimi, *Les consilia médicaux* (Turnhout: Brepols, 1994).

[20] See Nancy Siraisi, *History, Medicine and the Traditions of Renaissance Learning* (Ann Arbor: University of Michigan Press, 2007), 65–7. For an older but still useful discussion of *consilia*, see Pedro Laín Entralgo, *La historia clinica: historia y teoría del relato patográfico* (Madrid: Consejo Superior de Investigaciones Cientificas, 1950). For the related genre of medical *observationes* and *curationes*, see Gianna Pomata, "*Praxis historialis*: The Uses of *Historia* in Early Modern Medicine," in Gianna Pomata and Nancy G. Siraisi, eds., *Historia: Emprícism and Erudition in Early Modern Europe* (Cambridge, MA: MIT Press, 2005), 105–46. See also Brian Nance, "Wondrous Experience as Text: Valleriola and the *Observationes Medicinales*," in Elizabeth Lane Furdell, ed., *Textual Healing: Essays on Medieval and Early Modern Medicine* (Leiden: Brill, 2005), 101–18.

[21] On this edition and its significance, see Ian Maclean, "The Medical Republic of Letters before the Thirty Years' War," *Intellectual History Review* 18 (2008): 15–30, 21. For a basic introduction to the genre in the sixteenth and seventeenth centuries, see Martin Stuber and Hubert Steinke, "Medical Correspondence in Early Modern Europe: An Introduction," *Gesnerus* 61:3 (2004): 139–60.

[22] Siraisi, *History, Medicine and the Traditions of Renaissance Learning*, 67.

proved years ago, Angelo Poliziano revolutionized European intellectual culture by promoting and popularizing monographs that tackled specific subjects as opposed to the line-by-line commentaries that previously dominated classical scholarship.[23] This transformation in literate Italian culture had a strong impact on medical writing.

Because they evolved to address such a diverse range of material, *consilia* encouraged digression. In addition to routine advice concerning common medical problems such as headaches, dizziness, menstrual irregularities, fevers, and respiratory difficulties, Portaleone wrote about optics, the Greek language, thermal baths, deafness in the ancient world, and the connections between mood and health – he even lauded the salubrious effects of chicken soup.[24] As Ian Maclean has pointed out, the wide range of material contained in late sixteenth-century medical letters indicates that they were intended for a broad readership that consisted not only of doctors but of natural philosophers and humanists, too.[25] Had they been published in print, Portaleone's *Responsorum et consultationum medicinalium liber* might have attracted the attention of contemporary men of learning as well as future historians. And that readership may well have been as eclectic as the work's contents. Regarding Girolamo Mercuriale's letters to the Protestant Theodor Zwinger, Nancy Siraisi stressed that they "reveal the circulation of humanistic medical learning, regardless of political – and indeed religious – boundaries."[26] Similarly, Giuseppe Olmi has argued that naturalists' letters "seemed to ignore all geographic, ideological, and religious barriers."[27] Portaleone's medical letters, which contain epistles to and

[23] Anthony Grafton, "On the Scholarship of Politian and Its Context," *Journal of the Warburg and Courtauld Institutes* 40 (1977): 150–88.

[24] For this last topic, see "Consilium Excellentissimi Patris de catharro et melancholia hyppochondriaca pro Domino Rachiello di Foa Regenti hebraeo," in Portaleone's *Responsorum et Consultationum Medicinalium Liber,* 133r–135r at 134v, where Portaleone recommends "il brodo del Gallo di 4 anni" for a variety of ailments. On the use of chicken soup as a hospital remedy in Renaissance Italy, see Katharine Park and John Henderson, "'The First Hospital among Christians': The Ospedale di Santa Maria Nuova in Early Sixteenth-Century Florence," *Medical History* 35:2 (1991): 164–88, 183.

[25] Ian Maclean, "The Medical Republic of Letters before the Thirty Years' War," *Intellectual History Review* 18 (2008): 15–30, 21 and literature cited there.

[26] Siraisi, "Mercuriale's Letters to Zwinger and Humanist Medicine," 94.

[27] Giuseppe Olmi, "'Molti amici in varij luoghi': studio della natura e rapporti epistolari nel secolo xvi," *Nuncius: annali di storia della scienza* 6:1 (1991): 3–31, 8.

from Catholic, Protestant, Italian, and German physicians, substantiate Olmi's and Siraisi's claim.[28]

While the digressive nature of Portaleone's *responsa et consultationes* may have been common in the late sixteenth and early seventeenth centuries, other aspects of them were not. Most significantly, the depth of Portaleone's intellectual and social relations with Christian colleagues would have been harder to imagine outside of Mantua. The political and social policies of that city, established by the Gonzaga family and promoted by its sixteenth-century scions Guglielmo and Vincenzo I, facilitated a closer degree of collaboration between Jews and Christians than most Italian cities, let alone other European municipalities.[29] Many Jews populated early modern Hamburg, for example, but they were forbidden to worship in public or perform circumcisions within city limits.[30] Additionally, Jews were barred from entering many guilds, and membership in the city's college of physicians was restricted to Christians.[31] Even closer to Mantua, in cities that were relatively tolerant of Jews such as Venice, the College of Physicians became increasingly orthodox and intolerant of religious minorities during the second half of the sixteenth century. In 1550 Apollonio Massa redrew its statutes to

[28] Most of these letters are to Catholic medical practitioners. Portaleone did exchange letters with at least one German Protestant: the philologist Joseph Lange. See *Responsorum et consultationum medicinalium liber*, 515r. Lange edited Martial's epigrams, compiled an index to Martial's writings, and collected adages. See, respectively, *M. Valerii Martialis Epigrammaton libri XV* (Strasbourg: Zetzner, 1595); *Index omnium vocabulorum quae in omnibus M. Valerii Martialis poematum libris reperiuntur* (Strasbourg: Zetzner, 1595); and *Adagia sive Sententiae proverbiales graecae, latinae, germanicae ex praecipuis autoribus collectae* (Strasbourg: Rihel, 1596). He also wrote to the German mathematician and physician Andreas Schato (1539–1603). See *Responsorum et consultationum medicinalium liber*, 142r.

[29] On the Gonzaga court and its Jewish physicians, see Adalberto Pazzini, "La medicina alla corte dei Gonzaga a Mantova," in *Mantova e i Gonzaga nella civiltà del Rinascimento* (Mantua: A. Mondadori, 1977), 291–351. For a list of sixteenth-century Jewish physicians allowed to practice on Christian patients, see Luigi Carnevali, *Il Ghetto di Mantova, con appendice sui medici ebrei* (Mantua: Mondovi, 1884). See also Roberto Navarrini, "Note sui medici ebrei attivi in mantova nei secoli xv–xviii," *Postumia: annali del museo d'arte moderna dell'Alto Mantovano* 6 (1995): 64–9.

[30] See Yosef Kaplan, "The Sephardim in North-Western Europe and the New World," in Haim Beinart, ed., *Moreshet Sepharad: The Sephardi Legacy,* 2 vols. (Jerusalem: Hebrew University Press, 1992), 2:240–87, 246.

[31] See Jonathan I. Israel, *Diasporas within a Diaspora: Jews, Crypto-Jews and the World Maritime Empires (1540–1740)* (Leiden: Brill, 2002), 36.

rescind progressive measures that had accreted earlier in the century.[32] Under the leadership of Nicola Abiaso and Francesco Froza in 1555 and again in 1567, Jews were firmly excluded from Venice's College of Physicians.[33] More than other Italian cities, Mantua promoted cordial relations between its Catholic majority and its Jewish minority.

As Portaleone's medical letters are firmly rooted in their geographic setting, they are also products of their temporal context: the late sixteenth century. The image of a Jewish scientist or antiquary with wide intellectual interests who carried on extensive correspondence with gentile associates is one we typically associate with ultra-alpine countries and later centuries. For example, Emanuel Mendes da Costa was a Jew who lived in eighteenth-century England. A clerk and fellow of the Royal Society as well as a fellow of the Society of Antiquarians, he maintained intellectual and social contact with some of the great scientific luminaries of England and Europe, including clergymen.[34] Even in the eighteenth century, according to recent work by David Ruderman, da Costa's position was unique.[35] Portaleone's correspondence with more than forty Christian physicians proves that sixteenth-century Italy, particularly Mantua, provided a context in which Jews and Christians carried on learned correspondence predicated on personal acquaintance.

In addition to scientific and antiquarian excurses, Portaleone's medical letters demonstrate deep engagement with the natural history of the biblical world. The Mantuan physician dedicated *consultationes* or portions thereof to wild animals such as the *monocerote*, or unicorn, and a certain kind of "holy wood" (*legno santo*) that acted as a panacea.[36]

[32] Girolamo Dian, *Alcuni ricordi della medicina al tempo della Repubblica veneta* (Venice: A. Pellizzato, 1909), 5.

[33] N. E. Vanzan Marchini, "Medici ebrei e assistenza cristiana nella Venezia del '500," *La Rassegna Mensile di Israel* 45:4–5 (April–May 1979): 132–61, 151.

[34] David B. Ruderman, *Jewish Enlightenment in an English Key: Anglo-Jewry's Construction of Modern Jewish Thought* (Princeton: Princeton University Press, 2000), 205–6.

[35] Ibid., 206.

[36] On the *monocerote*, see David B. Ruderman, "Unicorns, Great Beasts, and the Marvelous Variety of Things in Nature in the Thought of Abraham b. Hananiah Yagel," in Isadore Twersky and Bernard Septimus, eds., *Jewish Thought in the Seventeenth Century* (Cambridge, MA: Harvard University Press, 1987), 343–64; Ruderman, *Kabbalah, Magic and Science: The Cultural Universe of a Sixteenth-Century Jewish Physician* (Cambridge, MA: Harvard University Press, 1988), 59–73. On holy wood, another name for guaiac, a wood imported from the New World and believed to be a cure for *morbus gallicus*, or syphilis, see Siraisi, *History, Medicine, and the Traditions of Renaissance Learning*, 174.

Eleazar Gutwirth has shown that Amatus's *consilia* are significant as "models of certain cultural habits," namely translation, textual study, and polyglossia, and that one may read them to gain knowledge of their author and his "general world."[37] The same may be said for Portaleone: his *consilia* reveal his cultural habits, too. Portaleone quotes Hebrew texts and addresses the relationship between religious authorities and modern medical practitioners. The pages that follow analyze two sets of letters: one concerning an antiquarian topic and the other an issue of serious medical-philosophical import. Those letters underscore the affinities between scientific research and religious study in Portaleone's oeuvre. His Hebrew encyclopedia *Shiltei HaGibborim*, whose chapters on incense I analyze in the following chapter, is a form of religious inquiry supported by science. Many of Portaleone's medical letters signal the opposite trend: they show how university-trained Italian physicians supplemented their understanding of scientific issues by studying religious texts and traditions. They also indicate the applicability of canonical Jewish texts such as the Talmud to cutting-edge scientific research at the end of the sixteenth and beginning of the seventeenth centuries.

BREAD

On 25 January 1582, Portaleone responded to a letter that Giovanni Battista Cavallara had sent him inquiring about bread.[38] Unfortunately Cavallara's original letter has not survived, but Portaleone's response has.

[37] Eleazar Gutwirth, "Amatus Lusitanus and the Location of Sixteenth-Century Cultures," in David Ruderman and Giuseppe Veltri, eds., *Cultural Intermediaries: Jewish Intellectuals in Early Modern Italy* (Philadelphia: University of Pennsylvania Press, 2004), 227, 217.

[38] There is no reliable biographical survey of Cavallara. He was born in Mantua at an unknown date and earned a medical degree from the University of Padua. For a time he served as a physician to the Gonzaga family, in whose courts he likely met and worked with Portaleone. Cavallara died in 1587. He published several *Discorsi ... sopra le compositioni degli antidoti et medicamenti, che piu si costumano di dar per bocca* (Mantua: Francesco Osanna, 1586), as well as a treatise entitled *De morbo epidemiali ... discursus* (Naples: J. J. Carlinus, 1602). Cavallara also described Filippo Costa's natural history collection in Mantua: "Lettera dell'eccellentissimo Cavallara," *Discorsi di M. Filippo Costa* (Mantua: Francesco Osanna, 1586), sig. Ee. 3v et seq. Dario A. Franchini et al. published Cavallara's letter about giants' bones in *La scienza a corte: collezionismo eclettico natura e immagine a Mantova fra rinascimento e manierismo* (Rome: Bulzoni, 1979): 48–51. Cavallara may also have treated the poet Torquato Tasso. See Pierantonio Serassi, *La vita di Torquato Tasso* (Rome: Pagliarini, 1785), 386–7 and sources there.

The letter is titled "Discourse … on the number and nature of breads, and what 'aquatic' and 'lotus' bread might mean."[39] Other Renaissance physicians wrote at length about ancient grains and breads, normally in connection with modern remedies. For example, Orazio Augenio, in several letters to Giulio Picchino, attempted to identify the grains used in a certain decoction mentioned by Hippocrates and other ancient authors in order to prescribe them.[40] By contrast, Girolamo Mercuriale wrote a *consilium* about ancient breads without emphasizing their curative properties.[41] Portaleone's letter is after the fashion of Mercuriale rather than Augenio; it is an antiquarian treatise with three clear goals: to list as many ancient breads as possible and to identify lotus bread and aquatic bread. None of these tasks was easy. Portaleone remarked to Cavallara that "the differences between breads, most excellent sir, is extremely great, owing to the diversity of grain, of cultivation, shape, preparation, and cooking."[42] In fact, Portaleone went on to say, there are probably no fewer types of breads than there are varieties of wine. And lest he get overwhelmed with contemporary breads, Portaleone made it clear to Cavallara that he wished to "leave aside the great diversity of grains from which breads are made today – there is truly a considerable number of them."[43]

39 "Discursus Excellentissimi Patris de numero et differentia panum et quid sit panis lotus et aquaticus ad instantiam Excellentissimi Cavallarae Medici Serenissimi D. Ducis Mantuae etc.," in *Responsorum et consultationum medicinalium liber*, 462r–464r.

40 Nancy G. Siraisi, *Communities of Learned Experience: Epistolary Medicine in the Renaissance* (Baltimore: Johns Hopkins University Press, 2013), 69; 140 n. 24. See Orazio Augenio, *Epistolarum et consultationum medicinalium prioris tomi libri XII* (Venice: apud Damianum Zenarium, 1602 [1592]), vol. 1, book 7, letters 2, 4–6, 8, fols. 76v–77r, 79v–82v.

41 *Hieronymi Mercurialis Foroliviensis responsorum, et consultationum medicinalium tomus quartus* (Venice: apud Iuntas, 1604), consilium XX, 44–5. "Bernardino Castellano Medico, Hieronymus Mercurialis. S. De quibusdam difficultatibus propositis."

42 Portaleone, *Responsorum et consultationum medicinalium liber,* 462r: "tante sono, Illustrissimo e Eccellentissimo Signore, le differenze de i pani per la diversità de i grani, dell'arteficio, figura, preparatione, miscellanea e cottura." Mercuriale made similar remarks in his letter to Bernardino Castellano. See *Hieronymi Mercurialis Foroliviensis responsorum, et consultationum medicinalium tomus quartus* (Venice: apud Iuntas, 1604), 44: "de pano saligineo, et aliis copiose, ut ipse quoque asseveras scripserunt Athenaeus, Plinius, atque Galenus noster, ita ut mirari non debeas, si inter eos, aliquam discrepantiam invenias, quae facile potius oriri ob varietatem regionum et consuetudinis in faciendis panibus haud secus atque tempestate nostra videmus apud diversos populos, diversi modi panes confici."

43 Portaleone, *Responsorum et consultationum medicinalium liber*, 462v: "lassando star da parte diversi grani da quali hoggi di si costuma a farne pani – eccone qui un numero assai

Portaleone's was a historical investigation; he had no interest in analyzing contemporary bread-making techniques. Some of his contemporaries did, and they acknowledged that even humble bakers were often experts on grains, their provenance, and the best means to convert grain to flour. Tomasso Garzoni, for example, noted that the art of bread making required "no small intelligence."[44] Sixteenth-century Italians considered baking to be a complicated art, one that demanded not only technical competence but also agricultural insight. Still, Portaleone's investigation was antiquarian rather than practical. His chief concern, as he put it to Cavallara, was to seek "the truth regarding what the ancients said about many breads."[45] As I have already remarked, a desire to determine the "truth" about ancient items is a recurrent theme in many works this book examines. David de' Pomi, Ulisse Aldrovandi, and Andrea Bacci all cast their antiquarian and natural philosophic labors as quests to discover the truth about the biblical world.

Portaleone's task was not an easy one. Numbers, for one thing, were against him: in this letter alone Portaleone listed more than fifty kinds of bread that were baked and eaten in ancient times, a list he had assembled in the course of his energetic reading of classical literature. Portaleone focused on two terms: lotus and aquatic bread. The Mantuan physician explained to Cavallara that he needed to "differentiate the lotus bread of the doctors" from "Pliny's aquatic bread."[46] Those differences fell into three categories: their faculties, the manner in which they were made, and the accidents they followed.[47] As we saw in Chapter 2, imprecise terminology in Pliny's *Natural History* spurred Ulisse Aldrovandi and Melchior Guilandinus to offer new interpretations of Pliny's work

notabile." Though this volume has a Latin title and a Latin index, many of the letters, like this one, are written in Italian with frequent, and occasionally lengthy, Latin quotations.

44 See Garzoni's chapter "De' fornari, o panatieri, e confertinari e zambellari e offelari e cialdonari," in his *Piazza Universale di tutte le professioni del mondo*, ed. Paolo Cherchi and Beatrice Collina (Turin: Einaudi, 1996), 2:1352–5.

45 Portaleone, *Responsorum et consultationum medicinalium liber*, 462v: "e che sia il vero che gli Pani delli quali gli authori vechi parlano molti siano."

46 Mercuriale, in his letter to Castellano, also discusses lotus bread and mentions many of the same ancient and medieval authorities. See *Hieronymi Mercurialis Foroliviensis responsorum, et consultationum medicinalium tomus quartus* (Venice: apud Iuntas, 1604), 45.

47 "Faculties," or *facultà* in Portaleone's letter – see pages 462v and 463r – refers to the formal properties of something. Aristotle explains the concept of faculties [*dunamis*] with regard to nutrition in *De Anima* ii 4, 415b27–416a22; 416b20–23; and also in his *De generatione et corruptione* i 5.

by incorporating Hebrew scientific vocabulary into their investigations. Portaleone's exploration of ancient breads led him to do the same: his quest to understand Pliny stimulated him to seek confirmation of his ideas not only in scientific texts but also in Jewish works such as the Talmud. One reason the Talmud could help Portaleone identify and understand these breads was that Pesaḥim, its tractate concerning the laws of Passover, differentiated various types of bread. It did so in order to ascertain which could be consumed during the festival and which could discharge certain ritual obligations during the Passover seder. Neither lotus bread nor *pane buffetto* was baked; they were scalded or boiled in water. As such, these foodstuffs occupied a liminal position between bread as traditionally understood and other grain-based comestibles.

In his efforts to identify these food products, Portaleone first combed through ancient writings for mentions of lotus and aquatic bread, as any university-educated natural philosopher would have done. He cited passages of varying relevance from ancient and medieval Greek, Roman, and Arab physicians, such as Galen, Avicenna, Oribasius, Aetius, Paul of Aegina, and Celsus, regarding the medical uses of those two breads.[48] But none of those authorities really helped Portaleone grasp the "truth" about those breads. From Galen, Portaleone learned that patients sick with fever will experience relief from ingesting pearl barley gruel, broth made from wheat, and certain kinds of soft bread.[49] He also ascertained that patients recovering from illness require something soft in their stomach – they should eat barley broth, a juice extracted from horehound, or lotus bread.[50] Panis lotus, according to Portaleone's

[48] Portaleone read Greek but knew no Arabic. Avicenna's medical writings were available in Latin in numerous editions throughout the sixteenth century. See Nancy G. Siraisi, *Avicenna in Renaissance Italy: The Canon and Medical Teaching in Italian Universities after 1500* (Princeton: Princeton University Press, 1987).

[49] See "Galeni methodi medendi, id est de morbis curandis liber decimus Thoma Linacro Anglo interprete," in *Galeni septima classis artem morborum curatricem describit* (Florence: Giunta, 1541): "oportet autem quamprimum ptisanae cremore, et sorbitione ex alica nutritum, paneque post oblato, aquae frigidae potione hominem cures; quippe protinus extinguitur ac cessat omnino febris" (64v).

[50] See *Galeni omnia quae extant opera* (12 vols.), vol. 6: *Galeni librorum quinta classis* (Venice: Giunta, 1565), book II, chap. 13, "De lacte," 12v: "Contemplator enim utrumque in exemplis propositis videlicet, exempli causa, duobus hominibus, quibus similiter os ventris mordicetur, et qui pariter aut succum ptisanae aut chondrum aut panem lotum

reading of Galen, is soft and easily digested. From Avicenna, Portaleone learned that the nutritional value of bread that is soaked in water is high – even though some of its nutrients are blocked from nourishing the body.[51] Oribasius taught Portaleone that for robust people the more fermentation bread undergoes the healthier it is.[52] Aetius supplied Portaleone with a long list of ancient breads, which he drew upon in his letter to Cavallara, and informed him that porridge-like breads (those that bathe in water for too long) are devoid of nutritional value.[53] Paul of Aegina slighted lotus bread and claimed that it "nourishes very little."[54] The Roman physician Celsus anticipated Aetius and disapproved of bread soaked in water, which he considered "among

sumpserint, deinde alteri mordicationem restinctam, alteri vero inauctam ponito. Obsecro, nunquid succus ptisanae aut chondrus aut panis ex se mordax est, per accidens autem in altero hominum morsum non modo non inauxit, sed mitigavit, an quod ex se quidem erat mitigavit, per accidens vero in altero irritavit? Ego sane ex sua natura epicerasticum esse dico succum ptisanae et chondrum et panem et, per Iovem, lac quoque caeterum in altero homine morsum auxisse ... ex quo patet, per suam quidem naturam boni esse succi, verum interdum una cum iis succis, qui mordicationes excitant, corrumpi et ipsum augere symptoma."

[51] See *Avicennae principis et philosophi sapientissimi libri in re medica omnes qui hactenus ad nos pervenere: Id est libri canonis quinque, De viribus cordis, De removendis nocumentis in regimine sanitatis, De sirupo acetoso, et Cantica. Omnia novissime post aliorum omnium operam a Ioanne Paulo Mongio Hydruntino et Ioanne Costaeo Laudensi recognita* (Venice: Vicentium Valgrisium, 1564), chap. 573, p. 365. "Panis quid est? Oportet ut sit panis mundus, salitus, massam habens confectam, fermentatus, coctus bene in tanor ultimae una nocte permanens ... et panis quidem furni non est sicut panis altanor si suscipiet decoctionem ab utroque latere ... modus vero ablutionis eius est ut sumatur medulla panis qui iacuit una nocte et infundatur in aqua calida, deinde effundatur ab eo aqua quae super ipsum natat, et renovetur super ipsum aqua, donec ab eo removeatur virtus fermenti, et reliquorum, et consequantur finem suae inflationis ... et ille qui non decoquitur bene est plurimi nutrimenti et similiter parum habens fermenti, sed eius nutrimentum oppilat, nisi illos qui sunt plurimi exercitii et panis de patella est huius generis, eius nanque pars interior raro decoquitur bene. Et panis quidem ablutus parvi est nutrimenti elongatus a similagineo levis digestionis et ponderis. Et panis frumenti rari, in iudicio existit opiri." By *panis altanor* Avicenna means a bread that is boiled "from both sides." See ibid., 365 n. f: "cui advenit decoctio ex utroque latere."

[52] See *Oribasii medicinalium collectorum ad imperatorem Iulianum Caes. Aug. liber primus*, book 1, chap. 8: "De panibus triticeis," in *Medicae artis principes post Hippocratem et Galenum*, 2 vols. (Paris: Stephanus, 1567), 1:209.

[53] See *Aetii medici graeci contractae medicinae, tetrabibli primae, sermo secundus*, chap. 251, "quae parum nutriunt," in *Medicae artis principes* 2:106: "porrum, crudum quidem nullum penitus alimentum praebet, bis vero aut ter coctum, paucissimum."

[54] See *Pauli Aeginetae de re medica liber I*, book 1, chap. 78: "De frumentaceis," in *Medicae artis principes*, 1:369–70: "amylum parum nutrit, velut etiam panis lotus" (miscited by Portaleone as chapter 28).

the weakest of food."[55] In short, the physicians who wrote about the medical and nutritional properties of lotus bread and aquatic bread barely differentiated between them. Portaleone did, and made this difference the focus of his exchange with Cavallara.

Portaleone, unlike his medical predecessors whom he quoted, did not shy away from defining lotus bread. He stated that it was made from dough that is scalded in boiling water and then cooked.[56] The immersion in water penetrates not only the surface but also the interior of the dough, which becomes spongy and aerated.[57] Portaleone's identification of lotus bread derived only in small measure from what he read in classical and medieval medical texts; observing bakers at work, or perhaps even baking the bread himself, helped even more. Given his tendency to assemble antiquarian products from descriptions in classical literature, he may well have tried to bake this particular type of bread.[58] But Portaleone could only make an educated guess, as he did when he wrote to Cavallara, that "this, according to my opinion, might be lotus bread."[59] Still, more than classical literature, ancient medicine, or discussions with Mantuan bakers and mill operators, Portaleone's own Jewish tradition helped him identify lotus bread and understand its properties. The final source to which Portaleone turned for information regarding this spongy bread was an unlikely one in the context of a learned exchange about ancient bread: the Talmud.

Portaleone explained to Cavallara that "I am given to believe that this agrees with what our sages say in the book of Passover Rites [Pesaḥim] in the second chapter and its commentaries on *Padh Chaluta*: it is bread

[55] See *Aurelii Cornelii Celsi de re medica libri octo,* book 2, chap. 18: "qui cibi, potionesve, aut valentis, aut mediae, aut imbecillae materiae sint," in *Medicae artis principes* 2:37–8, 38: "aqua quoque madens panis imbecillissimis annumerari potest" (miscited by Portaleone as chapter 19).

[56] "Cooked," or *cotto*, is not a verb typically associated with bread making. The process Portaleone describes indicates that *pane lotus* resembled a dumpling or a form of fried dough rather than bread.

[57] Portaleone, *Responsorum et consultationum medicinalium liber*, 463r–v: "Ma il pane loto sarà il pan crudo brovato e poscia cotto, che per haver havuto in pasta quella gionta di aqua che non solo bagna la superficie, ma anco entra nella midolla, diviene spungoso e aereo."

[58] In the following chapter I explore Portaleone's reconstruction of ancient Israelite incense based on ingredients listed in the Bible and the Talmud.

[59] Portaleone, *Responsorum et consultationum medicinalium liber*, 463v: "questo dunque a mio giudicio sara il Pane loto."

dipped and scalded in water."[60] In the Talmudic tractate Pesaḥim there is a discussion about the meaning of the biblical expression "bread of affliction." The phrase is prominently placed in the Passover Haggadah in a section where Jews are enjoined to eat unleavened bread on the first night of the festival and commanded to recite the Aramaic declaration concerning the "bread of affliction that our ancestors ate in the land of Egypt."[61] Since Talmudic law stipulates that the *maẓah* consumed on Passover must resemble the "bread of affliction," subsequent discussions elucidate what is meant by that expression. In the Talmud, the category "bread of affliction" excludes *ḥalut* – the very type of bread to which Portaleone compared lotus bread.[62] Several medieval commentators to whom Portaleone likely had access clarify the Talmud's language and describe *ḥalut*. The eleventh-century French scholar Rashi explains that it is "bread that is boiled in hot water after it is baked."[63] A later glossator, the tosafist Rabbenu Tam, states that *ḥalut* refers to bread cooked and not baked at all.[64] In sum, medieval commentators stress that while *ḥalut* is a type of bread, it may not substitute for "bread of affliction." The tosafist glossators of the twelfth century left little room for doubt when they pronounced *ḥalut* "bread, but not the bread of affliction."[65] The Talmudic text and its medieval glossators helped Portaleone visualize a foodstuff that was scalded rather than baked, thereby aiding him in his effort to define lotus bread.

But the Talmud did more for Portaleone than inform him about bread making; he could have come upon that knowledge by reading any number of Latin or Italian texts or by speaking to a baker.[66] Shortly after the

60 Ibid., 463v: "mi dò a credere che conviene con quello che gli nostri savii nel libro de i Riti Pasquali al secondo capitolo e al comento dell'Aphorismo secondo Padh Chaluta chiamano, cioè pane sbrufato et brovato nell'aqua." Portaleone's transliteration of פת חלוטה as "padh chaluta" is typical of Italian Jews' tendency to transliterate the Hebrew letter ת as "dh." Twenty-first-century readers would transliterate פת חלוטה as "pat ḥaluta."

61 Passover Haggadah, הא לחמא עניא די אכלו אבהתנא בארעא דמצרים

62 BT Pesaḥim 36b: תנו רבנן לחם עני פרט לחלוט ולאשישה ("our rabbis taught that 'bread of affliction' excludes pudding and pan-cake"). My translations of חלוט and אשישה follow Marcus Jastrow, *A Dictionary of the Targumim, the Talmud Babli and Yerushalmi, and the Midrashic Literature* (London: Trübner, 1903), 128.

63 Rabbi Shlomo Yitzḥaki, d. 1105, commentary on BT Pesaḥim 36v, s.v. חלוט: לחם שלאחר אפיה חזר ונתבשל במים חמים

64 See the comments of Rabbi Jacob b. Meir Tam (d. 1171) in *Sefer HaYashar le-rabbenu Tam* (Jerusalem: Kiryat Sefer, 1985), sec. 47.

65 See Tosafot to BT Pesaḥim 36b, s.v. פרט לחלוט

66 See Marilyn Nicoud, *Les régimes de santé au Moyen Age: naissance et diffusion d'une écriture médicale, XIIIe–XVe siècle* (Rome: École française de Rome, 2007); Ken Albala, *Eating*

analysis of "bread of affliction," the Talmud defined *pat ḥaluta* in more precise language. In a discussion of breads that are exempt from *ḥallah* – the commandment to remove a portion of dough prior to baking – *ḥalut* is understood to be an alimentary product made by pouring boiling water over flour.[67] *Ḥalut*, according to the ancient rabbis, did not count as bread at all, since it did not need to be tithed. For Portaleone, lotus bread corresponded to the Talmud's *pat ḥaluta*. Both were either fried or scalded and were made with generous amounts of water. To understand a mysterious bread from classical literature, Portaleone borrowed a corresponding identity, and a detailed description, from Talmudic literature.

Regarding the second bread, the aquatic variety, Portaleone understood it to be a foodstuff with which he was familiar in his daily life. His mission was to understand one of Pliny's cryptic remarks, and his method was to privilege his own experience over his formidable erudition. Portaleone reflected that,

> as for Pliny's *pane aquatico*, he said "recently we had a bread introduced from Parthia, known as water bread, from a method of kneading, whereby the dough is drawn out by the aid of water, a process that renders it remarkably light, spongy, and full of holes. Some call this Parthian bread." I am sure that this is our *pane buffetto*. It corresponds in the stated conditions of its production as well as in its substance.[68]

Most likely, when Portaleone wrote "our bread," he meant a product from Mantua or its environs; in the Renaissance, Italian cuisine varied enormously from region to region, even from town to town.[69] Using a bread he might have found in a local bakery to clarify an enigmatic term

Right in the Renaissance (Berkeley: University of California Press, 2002); Maria Paleari Henssler, *Bibliografia latino-italiana di gastronomia*, 2 vols. (Milan: Chimera, 1998).

67 BT Pesaḥim 37b: המעיסה קמח שעל גבי מוגלשין החליטה מוגלשין שעל גבי קמח (*meisah* is [made by placing] flour upon scalding water; *halita* is [made by pouring] scalding water over flour). This distinction is clarified in *Entsiklopedya Talmudit* (Jerusalem: Mosad HaRav Kuk, 1947–), vol. 15, col. 535.

68 *Responsorum et consultationum medicinalium liber*, 463v: "Quanto poi al pane aquatico di Plinio quando disse: 'non pridem etiam e Parthis invecto, quem aquaticum vocant, quoniam aqua trahitur ad tenuem et spungiosam inanitatem, alii Parthicum,' tengo certo che sia il nostro pane buffetto, in cui mi pare che concurrano le condittioni detti tanto nel modo di farlo, quanto nella riuscita della sostanza." For the Pliny quotation, see *Natural History* 18:43.

69 See Franco Banchi, *Il pranzo di S. Giovanni: racconti da tavola del Rinascimento fiorentino* (Florence: LoGisma, 1997); Phillippe Gillet, *Par mets et par vins: voyages et gastronomie en*

in classical literature was a bold act, and Portaleone knew it. To protect his scholarly integrity, he confessed, "If it seems [to you] that I have erred in this matter, I would prefer to avoid your illustrious presence, and great embarrassment. In my place I boldly send this letter; after all, it cannot blush as I would."[70] Portaleone was not entirely confident in his analysis of these two types of bread. To define the aquatic bread that Pliny only vaguely described, Portaleone relied on his empirical knowledge of local, Mantuan cuisine. To understand lotus bread, a comestible that was harder to identify, Portaleone relied not on Latin or vernacular texts but on the Talmud. The fact that he did so provides an important example of how scientific and antiquarian culture of sixteenth-century Italy was capacious enough to assimilate all manner of unusual sources, including a foundational text of Judaism whose possession or study was officially proscribed to both Jews and Christians.[71]

In Portaleone's correspondence with non-Jewish physicians and naturalists, the Talmud adjudicated in a number of scientific and philosophical disputes. Some were antiquarian. Talmudic literature provided descriptions and listed characteristics of obscure breads that aided Portaleone's effort to distinguish between various ancient bread products. Occasionally classical Jewish texts served Portaleone and his readers in a more nuanced capacity. The Talmud weighed in on live, pressing philosophical and medical debates. In Portaleone's correspondence with Alessandro Magno about a monstrous birth, for example, Talmudic passages confirmed several of modern science's contentious findings and lent those findings an aura of spiritual credibility.

Europe (16e–18e siècles) (Paris: Payot, 1985); Luigi Firpo, ed., *Gastronomia del Rinascimento* (Turin: Unione tipografico-editrice torinese, 1974); Jean-Claude Margolin and Robert Sauzet, eds., *Pratiques et discours alimentaires à la Renaissance. Actes du colloque de Tours de mars 1979* (Paris: G.-P. Maisonneuve et Larose, 1982); Marie Viallon-Schoneveld, ed., *Le boire et le manger au XVIe siècle. Actes du XIe colloque du Puy-en-Velay* (Saint-Étienne: Publications de l'Université de Saint-Étienne, 2004).

70 Portaleone, *Responsorum et consultationum medicinalium liber* 463v: "se in tutto quello che ho detto in questa materia ad alcuno paresse che io errassi, mi giovarà di non essere alla presenza di Vostra Eccellenza per non haver tanta vergogna, e venga in luogo mio questa lettera sfacciatamente, chè ad ogni modo non può, per quel ch'io me ne creda, arossire in faccia."

71 On continuing Jewish study of the Talmud in Italy even after the burnings of 1553 and 1559, see Amon Raz-Krakotzkin, "On Burning and Printing, the Press and Culture" (Hebrew), unpublished typescript, pp. 5, 7. I would like to thank Professor Krakotzkin for sharing this typescript with me. The best survey of Italian Jews' reaction to the burning of the Talmud is Abraham Yaari's "The Burning of the Talmud in Italy," in his *Meḥkarei sefer: perakim be-toldot ha-sefer ha-'ivri* (Jerusalem: Mosad Ha-Rav Kuk, 1958), 198–234.

MONSTERS

On 28 January 1594, a certain Alessandro Magno wrote to Abraham Portaleone to tell him he had witnessed the birth of a monster. Magno, whose letter was sent to Portaleone from Luzzara, a small city in Emilia not far from Mantua, has left no known works to posterity. Standard biographical and medical reference texts do not mention him. Nor do the *rotuli*, or matriculation records, from the University of Bologna, Emilia's only medical school in this period, mention his name.[72] Still, Magno's inclusion on the list of Portaleone's correspondents, doubtless designed by Portaleone's son David to highlight his father's high professional status, creates the impression that Magno was a respected medical practitioner in his time – or, at the very least, that Portaleone wished him to be.[73] Even though Alessandro Magno's name is not well known to the history of Renaissance medicine, variations of it turn up in early modern sources. For example, Leonardo Fioravanti's 1582 collection of medical writings, *Il tesoro della vita humana*, includes a letter Fioravanti wrote in October 1568 to a certain "Alessandro Magnese Piacentino" on the topic of tertian fever.[74] This physician from Piacenza may have been the same person with whom Portaleone corresponded. And there is further evidence that the surname Magno or its Latin equivalent may have belonged to a family from Emilia with strong medical qualifications: records kept by the University of Bologna note that Alexander de Magnis lectured on medical topics on the arts faculty from 1645 until 1650.[75] This Alexander de Magnis may have been a descendant or relative of Portaleone's correspondent.

Portaleone and Magno appear to have had a close professional relationship. Magno's letter that describes the monstrous birth is signed

[72] See Umberto Dallari, *I rotuli dei lettori legisti e artisti dello studio bolognese dal 1384 al 1799*, 4 vols. (Bologna: Regia tipografia dei Fratelli Merlani, 1888–1924).

[73] Other well-known correspondents featured in Portaleone's *consilia* include Hieronymus Fabricius de Aquapendente, Girolamo Mercuriale, Marcello Donato, and Scipio Cassola.

[74] Leonardo Fioravanti, *Il tesoro della vita humana dell'eccellentissimo dottore et cavaliere M. Leonardo Fioravanti Bolognese* (Venice: Melchior Sessa, 1582), book 3, chap. 5: 224v–225v. "Al Magnifico Messer Alessandro Magnese Piacentino: dove si discorre sopra una sua infermità di febre terzana."

[75] In the 1645–6 academic year, as well as the following one, de Magnis lectured on logic during the first hour of morning classes; in the academic year 1648–9 he taught physics; and in 1649–50 he lectured on theoretical medicine. See Dallari, *I rotuli dei lettori legisti e artisti dello studio Bolognese dal 1384 al 1799*, 2:148–52.

"from [your] most affectionate servant,"[76] and Portaleone's response, dated 10 February 1594, praises Magno for his letter that was "not only filled but overflowing with medical and philosophical perspicuity."[77] There is evidence beyond this single exchange that Magno and Portaleone were close colleagues. In a letter written in 1604, Magno extolled Portaleone's *humanitas* and alluded to their many conversations and letters throughout the years, especially on gynecological matters.[78] Portaleone's elaborate relationship with Magno magnified Portaleone's legacy in his readers' eyes and, just as important, provided Portaleone an opportunity to explore the connections between science, tradition, and faith – a topic that engaged him during the final portion of his life.[79]

In his letter of 28 January, Magno devoted the most space and detail to the birth of a deformed infant; in turn, that case was the most interesting to Portaleone. In Italian laced with Latin quotations and allusions, Magno explained to Portaleone that

> a monster was born here on the seventeenth of this month, sick with many afflictions, since it was missing its neck and its entire brain. It was born dead and my opinion is that it could not have been born alive. Therefore I said that it could never have lived as an animal in the womb, because "that which cannot live outside the womb does not have animal life in the womb, [and] a fetus without a brain cannot live outside the womb." The first issue is proved because "if it [the fetus] cannot live outside, the cause of life within [the uterus] is through continuity of ligaments, which make it live the life of a plant, as in the case of a *mola*." The second matter seems clear to me, since "no one can live without the animal spirit that enters through the brain" if it lacks a medulla [brainstem]. You cannot say [it is

[76] Portaleone, *Responsorum et consultationum medicinalium liber*, 199r, "servitore affetionatissimo." On the topic of informality in medical letters, see Candice Delisle, "The Letter: Private Text or Public Place? The Mattioli-Gesner Controversy about the *aconitum primum*," *Gesnerus* 61 (2004): 161–76.

[77] *Responsorum et consultationum medicinalium liber*, 199v: "Solutiones ad quaesita proposita ab Excellentissimo Domino Alexandro Magno et sunt Excellentissimi Patris."

[78] Ibid., 33r–33v: "Epistola Excellentissimi Doctoris Alexandri Magni ad Excellentissimum Patrem, in qua nonnulla continentur dubia circa quaedam Hippocratis verba in libro de septimestri et octimestri partu."

[79] See Portaleone, *SG*, as well as Alessandro Guetta's discussion of its introduction in his "Avraham Portaleone, le scientifique repenti," in Gad Freudenthal, Jean-Pierre Rothschild, and Gilbert Dahan, eds., *Torah et science: perspectives historiques et théoriques. Études offertes à Charles Touati* (Louvain: Peeters, 2001), 213–27.

alive] because "everything flows in through the brain, and this is lacking in proportions that have to do with the spirit."[80]

Though Magno never poses a well-defined question to Portaleone, the implications of this case are clear. Magno wishes to know, first of all, if the fetus may have been viable after birth. Closely related to this, Magno is curious about how the fetus was nourished in the womb and how it received its vital spirit.[81]

Religious concerns inspired Magno's questions and shaped Portaleone's answers.[82] Magno wished to know when the spiritual soul enters the human body in order to determine whether or not the fetus was fit for baptism. Exploring related issues, Portaleone drew on Talmudic discussions of neonatal viability. Magno, weighing practical concerns, called upon classical philosophical and medical literature to shed light on the status of the newborn infant. Portaleone leavened his response with material drawn from his own tradition's canonical texts. In fact, exploring Magno's case study presented an excuse for Portaleone to demonstrate his religious erudition and establish that texts associated with a religious tradition are at least as instructive as modern scientific ones, if not more so.

MAGNO AND BAPTISM

Although Magno never explicitly states the reason for his interest in this case, it is probable that religious ritual was on his mind. One of the first things a Christian physician must have considered in the late sixteenth

[80] Portaleone, *Responsorum et consultationum medicinalium liber*, 199r–199v: "il secondo infermo è stato un monstro nato qui alli 17 di questo mese, infermo di morbo in numero, perchè gli mancava il collo et tutto il cervello. Naque, morto, nè vivo, secondo il mio parere, poteva nascere, perciò dissi ch' mai non visse come animale nel ventre, perchè 'quod non potest vivere extra uterum, non vivit vita animali in utero etc.,' 'foetus sine cerebro non potest vivere extra questo.' La prima si prova, perchè 'si non potest vivere extra, causa vitae intus est, tamen continuatio ligamentorum, quae facit ipsum vivere vita plantae quemadmodum mola.' La seconda mi par chiara, perchè 'nullus potest vivere sine spiritu animali, qui a cerebro influit,' se pur la medulla non supplisse, il che non si può dire perchè 'omnia habet a cerebro influente etc. et caret proportionibus quae pertinet ad spiritum.'"

[81] For more on Renaissance embryology and theories of the soul, see Katharine Park, "The Organic Soul," in Charles B. Schmitt and Quentin Skinner, eds., *The Cambridge History of Renaissance Philosophy* (Cambridge: Cambridge University Press, 1988), 464–84, 469.

[82] James J. Bono and others have studied how, in sixteenth-century medical writings, the meaning of *spiritus* enlarged to encompass Christian notions of the soul as well as Aristotelian ones. See Bono, "The Languages of Life: Jean Fernel (1497–1558) and Spiritus in Pre-Harveian Bio-medical Thought" (PhD diss., Harvard University, 1981), 58 and 237.

century – a time of high infant mortality and frequent contagion – was whether or not to baptize a newborn.[83] The doctor-clergyman Karl Franz Nicholaus Capellman, writing in the late nineteenth century, noted the importance of baptism as an issue that confronted physicians who attend monstrous births and remarked that a child was fit for baptism only if it possessed a head and a chest.[84] Well before Capellman's time, Catholic theologians and doctors debated baptism in the context of unusual births. Those debates illuminate the issues Magno and his peers may have considered and underscore the conspicuous relevance of religious ritual to medical life.

In the middle of the eighteenth century, the Sicilian theologian Francesco Emanuello Cangiamila wrote an entire book about the souls of fetuses and the obligation that priests have – in the absence of doctors – to deliver babies and baptize them, and even to perform emergency cesarean sections if necessary.[85] Cangiamila offered an elastic definition of one's capacity for baptism and proposed that even those fetuses with limited chances for viability undergo the procedure. The criteria for neonatal viability were likely more flexible in Magno's mind than they were for Capellman some three hundred years later. In late sixteenth-century Italy, baptism was fiercely debated, and those debates colored Magno's reaction to the monstrous birth he witnessed in Luzzara.

At midcentury, the Council of Trent's decrees were unambiguous in their insistence that infant baptism was an essential sacrament and unbending in their assertion that whichever individuals or groups denied this, such as Waldenses and Cathari, were heretics.[86] Baptism was a live issue at this time not only because of Tridentine deliberations but because of the emerging Protestant practices, mostly in German-speaking areas

[83] Daniel Schäfer, *Geburt aus dem Tod: der Kaiserschnitt an Verstorbenen in der abendländischen Kultur* (Hürtgenwald: Guido Pressler, 1999), 55–71.

[84] Karl Franz Nicholaus Capellman, *Pastoralmedizin* (Paderborn: Bonifacius Druckerei, 1920), 129.

[85] Francesco Emanuello Cangiamila, *Embriologia sacra, ovvero dell'uffizio de' sacerdoti, medici, e superiori, circa l'eterna saluta de' bambini racchiusi nell'utero, libri quattro* (Milan: Giuseppe Cairoli, 1751).

[86] See *Universum sacrosanctum concilium tridentinum oecumenicum, ac generale, legitime tum indictum tum congregatum* (Brescia: Iohannes Baptista Bozola, 1563), 34v, session VII, 3 March 1547, *De baptismo*, especially canons xiii–xiv. The canons do not stipulate these two sects, although they are the most conspicuous rejectors of the baptismal sacrament. A. W. Bates makes a similar point in his *Emblematic Monsters: Unnatural Conceptions and Deformed Births in Early Modern Europe* (Amsterdam: Rodopi, 2005), 144.

north of the Alps, that challenged Catholic tradition. Anabaptists, for example, rejected infant baptism on the grounds that such a crucial religious practice requires adult consent.[87]

Baptizing healthy infants was complicated enough, but whether or not to baptize developmentally disabled newborns was an even stickier subject. It was not until the middle of the eighteenth century that a Catholic theologian was to offer a clear ruling on this question. Pope Benedict XIV (pope from 1740 until 1758), in his *De synodo dioecesana*, urged midwives to baptize endangered fetuses while still in the womb, if they could reach the fetus with the aid of an instrument.[88] Even so, Benedict differentiated between absolute baptisms, where the midwife could reach the fetus's head, and conditional baptisms, where the midwife could access only another part of the body.[89] As Cangiamila observes in *Embriologia sacra*, common people believe that male fetuses do not possess souls until forty days after conception, and that female fetuses lack them until eighty or ninety days after conception. As such, abortion was often justified during the first month or two of pregnancy on the grounds that fetuses in the first trimester of pregnancy lacked human souls. Among the arguments Cangiamila marshals against this popular belief is the rabbinic legend that people's souls were created long before their bodies, so that all Jews were able to hear God's revelation on Mount Sinai.[90]

Early modern Catholic thinkers had much to say about baptizing monsters. The *rituale romanum*, standardized by Pope Paul V around 1614, was explicit on the matter, saying that, "with regard to monsters,

[87] See Winfried Glade, *Die Taufe in den vorcanisianischen katholishen Katechismen des 16. Jahrhunderts im deutschen Sprachgebeit* (Nieuwkoop: B. de Graaf, 1979); Hughes Oliphant Old, *The Shaping of the Reformed Baptismal Rite in the Sixteenth Century* (Grand Rapids, MI: Eerdmans, 1992); and Karen E. Spierling, *Infant Baptism in Reformation Geneva: The Shaping of a Community, 1536–1564* (Aldershot: Ashgate, 2005).

[88] Benedict XIV (Prospero Lambertini), *De synodo dioecesana libri tredecim*, 2 vols. (Ferrara: Giovanni Manfrè, 1756), 1:304, book 7, chap. 5.

[89] Ibid., 307.

[90] Cangiamila, *Embriologia sacra*, 20: "Molti de' Rabbini favoleggiarono, tutte le Anime degli Uomini essere create assai prima de' Corpi, e che tute si ritrovarono nel Monte Sinai per udire la promulgazione della Legge, senza la quale promulgazione non sarebbero ora tenute all'osservanza de' Precetti." The belief in ensoulment at forty days for male fetuses and at eighty days for female fetuses has a long history that was as learned as it was popular. See E. Amann, E. Mangenot, and A. Vacant, eds., *Dictionnaire de théologie catholique*, 15 vols. (Paris: Letouzey et Ané, 1903–50), s.v. "animation," 1:1305–20, esp. 1306–11.

they should certainly be baptized." However, there was a proviso: "If the monster itself is not considered to be human, it ought not to be baptized, or, if there is doubt, baptized under this condition: 'If thou art a Man, I baptize thee.'"[91] The precise meaning of the phrase "if the monster itself is not considered to be human" was open to debate. Cangiamila summarizes a considerable body of seventeenth-century scholarship attentive to the issue of precisely which deformed infants merited baptism. Massimiliano Dezza, in his *Rituale di Paolo V*, argued that if the infant is able to move it must be baptized. Girolamo Fiorentini of Lucca (1602–78) went even further in his *De hominibus dubiis, sive de baptismo abortivorum*, suggesting that the fetus does not even need to display movement; it merely needs "the instruments" of motion, which are "arms, thighs, and calfs."[92] During the middle of the seventeenth century, when Dezza, Fiorentini, and others wrote, Catholic theologians systematically expanded the definition of which infants are capable of undergoing baptism. By the middle of the eighteenth century, Cangiamila was confident enough about the importance of baptism to say about a monstrous infant that "if you are not certain, and it might be a beast, baptize *sub conditione*."[93] Magno's concern about whether or not to baptize the infant echoed debates in early modern Catholic theology.

Still, baptism was not merely a practical concern for a Christian physician of Portaleone's time such as Magno; it was a matter of faith. Various legends pertinent to the topic existed: some described monstrous fetuses who were miraculously rehabilitated and subsequently went on to illustrious careers in the church. Cangiamila reports a well-known one about Saint Elzeario of Ariano (d. 1323), clearly designed to warn young mothers about the foolhardiness of abortion.[94] According to the story, Anfisibia, the wife of Grimaldo, gave birth to a frightful monster that lacked human form. Saint Elzeario subsequently

[91] *Rituale romanum Pauli V Pontificis maximi jussu editum, et a Benedicto XIV auctum et castigatum cum cantu emendato* (Mechelen: P. J. Hanicq, 1854), 11: "In monstris vero baptizandis, si casus eveniat, magna cautio adhibenda est, de quo, si opus fuerit, Ordinarius loci, vel alii periti consulantur, nisi mortis periculum immineat. Monstrum, quod humanam speciem non prae se ferat, baptizari non debet, de quo si dubium fuerit, baptizetur sub hac conditione: 'si tu es homo, ego te baptizo.'"

[92] All quoted by Cangiamila, *Embriologia sacra,* 52–3.

[93] Ibid., 92: "quando non è certo, che sia di Bruto, battezzarsi sotto condizione."

[94] On Saint Elzeario, see Jacques Campbell, *Vie occitanes de saint Auzias et de sainte Dauphine* (Rome: Pontificium Athenaeum Antonianum, 1963).

appeared, prostrated himself, and prayed and cried with such fervor that the shapeless pile of flesh was transformed into an angelic infant. Not content with his accomplishment, the saint prophesied that the baby would one day become pope, and indeed the baby grew up to be Pope Urban V. Appropriately, Cangiamila's only addendum to this story is "it must be said that the aforementioned pile of flesh had *some* human characteristics, however imperfect, at least internally, so that it could receive a rational soul."[95] The anecdote proves, to the credulous reader at least, that monstrous infants may not only be viable but can grow up to be saints or even popes. Versions of this legend or similar ones may have circulated during Portaleone and Magno's time. At the very least, the pervasiveness of stories like this one establishes that baptizing "monsters" was not merely a juridical concern but also fodder for moral fables that demonstrated the power of faith to transform monsters into men.

PORTALEONE AND JEWISH CONCERNS

Christian physicians like Magno had a clear problem to confront when faced with abnormal births. Jews such as Portaleone did as well. Whether or not to circumcise a child was the most pressing concern on the minds of Jewish thinkers in the early modern period. Although Portaleone does not directly address the issue, several of his contemporaries did. From their surviving letters and legal opinions, which likely represent only a few of the original discussions of this matter, we learn how rabbis and doctors alike had a stake in the assessment of newborn monsters.

[95] Cangiamila, *Embriologia sacra,* 92–3: "Anfisibia moglie di Grimaldo della prima nobiltà di Provenza, e Signore di Grisato, dopo atrocissimi dolori partorì uno spaventoso mostro, cioè una massa di carne, che col suo continuo moto apportava orrore a chiunque la mirava. Non pareva Uomo, perchè non aveva figura umana, e non sembrava neppure una bestia, perchè non aveva sembianza di Bruto, e non aveva in somma alcuna effigie. S. Elzeario Parente de' Genitori, e che si ritrovava presente, mosso dalle lagrime di quelli, inginocchiossi: ed orando con gran fervore, cambiò prodigiosamente quella massa di carne in un Puttino di rara bellezza, a cui vagiti accorsero tutti d'un subito per ammirare il portento divino. Profetizzò ancora il Santo, che questo Bambino sarebbe un giorno Sommo Pontefice, e lo fu di celebre memoria sotto nome di Urbano V. Bisogna dire, che la detta massa di carne aveva qualche configurazione umana, quantunque imperfetta, almeno interna, bastante ad accogliere Anima ragionevole."

Circumcision of deformed infants was perhaps early modern rabbis' chief consideration in the event of a monstrous birth.[96] When Siamese twins were born in the Venetian ghetto in the spring of 1575, at least one rabbi took up his pen to address the topic. Abraham Carmi of Cremona wrote to his teacher David Samuel Pescarolo of Vercelli that same year and told him about a bizarre birth; his original letter even included a drawing, now lost.[97] Carmi told Pescarolo that, given the complications at birth, the infants could not have lived long enough to endure a circumcision and confessed that he was perplexed about what to do regarding that ritual.[98] Finally, he states that he would have treated the case as one of a child too sick to undergo the procedure – in such an instance one waits until the child is healthy enough to be circumcised.[99] Even more significantly, Carmi mentions a Talmudic debate about the ritual impurity of the mother, ruling that had the child lived, the mother would have been considered impure, thus confirming the human status of the child.[100] The ritual status of a postpartum woman in the aftermath of a monstrous birth was something rabbis had to consider.[101] Abraham Carmi's letter serves as a bridge between Talmudic debates and sixteenth-century concerns and proves that Italian Jews of Portaleone's generation took questions of maternal ritual purity and infant circumcision seriously.

96 Toaff, *Mostri giudei: l'immaginario ebraico dal Medioevo alla prima età moderna* (Bologna: Il Mulino, 1996), 163. Toaff cites several examples of rabbis debating this, though most of his cases date from the middle of the seventeenth or the beginning of the eighteenth century.

97 Yaakov Boksenboim, ed., *Iggrot Bet Carmi* (Tel Aviv: Hayim Rozenberg, 1983), 162–3. Carmi told Pescarolo about the צלם ודמות אשר יצוייר למטה For an Italian summary of this letter, see Toaff, *Mostri giudei*, 143–4.

98 Boksenboim, *Iggrot Bet Carmi*, 163: ואאמין כי לא יוכלו להאריך לחיות זמן רב. וכן היה

99 Ibid.: וע"ד המילה נסתפקתי דלא גרוע מחולה שאינו נמול בזמנו. אכן אם יחיו זמן מה אאמין כי יחול עליהם חובת מילה ואמם ודאי טמאה עליהם טומאת לידה

100 Mothers who gave birth to monstrous infants were considered ritually impure and forbidden for a specified time period from performing certain ritual acts.

101 Curiously, in medieval Hebrew gynecological texts, of which Ron Barkai gives a helpful sampling in his *A History of Jewish Gynaecological Texts in the Middle Ages* (Leiden: Brill, 1998), although stillbirths are a worry, such texts were concerned mostly with how to remove them from the uterus and birth canal and how to treat the mother after such a difficult birth (205–6). See, respectively, a Hebrew translation of *Liber de symptomatibus mulierum* (title page missing, no official title) Jews' College, Ms. Montefiore 440, fols. 60r–62r, printed in ibid., Hebrew text 181–4; English translation 184–91, 188; and *Medicament for Pregnancy Called the Head Shield* (תרופות להריון נקרא מגן הראש), Oxford, Bodleian, Ms. Or. 2142, fols. 251v–257v, printed in ibid., Hebrew text, 192–8; English translation, 198–211, 205.

As in his letter to Cavallara on bread, much of Portaleone's answer to Magno's query drew from his knowledge of ancient Greek philosophy and medieval medical theories. But he also introduced an unlikely source for a discussion about postpartum fetal viability: the Talmud. Just as practical religious concerns attended this monstrous birth in Magno's mind, they did so in Portaleone's as well. But he merely alludes to them rather than directly addressing them. While sorting out the real-life ritual issues the monstrous birth brought up, Portaleone waded into the *mare magnum* of the Talmud. He wrote to Magno:

> I know that you are curious and that you never tire of hearing [from] doctors. But you should desire to hear that learned theologian, who certainly tells the truth. I shall point out to you the place, and the magnificent gentleman Gratiadio Rieti, our mutual friend, will tell you the whole matter in his native language. The place is in the great volume of the Talmudic Masters, which deals with purification, that is Tahorot, in the part on menstrual separation, that is tractate *niddah*, the chapter [that describes] which partial births are permitted, *perek hamapelet*, under the heading "Rabbi Samlai said." That section analyzes the position of the fetus in the uterus, nutrition, and other things perhaps better than what most modern anatomists say.[102]

Rabbi Samlai's thoughts on fetal nourishment and positioning come as a part of a digression from the topic of miscarriages; the Talmudic chapter concerns women who give birth to severely deformed children, or even parts of a fetus.[103] The main question the Talmudic rabbis are trying to resolve in this chapter is the mother's ritual impurity – how long must she wait after discharging incomplete fetuses before she may

[102] Portaleone, *Responsorum et consultationum medicinalium liber*, 204r: "perchè so che sete curioso, che non vi bastava di udir li medici, ma vorrete ancora sentir quel dotto theologo che dice di certo la verità, vi segnarò anco il luoco e il Magnifico Signor Gratiadio Rieti nostro commune amico vi dichiararà in materna lingua tutta la sentenza. Il luoco è in magno volumine Domines Thalmudistarum, ubi agitur de Purificatione, id est טהרות, in dictione de menstrua separatione, id est in מסכת נדה capitulo 'quae abortum patitur' id est פרק המפלת sub illa lynea 'dixit Rabi Samlai'; in quel luogo si tratta del sito del foeto nell'utero materno, della nutritione e de altri particolari forsi meglio di quello che ne dicino i più de' moderni Anatomaci." I identify Rieti in the following section.

[103] The first *mishnah* of this chapter discusses procedures for women who discharge "things resembling fish, locusts, crawling insects, or worms … a domesticated animal, a wild animal, or a bird." However, the passage concludes that "anything that does not have human form is not a child." See BT Niddah 21a.

immerse herself in a ritual bath and become pure. The discussion affords the participants ample opportunities to veer from the subject at hand and deliberate other matters pertinent to neonatology and embryology. The Babylonian Talmud Niddah (30b) records Rabbi Samlai's words as follows:

> Its two hands rest on its two temples; its two armpits on its two ankles; its two heels rest against its two buttocks; and its head lies between its knees. Its mouth is closed and its navel is open, and it eats of what its mother eats and drinks of what its mother drinks but it does not discharge excrement, for were it to do so it might kill its mother. Once it is born and it emerges into the air of the world, that which was closed opens and that which was open closes; for were it not so the fetus would not be able to survive even for a moment.[104]

Portaleone is interested in two aspects of Rabbi Samlai's comment: his insistence on umbilical nourishment in utero, and his description of fetal placement in the womb. Ultimately, Portaleone is more interested in the latter topic and praises Samlai for saying things "better than what the modern anatomists say." As we shall see, Samlai's statements about fetal placement constitute only one node in an extensive web of statements about unusual births, embryonic health, and the religious ramifications of parturition, all of which Portaleone would have encountered in the few pages around Rabbi Samlai's commentary. Portaleone's belief in Samlai's scientific prescience is a matter I will discuss presently. But to whatever degree Rabbi Samlai was correct regarding fetal positioning, we must first ask whence came his – and by extension other Jewish savants' – knowledge of recondite scientific information.

Thankfully, there has been significant work dedicated to explicating the scientific acumen of Talmudic rabbis. Julius Preuss, in his *Biblical and Talmudic Medicine*, points out passages in late antique exegetical literature as well as the Talmud that touch on fetal nourishment and positioning. The Midrashic work Song of Songs Rabbah 7:3, for example, observes that as long as a fetus is in its mother's womb, it receives nourishment only through its navel.[105] In addition to the preceding

[104] Translation is taken from the Soncino edition of the Talmud.

[105] Julius Preuss, *Biblical and Talmudic Medicine*, ed. and trans. Fred Rosner (New York: Sanhedrin Press, 1978), 388.

passage concerning Rabbi Samlai, Preuss points out that Rabbi Eleazar (BT Niddah 31a), Abba Saul, Rabbi Nahman, and Abbaye (BT Niddah 25a) all discuss the position of the fetus inside the womb.[106]

From the work of Preuss and his predecessors, we know a considerable amount about Rabbi Samlai's and other rabbis' knowledge of human anatomy and fetal embryology. A. H. Israëls's discussion of Talmudic gynecology, while dated, is the best work we have on the topic.[107] In a remark Portaleone would have approved of, Israëls notes that "in [embryological] writings there exists a great amount of confusion regarding the evolution of the embryo that may be attributed to Hippocrates."[108] Regarding the rabbis' familiarity with Greek medicine, Israëls observes that while the rabbis were not experts in Greek science, they were certainly familiar with it.[109] More specifically, Israëls maintains that rabbis were especially well versed in obstetrics.[110] This refined knowledge, Israëls argues, derived from the rabbis' awareness of the fact that one cannot deduce anatomical data about humans from animal anatomy. Quoting a passage from Ḥulin, a tractate in the Babylonian Talmud that outlines the requirements of animal slaughterers and the fitness of animals for human consumption, Israëls notes that the rabbis knew that "one cannot conclude anything about men from beasts." Citing the well-known fact that Galen performed his dissections on animals and not on humans, and indulging in apologetic exaggeration, Israëls muses that "had Galen known what the rabbis knew, he would not have committed so many errors."[111]

[106] Ibid., 389. Abba Saul's remark is quoted in A. H. Israëls's work on Talmudic gynecology, *Tentamen historico-medicum, exhibens collectanea gynaecologica, quae ex Talmude Babylonico depromsit A. H. Israëls* (Groningen: P. van Aweeden, 1845). Sotah 45b: "nam infans quum formetur ex medio suo formatur." (Quoted in Israëls, 46.)

[107] Israëls, *Tentamen historico-medicum*. More recently Ron Barkai has also written about gynecology in ancient and medieval Jewish traditions. See his *Les infortunes de Dinah: le livre de la génération: la gynécologie juive au Moyen Âge* (Paris: Cerf, 1991); Barkai, *A History of Jewish Gynaecological Texts*.

[108] Israëls, *Tentamen historico-medicum*, 48.

[109] Ibid., 28.

[110] Ibid.

[111] Ibid., 42: "Nolunt Rabbini semper concludi a brutorum corporis fabrica ad hominis formationem, et praesertim non, quod attinet ad partes genitales. Dicunt enim (Chulin 68a) 'a bestia ad hominem non est concludendum; nam bestiis non est vestibulum; et ab homine ad bestiam non est concludendum, quia vultui (hominis) inest quid honorabile.' Sensus est: corporis humani fabrica longe alia est, quam fabrica brutorum; et hanc ob rem ea quae sectionibus brutorum inveniatur, non omnino ad humanum corpus possunt applicari."

Apart from the child's fitness for circumcision, and its mother's ritual purity, another issue that arose in connection with classifying unusual infants as human or subhuman is whether or not the parents of the newborn are required to redeem it. Scripture (Exodus 13:13; Numbers 8:17) demands that parents redeem their firstborn child by bringing a token contribution to a priest, and rabbinic law expands upon the particulars of the obligation. The rabbis conclude that only a fetus of human form that is truly viable required redemption in conformity with biblical and Talmudic law.[112]

The Talmud's discussion in Niddah is decisive on the subject of what forms of new life the rabbis considered human. Evaluating the status of a creature born with an animal's body and a human face, the rabbis conclude that the mother of the infant does not need to purify herself unless the creature has "a forehead, eyebrows, eyes, cheeks, and a chin."[113] This remark implies that the infant must, after all, have a head. The most definitive ruling on this issue comes when the Talmudic rabbis discuss a fetus that emerges in human form but is missing essential parts. After deliberating how much of the lower body is necessary for survival, the topic shifts to the cranium. There is little debate here, and the Talmud concludes that even if a portion of the skull is missing, the mother is considered ritually pure – that is, the creature born to her was not a human being.[114]

Rabbi Samlai, whom Portaleone designated "a theologian," is the only Talmudic authority Portaleone singled out from these extensive juridical debates. It is remarkable that Portaleone labeled Rabbi Samlai a "theologian"; elsewhere in his Latin and vernacular writings he uses less specialized language.[115] His application of Christian religious terminology to a Jewish authority shows how comfortable Portaleone was describing Jewish intellectual traditions with the vocabulary of a

[112] See BT Niddah 23b for this discussion and Numbers 18:15–16 and Deuteronomy 21:17 for the scriptural sources.

[113] BT Niddah 23b.

[114] BT Niddah 24a.

[115] Abraham Portaleone, *De auro dialoghi tres* (Venice: apud Iohannem Baptistam à Porta, 1584), 170, "sapientes nostri." For discussion of this passage, though not of this terminology, see Gianfranco Miletto, *Glauben und Wissen im Zeitalter der Reformation: Der salomonische Tempel bei Abraham Ben David Portaleone (1542–1612)* (Berlin: de Gruyter, 2004), 253–5.

common language. It is even more noteworthy that Portaleone labels Graziadio Rieti as our "mutual friend." Graziadio (Ḥananel) Rieti and his brother Vitale (Yeḥiel) were prominent bankers in Mantua at the end of the sixteenth century.[116] It is not clear how exactly Magno might have known him, but given Rieti's banking connections, it is not surprising that they knew each other or implausible that they might have. Most unusual in this passage is Portaleone's use of the Talmud as a historical and scientific source in a discussion about fetal nourishment and embryonic placement.[117] The fact that Portaleone – or, at the very least, David, his son – was willing to write the name of the order, the tractate, and the chapter in Hebrew suggests either that Magno was able to read enough of the language to decipher a citation or, just as likely, that he had recourse to a learned acquaintance who could.

PORTALEONE AND GALEN/RUFUS

Portaleone did more than simply evoke a Talmudic authority; he juxtaposed that authority to an ancient Greek physician. As he did years later in his Hebrew encyclopedia *Shiltei HaGibborim*, Portaleone uses Greek medicine to confirm Talmudic truths. After concluding his praise of Rabbi Samlai's ingenious remarks, Portaleone deems it time to "move on to the doctors." He adds, "Rufus says in his eleventh chapter of *The Introduction to Medicine*, confirming Rabbi Samlai, that the fetus is nourished by the umbilical cord and is therefore able to live in the uterus."[118] Here Portaleone shifts his focus to fetal nourishment. In ancient medical traditions there was considerable discussion of how

[116] Simonsohn, *History of the Jews in the Duchy of Mantua* (Jerusalem: Kiryat Sefer Ltd., 1977), 357 n. 133. Graziadio Rieti was also a friend of Abraham Yagel. See David B. Ruderman, *Kabbalah, Magic and Science*, 16–18, 176.

[117] In the seventeenth century and in Northern Europe, scholars such as Isaac Casaubon and John Selden incorporated Talmudic citations into their works on a variety of topics. But examples are lacking of sixteenth-century Italian Jews including Talmudic citations in their letters to gentile correspondents.

[118] Portaleone, *Responsorum et consultationum medicinalium liber*, 204r: "Solutiones ad quaesita proposita ab Excellentissimo D. Alexandro Magno et sunt Excellentissimi Patris." "Ma passiamo alli medici, Ruffo nell'Introduttorio seu Medico al capitolo xi s'accorda con Rabi Samlai, quando disse: 'ab umbilico autem venae ad iecinoris portas sanguinem in foetibus transmittunt,' dove par che voglia che per questa via sola e non per altra il foeto si nutrisca nell'utero."

fetuses ingested nutrients. Some authorities held that the umbilical cord provided needed nourishment, while others insisted that an infant used its mouth to suckle; still others tentatively argued that the mouth and umbilical cord acted in concert.[119]

Portaleone's use of an ancient Greek physician to confirm the teachings of a Talmudic rabbi who lived a century and a half later seems anachronistic and baldly apologetic to modern sensibilities. But in the Jewish community Portaleone inhabited, sacred authorities, among whom Talmudic rabbis ranked very high, held considerable sway over Christian or pagan ones.[120] Much more noteworthy from the perspective of the history of medicine is Portaleone's attribution of this medical insight to Rufus. Rufus of Ephesus was a prominent physician who flourished late in the first century AD.[121] His works were just beginning to be studied seriously in the sixteenth century. While some of Rufus's works were known in the late Renaissance, and many more have been discovered since, the *Introduction* that Portaleone quotes in the preceding passage has never definitively been attributed to Rufus.[122]

The passage that Portaleone quotes regarding fetal nourishment may be found in the 1565 edition of Galen's *Opera Omnia*. The *Introduction* that Portaleone refers to, then, was considered one of Galen's works in mid-sixteenth-century editions. In the 1541 Giunti edition of Galen's *Opera Omnia*, there is discussion of Galen's spurious works; the *Introduction* was considered to be among these. However, none of the scholars who worked on either the 1541 or the 1565 edition of Galen's works, each of which Portaleone would have had access to as a medical student and a mature practitioner, attributed the *Introduction* to Rufus.

119 Some of these debates are summarized in Luc Brisson, Marie-Hélène Congourdeau, and Jean-Luc Solère, eds., *L'embryon: formation et animation: antiquité grecque et latine, traditions hébraïque, chrétienne et islamique* (Paris: Vrin, 2008).

120 On the nature of rabbinic authority in Renaissance Italy, see Robert Bonfil, *Rabbis and Jewish Communities in Renaissance Italy*, trans. Jonathan Chipman (Oxford: Littman Library, 1990).

121 The best discussion of Rufus of Ephesus may be found in Vivian Nutton, *Ancient Medicine* (London: Routledge, 2004). See bibliography there.

122 The best modern collection of Rufus's writings is C. Daremberg and C. Émile Ruelle, *Oeuvres de Rufus d'Ephèse* (Paris: Imprimerie nationale, 1879). It contains the complete Greek text with a facing French translation. Caroline Petit has conducted a thorough survey of Rufus's works and their reception in later periods. According to her *Galen, Le médecin, introduction* (Paris: Belles Lettres, 2009), no one ever attributed the *Introduction* to Rufus.

This appears to have been Portaleone's original contribution to source criticism. The sentence Portaleone quotes reads "veins transmit blood to fetuses through the umbilical cord to the entrances of the liver."[123] Portaleone does not offer his reasons for attributing the work to Rufus; his offhand remark belies any careful consideration of textual or historical reasons Portaleone might have called upon to make this assessment. His may have been the first attribution of the *Introduction*, commonly thought to be Galen's, to Rufus.[124]

But Portaleone's chief interest in his correspondence with Magno was not in textual attribution but in medical science. As we have seen, ancient authorities were divided on the issue of how fetuses were nourished in the womb. Portaleone himself provides a helpful introduction to these debates. He reminds Magno that "Hippocrates, in *De carnibus*, wants to say that the child is nourished through its mouth, but in reality he says that an infant's lips are pressed together in the womb, so it receives food and spirit from the mother through a cord."[125] That is to say that Hippocrates, according to Portaleone, contradicts himself, wishing to say one thing but providing evidence to the contrary.[126] The Mantuan

[123] See Galen, "Introductio, seu medicus," chap. 11 in *Galeni Isagogici libri* (Venice: Giunti, 1586), 54v: "ab umbilico autem venae ad iecinoris portas sanguinem in foetibus transmittunt: arteriae vero iuxta vesicam, crassiori arteriae: nervuus hic spinae insertatur."

[124] Petit, *Galen*, demonstrates that attributions of Galen's *Introduction seu medicus* to Rufus occurred only in the modern period. I have not been able to examine Dr. Petit's work. I wish to thank Nancy Siraisi for corresponding with me on this matter.

[125] Portaleone, *Responsorum et consultationum medicinalium liber*, "Solutiones ad quaesita proposita ab Excellentissimo D. Alexandro Magno et sunt Excellentissimi Patris," 204r–204v. "'Non enim ab ea solum, quae per umbilicum ad portas in iecur e secundis fertur materia, nutrivi putatur. Etenim per has quoque vias alitur, maxime vero per eas, quae perfectiores sunt et per quascunque defertur, nutrimento fruitur. Neque enim putabis Hippocratem dicentem, quod antiquius est nutrimentum per abdomen, qua umbilicum est, invehi, ignorasse num id ore nutriatur. Etenim de hac quoque via locutus est etc.'; e perchè gli pare che non accade a provar che 'per umbilicum nutriatur fœtus,' si volta all'altra, et adduce due raggioni tolte però da Hippocrate nel libro detto di sopra cioè de Carnibus."

[126] See Hippocrates' remarks in *Magni Hippocratis medicorum omnium facile principis opera omnia quae extant* (Frankfurt: apud heredes Andreae Wecheli, 1596), section III, *De carnibus,* 209: "At vero puer dum in utero est, compressis labris ex matris utero tum alimentum sugit, tum etiam spiritum, qui in puero caldissimus est, ubi sane mater respirat, in cor attrahit.... Quod si quis roget, unde hoc quis noscit, quod puer in utero trahat et sugat, hoc illi respondere licet. Pueri cum in lucem prodeunt, stercus in intestinis habere conspiciuntur, et simul ac in lucem editi sunt, tum homines, tum percora, id iis per ventrem secedit. Atqui neque stercus haberet, nisi in utero sugeret, neque; ut primum puer natus est, ubera sugere nosset, nisi in utero suxisset."

physician points out that "Hippocrates says that in order for an infant to receive nourishment through the mouth after it is born it must be able to use its mouth when it is in the womb" and glosses this by exclaiming "O beautiful reason! O true and overblown conjecture! Since a kid is born and immediately begins to walk, run, and jump, surely therefore it walked and jumped inside the womb of the nanny goat!"[127] Resuming a more solemn tone, Portaleone writes, "Signor Alessandro: whoever reads these books uncritically without thoroughly considering the truth of things often finds himself deceived and that these writers are not deserving of the trust he has [in them]." In conclusion, he maintains that "it is not true that the fetus nourishes itself through the mouth while in the uterus, as these fathers of medicine say."[128] Having ridiculed Hippocrates, whose authority was nearly beyond reproach in mid-sixteenth-century Italy, Portaleone asserted his own intellectual independence. Not wishing to leave Magno utterly confounded, he urges his correspondent to "read Realdo Colombo in his book on the formation of the fetus ... [the fetus] receives nourishment through the umbilical vein."[129]

PORTALEONE AND COLOMBO

Abraham Portaleone had a habit of enthusiastically endorsing modern scientific works. In the middle of a thorny discussion about the herb balsam in his Hebrew encyclopedia *Shiltei HaGibborim,* Portaleone advised his readers to "go read the books of Prospero Alpino."[130] Alpino

[127] Portaleone, "Solutiones ad Quaesita proposita ab Excellentissimo D. Alexandro Magno et sunt Excellentissimi Patris," in *Responsorum et consultationum medicinalium liber*, 204v: "Quod vero in utero ore nutrimentum summat, testis est post partum protinus mammae appetitum, neque non nisi antea huic viae assuetus esset, tam cito ad mammam ferretur, che risponde a quelle parole de Hippocrate imo neque mamma statim ut natu est sugere noscet si non in utero suxisset. O bella ragione, o vera e arteficiosa coniettura, il capretto subito nato camina, corre e salta, dunque ha caminato certo e saltato nel ventre della capra."

[128] Ibid., 205r: "Signor Alessandro chi legge i libri oscitantemente, senza considerar bene la verità delle cose, si trova spesse volte ingannato, nè vale la fiducia che si ha alla gravità de' scrittori, perchè ancor essi, come homeni, pono declinare dalla verità e dalla via retta disputtando delle cose incerte. Non è vero che'l foeto si nutrisca per la bocca, mentre sta nell'utero, come dissero questi padri della medicina."

[129] Ibid., 205r: "Legete Realdo Colombo nel suo trattato de formatione foetus che da lui come da authore più esperto che non furono Hippocrate e Galeno in questa parte, intenderete che non si puo nutrire per quella via se non con la sua morte ... non è perciò che si sia nutrito per la bocca, ma per la vena umbelicare."

[130] Portaleone, *SG*, 95v.

resolved many of the difficult issues with which Portaleone struggled. On the topics of fetal nourishment and positioning, Portaleone turned to Realdo Colombo's works. Colombo filled in the gaps of Portaleone's understanding on those two issues, but he also appealed to Portaleone for another reason: he emphasized the inherent difficulty of embryology as a subject and underscored its quasi-divine status in relation to other areas of scientific inquiry. A group of sixteenth-century anatomists anticipated and echoed Colombo, including Gabriele Fallopia, Andreas Vesalius, and Conrad Gesner. Because of his scientific respectability, and his insistence on the connections between science and faith, Colombo was an ideal author for Portaleone to invoke as a modern mouthpiece for Rabbi Samlai.

First published in 1559, Realdo Colombo's *De re anatomica liber* was widely known in the second half of the sixteenth century.[131] Originally hailing from Cremona, Colombo taught anatomy in Rome while he wrote his great anatomical work. Near the beginning of his remarks on embryology, Colombo stressed the subject's seriousness. "It must be noted before all else," Colombo observed, "prudent and pious reader, that one cannot think anything more astonishing than the generation of man, or rather the fetus. Nothing else seems to be equal in nature to a miracle, and nothing else inflames men to love of divine providence and wisdom." The subject, Colombo continued, "represents something you can better admire than praise, and praise more than you are able to discern precisely."[132] Before beginning his scientific exploration of the topic, Colombo warns his readers of the complexity of the task at hand.

Portaleone learned much from Colombo's treatment of embryonic nourishment. Proclaiming that the umbilical cord is the sole medium through which an embryo obtains nourishment, Colombo criticizes

[131] *Realdi Columbi Cremonensis De re anatomica libri XV* (Venice: ex typographia Nicolai Beuilacquæ, 1559). On Colombo, see *DBI* 27:241–3. I have used the 1562 edition: *De re anatomica libri XV* (Paris: Aegidium Gillium, 1562).

[132] Realdo Colombo, *De re anatomica libri XV* (Paris: Aegidium Gillium, 1562), book XII, *De formatione foetus, ac de situ infantis in utero*, 451: "qua in re illud primum admonendus est prudens, piusque lector, hominis generatione, foetus inquam, formatione nihil admirabilius excogitari posse, nihil quod aeque naturae miraculum videatur esse, nihil quod humanum genus divinae providentiae, sapientiaeque amore magis inflammet. Ea enim arte effictus est, atque efformatus hominis foetus, ut illam admirari magis, quam laudare, laudare magis, quam exacte introspicere omnia possis."

Hippocrates for his shortsightedness: "The fetus receives nourishment through the power of the umbilical vein when it is in its mother's uterus. What the great Hippocrates, who alone could not know everything, said about the nourishment of children in the womb is pure fantasy, namely that the fetus suckles through its mouth. Evidently many men were led into error, such that I cannot stop marveling at it." Colombo finishes his critical remarks with a simple declaration: the fetus "is nourished through the umbilical vein."[133] This argument for fetal nourishment, as well as Colombo's strongly critical stance against Hippocrates, would have appealed to Portaleone and served him well in his quest to persuade Alessandro Magno.

Colombo's discussion of embryonic placement, which figures even more prominently in *De re anatomica*, helped Portaleone even more. Denouncing all previous attempts to understand fetal positioning, Colombo boldly advises his "candid reader" to "skip past other works, for they do not see the thing itself but rather a version of it, and that is what they end up writing about." Colombo, of course, pursues a different strategy. "I am not like that," he asserts, "for very often I have observed not dead fetuses, but living ones, which I have extracted with my very own hands from the mother's uterus; then I take proper note of its placement in the uterus." As a result of these numerous experiences, Colombo boasted, "I could easily tell how different [fetal placement] is from some pictures of the anatomists, such that I could not help marveling at their temerity, given that they were wrong, and that [their drawings] went far beyond sense – they were not even ashamed to leave [these] written [matters] to posterity."[134] Colombo's position is clear: other anatomists

[133] Ibid., 459–60: "Foetus in matris utero alimentum per umbilicum suscipit, venae umbilicalis ope: fabulaeque sunt, quas magnus Hippocrates, qui omnia scire non potuit solus, de pueri nutrimento in alvo matris dixit: quod scilicet per os exugat: et profecto tanti viri errorem tam crassum nequeo satis mirari. Nam inter os foetus, matricisque substantiam multum interest sed fac nullum inter haec spatium dari: age, os foetus uteri corpus attingat: quo pacto succum, qui vel in matris ventriculo est, aut in intestinis, exugere posset optime Hippocrates? Quamobrem haud dubie scias candide lector, foetum nihil prorsus per os assumere. Quod si assumeret, suo ipsius sudore hausto obrutus non interire non posset: sed per venam umbilicalem duntaxat nutriri, nutriri inquam bono sanguine, atque adeo perfecto qui per vasa seminaria defertur: quod idcirco factum fuit, ut materiam una cum sanguine continenter deorsum ferrent, tanquam auxiliares copias, si quandoque sanguis deesset."

[134] Ibid., 463: "de foetus formatione satis multa hactenus dicta sunt: nunc de situ eius in utero dicamus. Quam partem libentius, ut opinor, lector candidus percurret, quod alii non rem

have observed only dead fetuses, or no fetuses at all, and have based their illustrations on either aberrations or fantasies, and have permitted themselves to write on the basis of false conjecture. He, on the other hand, had direct experience examining fetal positioning, and as a result his readers should take his findings more seriously.

Colombo's discussion of uterine fetal positioning is more nuanced than Rabbi Samlai's; still, in Portaleone's reading it substantiates the Talmudic master's embryonic expertise. In contrast to Rabbi Samlai, who described one typical position, Colombo discerned three. "There are three positions in the uterus that I acknowledge having observed." "The first," Colombo notes, "is where the head is tilted downward, and this is the most frequent. The second is where the head is tilted upward, and this is seen only rarely. The third is a transverse lie, but this is even more rare."[135] Beyond these specificities, Colombo offers some general observations that are much more detailed than those of Rabbi Samlai:

> The infant is in a globe or a sphere, an oblong sphere ... the right arm is bent, the outer hand has its fingers extended, below the ear and above the neck. The left arm is not extended above the right part of the chest, and certainly not above the face (since the head is tilted in the uterus) ... the left arm supports the right elbow with its fingers semiextended, with the thumb pointing downward. The legs are very carefully brought upward, and they are bent, such that [the fetus] is on its head – it is a most beautiful thing to see and is admirable. The femur, the tibia, and the right foot are bent, such

ipsam, sed quod verisimile cuique visum est, ita scriptum reliquerunt: omnes tamen a rei veritate tam aberrarunt, quam qui maxime. Ego vero non semel, sed saepius non modo mortuos foetus, sed vivos etiam e matris utero hisce manibus extraxi quod dum efficerem, situm eius in utero diligenter observavi, quem a quibusdam Anatomicorum picturis adeo diversum esse facile perspexi, ut non potuerim eorum temeritatem non valde mirari, qui quod falsum est, cuius oppositum sensu deprehendi potest, posteris scriptum relinquere non erubuerint." Colombo may have had in mind such treatises as Jakob Rueff's *De conceptu et generatione hominis, et iis quae circa haec potissimum considerantur, libri sex* (Zurich: Christophorus Froschoverus, 1554), which featured highly schematic illustrations. I thank Nancy Siraisi for pointing this out to me.

135 Colombo, *De re anatomica libri XV*, 463–4: "Tres igitur foetus in utero situs observasse fateor, et profiteor, praeterea nullos, quorum prior est caput deorsum versum, hicque est situs omnium frequentissimus. Secundus capite sursum elato, quo situ raro videntur infantes in utero. Tertius transversim iacet, atque hic est secundo rarior, propterea priore situ infantes capita praeeunte [*sic*: praevente] in lucem prodeunt. Secundi pedibus, qui et agrippae vocantur. Tertii natibus, facie omnes coccygem matris versus respiciunt."

that they are touching the femur and the abdomen, with the knee touching the umbilical cord. The tibia is bent downward, and the sole of the left foot is touching the buttocks, and the foot is elevated, the private parts are hidden, so that half of the thumb and the tibia are turned above the abdomen and the thorax, and are below the outer arm. The foot is turned outward, attached to the right elbow and the left metacarpus. The back is in the anterior position, such that [the fetus] can escape from its elongated global sphere.[136]

Colombo was confident enough in his findings to share them with esteemed colleagues. Colombo boasted that "this is the true and legitimate positioning of the human fetus in the uterus, which I showed to Giacomo Antonio Buoni of Ferrara, the eminent physician, who teaches medical simples in the Roman Academy, as well as anatomy, and is very accomplished in all the other noble arts and sciences."[137] At the end of his thoughts on embryology, Colombo closes with a pious salutation: "Who, contemplating the generation, nutrition, and positioning of the human fetus, is not astonished? Who is able to praise God sufficiently in his infinite goodness? It is enough to trust in these matters, and to say

[136] Ibid., 464–5: "quocunque autem situ ex hoc triplici toties euumerato [*sic*: enumerato] nos uterus exceperit: in globum atque orbem excipimur, sphaericusque est omnis situs infantis in utero: sphaericus inquam in oblongum vergens, et ut privatim res magis innotescat, dexterum brachium nobis tunc flectitur, manus autem extrema una cum digitis extenditur, qui digiti sub aure dextera, superque cervice positi sunt: sinistrum vero brachium tantum non extenditur, supraque sinistram mammam, necnon supra faciem (caput nanque in utero ita flectitur, ut mentum ad thoracem perveniat): sinistrum itaque brachium medio cubito dextero fulcitur digitis semiextensis, pollice deorsum. Crura tanta arte sursum feruntur, et incuruantur, quasi in arcum ut dicu, visuque res pulcherrima, et admirabilis existat. Femur, tibia, pesque extremus dexter nobis eo tempore flectuntur, adeo ut a femore abdomen attingatur, a genu umbilicus, deinde tibia deorsum flectitur, calceque sinistras nates attingit, extremum elevans pedem, pudendaque occultans, adeo ut pollice dimidium, tibiam ipsemet tangat, sinistrum crus ipsum quoque semiflectitur, femur ventrem imum tangit, tibia supra abdomen, thoracemque vertitur, et sub extremum brachium. Pes autem extremus sursum voluitur dextrum ὠλέκρανον attingens, sinistrique brachii μετακάρπιον. Dorsum deinde in anteriora fertur, adeo ut ex his omnibus globus sphaericus oblongus evadat."

[137] Ibid, 465: "Atque hic est verus, et legitimus situs humani foetus in utero, quem ego Iacobo Antonio Bono Ferrariensi Medico praecellenti, qui simplicia medicamenta in Romana Academia publice profitetur, estque rei Anatomicae, reliquarumque bonarum artium, et scientiarum tam studiosus, quam qui maxime, cum eum unicè diligam, primum lubens ostendi." Bono, or Buoni, was the author of *Del terremoto dialogo* (Modena: Paolo Gadaldini et fratelli, 1571), which Azariah de' Rossi quotes several times in his *Me'or Enayim*. See Azariah de' Rossi, *The Light of the Eyes*, trans. and ed. Joanna Weinberg (New Haven: Yale University Press, 2001), 14, 22, 301–2, and 659.

little."[138] Colombo's pious packaging of his anatomical investigations met with Portaleone's approval and provided another reason for him to use Colombo's text to corroborate the words of his rabbinic predecessor.

CONCLUSION

Jacques Roger has shown how up until the end of the eighteenth century religious questions played an important role in the development of the natural sciences.[139] Issues of faith and the scrutiny of religious texts played significant roles in prompting and directing medical explorations of the antiquarian and the anomalous. Renaissance doctors drew on sacred texts to enlarge their understanding of medical arts. Talal Asad has persuasively argued that religious texts, beliefs, and suppositions can instigate decidedly nonreligious explorations.[140] Portaleone's letters underscore Asad's point: they constitute scientific excurses catalyzed by religious concerns.

In the late Renaissance Jews drew attention to classical Jewish sources, which were then absorbed by Christians who wished to supplement their scientific learning. The foregoing material underscores how Jews, and not merely Jewish texts, had a unique role to play in Christian use of classical Jewish texts. Contemporary scholarship insists that Christians were mainly interested in Jewish books, and less so in Jews themselves, to confirm Christian doctrines or convert Jews.[141] Similarly, historians have not recognized that Jews freely shared their religious and intellectual resources with Christians with no ulterior motive beyond

[138] Colombo, *De re anatomica libri XV*, 465: "Quis enim foetus humani generationem, nutritionem, situmque contemplatus non obstupescat? Quis Dei infinitam bonitatem satis laudet? Equidem de his silere satius est, quam pauca dicere."

[139] Jacques Roger, *Les sciences de la vie dans la pensée française du XVIII siècle* (Paris: A. Colin, 1963). For an earlier adumbration of this view, see Walter Pagel, "Religious Motives in the Medical Biology of the XVIIth Century," *Bulletin of the Institute of the History of Medicine* 3 (1935): 97–128, 213–31, 265–312. Reprinted with original pagination in Marianne Winder, ed., *Religion and Neoplatonism in Renaissance Medicine* (London: Variorum, 1985).

[140] Talal Asad, *Formations of the Secular: Christianity, Islam, Modernity* (Stanford: Stanford University Press, 2003).

[141] See, for example, Alba Paladini's *Il* De arcanis *di Pietro Galatino: traditio giudaica e nuove istanze filologiche* (Lecce: Congedo, 2004). For an important exception, see Anthony Grafton and Joanna Weinberg, *"I Have Always Loved the Holy Tongue": Isaac Casaubon, the Jews, and a Forgotten Chapter in Renaissance Scholarship* (Cambridge, MA: Harvard University Press, 2011), chap. 5.

the advancement of scientific knowledge. Christian physicians such as Alessandro Magno and Giovanni Battista Cavallara asked Jews about topics that they presumed Mosaic tradition could help inform, and Jews such as Portaleone distributed their faith's intellectual resources in order to aid natural philosophical investigations.

Portaleone saw his Christian colleagues as true intellectual partners and considered himself part of their professional society. There is no better proof of this than the way he describes his fellow members of Mantua's College of Physicians. In a postscript to his Hebrew encyclopedia, Portaleone recollected how "in the year 1566, on the 19th of Elul, the third of September, the week of the pericope *atem nitzavim* (Deuteronomy 29:9–30:20), the College of Physicians of Mantua accepted me [as a member]." He went on to observe that "at the time there were thirty-five doctors, all wise and men of understanding. They permitted me to practice medicine like their other physicians in Mantua and its environs."[142] Writing in Hebrew for Jewish readers, Portaleone boasted of his membership in Mantua's medical community and his participation in Christian society. His Latin and vernacular correspondence with Christian physicians confirms his claims, and his free dispensation of Talmudic learning to contribute to their scientific investigations is direct proof of the close connections between Portaleone and his gentile colleagues, as well as those between religious studies and medical science at the end of the sixteenth century.

[142] *SG*, unnumbered folio corresponding to 185v: ובשנת ש"כו י"ט אלול ג' סיטימברי פרשת אתם נצבים קבלוני רופאי הקולוגיאו במנטובה שהיו אז שלשים וחמשה כלם חכמים ונבונים והרשוני לרפאת כשאר רופאיהם במנטובה וחוצה לה

5

"I Seek the Truth from Whomever Pronounces It"

Abraham Portaleone and Ancient Israelite Incense

Ulisse Aldrovandi's hunt for biblical *manna* in the Dolomite foothills and David de' Pomi's insistence that the biblical stone *tarshish* could be found in Venetian marketplaces exemplify a shift in how Italian physicians studied the natural philosophy of the biblical world at the close of the sixteenth century. They no longer believed that the best way to understand the Bible was by clarifying its obscure passages with material drawn from other ancient texts. Instead they sought out modern books and material objects that could supplement and transform their understanding of the Bible's natural details. Aldrovandi and de' Pomi were hardly alone; Abraham Portaleone's study of ancient Jewish antiquities bears witness to a similar approach to biblical naturalia. *Shiltei HaGibborim* (Shields of the mighty), Portaleone's self-published Hebrew encyclopedia printed in Mantua by Moses Elishama ben Israel Zifroni of Guastalla in 1612, contains a lengthy excursus on biblical incense.[1] Portaleone's encyclopedia was framed as a hortatory address

[1] The best introduction to *SG* is *Die Heldenschilde. Vom Hebräischen ins Deutsche übersetzt und kommentiert von Gianfranco Miletto*, 2 vols. (Frankfurt: Peter Lang, 2002), 1:21–75. According to its title page, the book was printed "by his [Portaleone's] commission and in his house," במצותו ובביתו For more, see Miletto, *Glauben und Wissen im Zeitalter der Reformation: der salomonishce Tempel bei Abraham ben David Portaleone (1542–1612)* (Berlin: de Gruyter, 2004), 15 and notes there. Recently David Garber and Yo'el Katan published an edition of *SG* with some explanatory notes (Jerusalem, 2009). See also Miletto, *La biblioteca di Avraham ben David Portaleone secondo l'inventario della sua eredità* (Florence: Olschki, 2013). Unfortunately, Dr. Miletto's book was published after I had submitted the

A portion of this chapter previously appeared as "Judah Moscato, Abraham Portaleone, and Biblical Incense in Late Renaissance Mantua," in Gianfranco Miletto and Giuseppe Veltri, eds., *Rabbi Judah Moscato and the Jewish Intellectual World of Mantua in the 16th–17th Century* (Leiden: Brill, 2012), 105–19.

to its author's children and structured as a study of Solomon's Temple. It charts the dimensions of that edifice, describes the details of its construction, and studies the practices associated with the ancient sacrificial cult, including the assembly and burning of incense. Its chapters on incense have two goals: to identify the elements of biblical incense, only some of which are specified in scripture, and to instruct readers how to make a vital component of the incense mixture – the anointing oil. *Shiltei HaGibborim*'s study of incense accomplishes those goals by transposing trends new to sixteenth-century botany, and natural philosophy more generally, to the study of Jewish texts. Among these trends were a preference for modern scientific writings rather than classical ones and an openness to nonbookish sources of knowledge, chiefly artisanal expertise. The transposition of habits of thought characteristic of the medical profession and the natural philosophic community to the study of religious texts engendered a critical stance toward received tradition – rabbinic and scientific alike.

Modern scholarship has not recognized the important role of Portaleone's medical education and practice in his encyclopedic work. Though contemporary evaluations of Portaleone's writings have moved away from Cecil Roth's diagnosis of Portaleone as "discursive to the verge of eccentricity,"[2] very little recent work has endeavored to measure Portaleone's scholarly reach or assess his scientific achievement. A few studies have mentioned Portaleone's interest in incense. Alessandro Guetta and Samuel Kottek, in essays focused on other aspects of *Shiltei HaGibborim,* each note Portaleone's treatment of the subject.[3] Gianfranco Miletto devotes several pages of his book on Portaleone to incense in the ancient temple.[4] Most recently, Peter Miller has flagged

final version of this typescript, and I was unable to consult it. For more on Moshe Elishama ben Israel Zifroni of Guastalla, see the literature cited in Chapter 3, note 48.

2 Cecil Roth, *The Jews in the Renaissance* (Philadelphia: Jewish Publication Society of America, 1977 [1959]), 318.

3 Alessandro Guetta, "Avraham Portaleone, le scientifique repenti"; Guetta, "Abraham Portaleone From Science to Mysticism," in Judit Targarona Borrás and Angel Sáenz-Badillos, eds., *Jewish Studies at the Turn of the Twentieth Century*, vol. 2: *Judaism from the Renaissance to Modern Times* (Leiden: Brill, 1999), 40–7; Samuel S. Kottek, "Jews between Profane and Sacred Science in Renaissance Italy: The Case of Abraham Portaleone," in Jurgen Helm and Annette Winkelman, eds., *Religious Confessions and the Sciences in the Sixteenth Century* (Leiden: Brill, 2001), 108–18.

4 Miletto, *Glauben und Wissen*, 226–38.

Portaleone's digressive treatment of natural history and the spice trade as emblematic of an early modern, encyclopedic disposition.[5] In spite of this awareness of the role of botany in *Shiltei HaGibborim*, there is no article-length treatment of Portaleone's study of the composition of ancient incense, the precise details of which, according to rabbinic tradition, were transmitted to Moses by God himself on Mount Sinai.[6] Similarly, scant scholarship addresses the centrality of medicine in his printed oeuvre.

Abraham Portaleone's work on the ancient Jewish incense mixture is a significant achievement of Renaissance scholarship and an unusual contribution to premodern Jewish thought. *Shiltei HaGibborim*'s eleven chapters on incense, which comprise more than 12 percent of the total work, are especially notable for two reasons. First, they advocate and enable reconstruction of the ancient incense mixture, which was proscribed in Jewish law. Second, they are highly critical of Portaleone's rabbinic forbears. A central theme emerges from an examination of Portaleone's work on incense: to the mind of an early modern Jewish physician, rabbinic knowledge of natural history is deficient. In his chapters on incense, Portaleone routinely censures rabbinic authorities ranging from Talmudic redactors to medieval and early modern luminaries such as Rashi, Gersonides, Ibn Ezra, Radak, Sforno, and Abravanel.[7] Although Portaleone respects his rabbinic forbears, he disparages their scientific acumen.

Portaleone's critical stance toward rabbis' botanical knowledge runs parallel to, and was stimulated by, his dissatisfaction with ancient Greek and Roman botanical authorities. As such, his negative evaluation of rabbinic literature must be understood as an adaptation of Renaissance debates about the fallibility of ancient and medieval scientific sources.[8] *Shiltei HaGibborim*'s exploration of ancient incense relies much more on the work of fifteenth-century explorers, sixteenth-century botanists, and contemporary pharmacists than on either ancient scientific authorities

[5] Peter N. Miller, "Lost and Found," *Jewish Quarterly Review* 97:4 (2007): 502–7.

[6] See BT Keritot 6v.

[7] Rashi: Rabbi Solomon Yitzhaqi, 1040–1105; Gersonides: Rabbi Gerson ben Levi, 1288–1344; Ibn Ezra: Abraham ibn Ezra, 1092–1167; Radak: Rabbi David Kimḥi, 1160–1235; Sforno: Rabbi Ovadiah ben Jacob, 1475–1550; Abravanel: Isaac Abravanel, 1438–1508.

[8] For a summary in the context of Renaissance botany, see Brian Ogilvie, *The Science of Describing: Natural History in Renaissance Europe* (Chicago: University of Chicago Press, 2006).

or Portaleone's Jewish predecessors. Analyzing Portaleone's working methods and his encyclopedia's critical features tells us not only about one particular premodern Italian Jewish thinker but also about the study of religious texts by early modern physicians.

WHY INCENSE?

Incense was an important part of cultural and religious life on the Italian Peninsula during the second half of the sixteenth century. The twenty-second session of the Council of Trent, held on 17 September 1562 under the aegis of Pope Pius IV, affirmed the centrality of incense as a component of Catholic worship that would "excite the minds of the faithful" and assist them in the "contemplation of those most sublime things that are hidden in this sacrifice."[9] The role of incense as an aid to worship even plays a part in popular fiction concerned with this period: Maria Bellonci's *Segreti dei Gonzaga* depicts the young Vincenzo, Duke of Mantua from 1587 until 1612, praying in churches saturated with the odors of incense.[10] Beyond its everyday use in church ceremonies, early modern Italians were also interested in the incense of the ancient world. David de' Pomi, whose work was the subject of Chapter 3, includes in his Italian definition of the Hebrew term for "Lebanon" the following observation: "Everyone who passes by that mountain affirms that they smell a fragrance of marvelous quality, and attests that the scent is still present two hundred fifty miles from the mountain." He goes on to add that the cedar wood used to build the ceiling beams of Solomon's temple "is extremely durable and knotted and does not putrefy. It is no wonder that Salomon put this [wood] to use in building the Temple, which, owing to its material and its divine composition, might still be found today in its pristine state."[11] Indeed, the oil (or resin) from trees that grew upon

9 Council of Trent, session 22, 17 September 1562, chap. 5, "De Missae caeremoniis et ritibus." The relevant passage reads "ut mysticas benedictiones, lumina, thymiamata, vestes aliaque id genus multa ex apostolica disciplina et traditione … et mentes fidelium per haec visibilia religionis et pietatis signa ad rerum altissimarum, quae in hoc sacrificio latent, contemplationem excitarentur." See A. L. Richter, *Canones et decreta concilii tridentini* (Leipzig: typis et sumptibus B. Tauchnitii, 1853), 126.

10 Maria Bellonci, *Segreti dei Gonzaga* (Milan: Mondadori, 1947), 14.

11 David de' Pomi, *צמח דוד*, *Dittionario novo Hebraico* (Venice, 1587), 70b, col. 1: "Chiunque passa per quel monte dicono sentire una refraganza di odore maraviglioso, affermano

Mount Lebanon in the Queen of Sheba's fabled realm yielded two of the four incense elements specified in scripture: frankincense and myrrh.

Ancient incense and its modern derivatives attracted more than just episodic attention from sixteenth-century European scholars, Portaleone being one of them. There are at least two reasons the Mantuan physician might have been interested in incense. One is that some Jews in Portaleone's time believed that reciting liturgical passages containing the incense mixture could obviate and even eliminate the effects of the plague.[12] The second is that Portaleone's training in medicine, and his practice as a physician in Mantua, accustomed him to study spices and herbs. Apart from the administration of herbs as medicaments, Portaleone would have learned how to describe plants and compare samples with accounts of them in ancient botanical texts as part of his education in medical "simples" at Padua.[13] Portaleone's botanical education, medical practice, and familiarity with Jewish liturgy stimulated him to investigate this antiquarian topic.

IDENTIFYING THE ELEMENTS OF INCENSE: PORTALEONE'S CRITICISM OF RABBINIC SOURCES

Portaleone's work on incense may be divided into two sections: a preliminary one in which he identifies elements of ancient incense and a later one in which he constructs a portion of it.[14] Both show signs of

parimente esser di lunghezza più di 250 miglia. Li arbori di cedro non patiscono corrottione, essendo legno durissimo e nodoso, laonde non è meraviglia se Salomone lo mise in opera per l'edificio del Tempio, il quale, ancor che per la materia e per la Divina compositione fosse stato possibile che hoggidì se ritrovasse nel suo pristino essere, tuttavia (per i nostri peccati) non pasò 410 anni dopo l'esser edificato che andò in rovina e l'altro rifatto non arrivò alli 420. Dicono anco di quel legno cavarsene un'olio, il quale non lassa putrefar cosa unta con esso."

12 S. D. Luzzato, *Mavo le-maḥzor benei Roma* (Livorno: S. Beleforti, 1855) (reissued by Daniel Goldschmidt, ed. [Tel Aviv: Devir, 1965]). Portaleone's younger Mantovano coreligionist Abraham Catalano clearly believed in the benefit of reciting an enumeration of the biblical *pitom qetoret*, or incense mixture. In his 1631 work *Olam Hafukh* (for full citation, see Introduction, note 50) Catalano writes that the Jewish community of Pisa would chant the *pitom qetoret* liturgy every Monday and Thursday in the synagogue. See *Olam Hafukh*, 74.

13 Courses in botany and medical "simples" were given at Padua from the 1540s on. See Paula Findlen, "The Formation of a Scientific Community: Natural History in Sixteenth-Century Italy," in Anthony Grafton and Nancy Siraisi, eds., *Natural Particulars: Nature and the Disciplines in Renaissance Europe* (Cambridge, MA: MIT Press, 1999), 369–400, 370.

14 For a list of ingredients mentioned in the Bible and Babylonian Talmud, see Appendix I.

his critical engagement with Jewish tradition and creative importation of natural philosophy into sacred studies. Current scholarship on Portaleone emphasizes his fidelity to Jewish traditions. However, it is clear from an examination of *Shiltei HaGibborim* that its author routinely moves away from rabbinic teachings and privileges other sources of scientific knowledge. Gianfranco Miletto, the chief authority on Portaleone, maintains that "Portaleone's description of the temple faithfully follows biblical and rabbinic texts."[15] The following remarks investigate Portaleone's scholarly criticism of rabbinic natural science and show that Portaleone's work was more serious – and more subversive – than historians acknowledge.

There is a considerable gap between Portaleone's professed method for his botanical research and his actual practice. Well into the series of chapters that constitute his work on incense, Portaleone describes his research method. Discussing the identity of *yein qaprisin*, one of the elements in ancient incense not specified in the Bible and often understood by postclassical commentators as Cypriot wine, Portaleone pauses and previews his method for this investigation. In fact, it may be applied not only to *yein qaprisin* but to his whole project of identifying incense: "First of all I shall investigate if anyone among our sages of former generations has told us what this *yein qaprisin* is. After this I shall inform you what my heart has already indicated to me about the matter … and finally I shall report why I have deviated from the long-established learned tradition."[16] Conspicuously absent from this summary of his method is any mention of Greek or Roman scientific works; in fact, Dioscorides, Pliny, and Theophrastus are cited in these chapters nearly as often as Talmudic rabbis and their postclassical successors. More significantly, his statement does no justice to the frequency with which he quotes modern authors or confesses to having learned from pharmacists and Mantuan artisans.

[15] Miletto, *Glauben und Wissen*, 264.

[16] *SG*, 91b: קודם כל דבר אחקור אם יש בחכמינו הקודמים מי שאמר לנו מה הוא היין קפריסין הלזה. אחרי כן אגיד לכם מה שבשכבר לבי אמר לי עליו ... וסוף סוף אכתוב מפני מה נטיתי מהגרסא הנהוגה מימי עולם David Ruderman has shown how in the middle of the eighteenth century the Ferrarese rabbi and physician Isaac Lampronti articulated a similar position in his writings on the permissibility of killing lice on the Sabbath. See Isaac Lampronti, *Paḥad Yiẓhak* (Lyck: Mekitse nirdamim, 1874 [1750–]), 21r–22v, and David B. Ruderman, *Jewish Thought and Scientific Discovery in Early Modern Europe* (New Haven: Yale University Press, 1995), 256–72. For Cyprus wine, see Appendix I.

At the beginning of his cluster of chapters on incense, Portaleone is pessimistic about his chances of successfully identifying all the spices in the ancient incense mixture. He notes that scripture specifically states what only four of the elements in that mixture are, leaving eleven ingredients that need to be researched. The prospects of identifying the others are dim, especially since, as Portaleone notes, all the commentators differ from one another when it comes to identifying spices. He laments that

> in the explanation of spices for the incense all of the commentators are perplexed. This one says one thing, and another says something else, according to their imagination and dreams. Until now I have not seen one among them who arrived with certainty at the truth about the essence of incense. Therefore I shook out the bosom of my garment (Nehemiah 5:13) and toiled in order to find useful sayings and truthful words; I shall offer them up in print for everyone's acceptance.[17]

This passage expresses Portaleone's determination to discover the truth about the ancient incense mixture and announces that he is doing so because of the lack of quality studies on the topic in medieval rabbinic literature. In his investigation of *tzori* (balsam), Portaleone expresses faith that God will assist him in his unprecedented efforts. Instead, he turns to a more earthly source, transcribing the Greek botanist Dioscorides' full description of that plant.[18]

This devotion to Dioscorides as a principle source is indicative of Portaleone's intellectual proclivities. Early in his work, he relies on ancient Greek works to identify biblical and Talmudic botanical terms and fill in the gaps in rabbinic analyses. As a prerequisite to identifying the elements of the spice mixture Portaleone convinces his readers that what the rabbis wrote is insufficient. The most common method Portaleone employs to achieve this is to ridicule medieval rabbis' knowledge of Greek botanists and the Greek language. After a discussion about the medicinal properties of balsam, Portaleone highlights the similarities

[17] *SG*, 81a: הנה בפירוש סממני הקטרת נבוכו המפרשים כלם זה אומר בכה וזה אומר בכה כפי דמיונם וחלומותם ולא ראיתי עד הנה מי שבא על נכון על אמתת מהותם. לכן נערתי את חצני ויגעתי למצא דברי חפץ קושט דברי אמת אעלם על ספר לרצון כולם

[18] Christian naturalists were also interested in finding "true balsam," both the biblical product and the medicament known to Dioscorides. See Richard Palmer, "Medical Botany in Northern Italy in the Renaissance," *Journal of the Royal Society of Medicine* 78:2 (February 1985): 149–57, 152.

and differences between various sap-producing trees. While describing one particular type of tree that yields sap when tapped, Portaleone states that the rabbis, owing to their lack of familiarity with Greek, misidentified the tree. Regarding trees that release sap, Portaleone informs his readers that

> the choicest tree among them is called *xilobalsamo* (*xilon* in Greek means "tree" – and not *aqsil*[19] – as they wrote in our sacred books). Those men did not know the particulars of that language [Greek], and they wrote this Greek word not with the letters that are read in their [the Greeks'] language (*kappa* or *chi* and *sigma*) but rather with the letter that was familiar to them, *xi*, which is the fourteenth letter in their alphabet. That fine wood is fresh, reddish, and fragrant, since its aroma resembles its sap, and furthermore its wood and branches are thin.[20]

Portaleone's most trenchant condemnation here is that the rabbis, more accustomed to the sound of the letter *xi* (presumably because of its phonetic proximity to the Hebrew letter *khaf*) misread a word where the actual spelling called for a different letter entirely. For Portaleone, basic familiarity with Greek is a prerequisite for botanical – and also rabbinic – research. Knowledge of that language provides a clear point of demarcation between Talmudic learning and medieval expositors. Referring to the rabbis of the Talmud, Portaleone wrote: "With my heart I decided to remind you that our rabbis, of blessed memory, also used Greek, and desired the beauty of Japheth to dwell periodically in the tents of Shem. As such, I came across many Greek words in my books since our sages, of blessed memory, spoke them."[21] The poverty of many medieval rabbis'

[19] אקסיל, paired with אלואון, is used in the Targum to Psalm 45:9. Together they mean "pieces of bitter aloe wood." The Targum is translating אהלות, the very term that exercised Lusitanus in his commentary on Dioscorides' *De materia medica*.

[20] *SG*, 81b: ואולם העץ המובחר ממנו הנקרא גסילובאלסאמו (גסילון בלשון יון רוצה לומר עץ לא אקסיל כמו שכתבו בספרינו הקדושים האנשים ההם שלא ידעו בטיב הלשון ההוא וכותבין המלה הזאת היונית לא אם האותיות שקוראין בלשונם קאפה או כי וסיגמה אלא עם האות הנקראת אצלם גסי שהיא האות הארבעה עשר מהאלפא ביתא שלהם) העץ ההוא הטוב הוא הרטוב האדום והמבושם שיהיה ריחו דומה לשרף שלו ושיהיו עציו וענפיו דקים

[21] *SG*, 4r: עם לבבי אמרתי להזכיר לכם כי רבותינו ז"ל נשתמשו גם הם בלשון יוני ונתרצו שיפיפותו של יפת ישכון לפעמים באהלי שם. ועל כי נזדמנו לי בחבורי מלות רבות בלשון יון שדברו בם חכמינו ז"ל Further evidence of Portaleone's knowledge of Greek abounds in his unpublished medical *consilia*. See, for example, *Abrahami Portaleonis Medici Mantuani hebrei responsorum et consultationum medicinalium liber,* Paris, Bibliothèque nationale, Ms. Latin 13004, "Consilium excellentissimi patris de histerica passione pro mulieri hebraea. Excellentissimo Legum Artiumque Doctori D. Abrahae Provinciali Hebreo," 293r–298v, esp. 293v. For a discussion of Jewish

knowledge of Greek is a complaint that Portaleone reiterates time and again in his work on incense and is a basic criterion he uses for assessing botanical competence.

Another example that illustrates this is Portaleone's censure of a group of Jewish sages who fail to identify the spice *qetzi'ah* (cassia). He states that with regard to "the definition of this spice we cannot establish its true nature from the remarks of the commentators. In his commentary on the Torah (Exodus 30:23), Rashi, of blessed memory, writes that *qidah* is an herbal root that the sages refer to as *qetzi'ah*."[22] For Portaleone, this sort of tautological identification of a spice is insufficient: since there is no referent beyond scriptural terminology, there is no way to establish the true nature of the element. After reviewing the identifications proposed by Abravanel, Radak, and Saadiah Gaon and pronouncing them inaccurate, Portaleone turns his attention to the author of the *Arukh*[23] and questions his identification of *qetzi'ah* with the Greek spice *cassia*. This time the issue is not the *Arukh*'s lack of Greek vocabulary but his unreliable classificatory memory. Portaleone gently points out that "here, in my humble opinion, both the author of the *Arukh* and the Latin translator did not arrive at the true meaning of *qezi'ah* since *qillufah* [another of the spices in the incense] is indeed *cassia*. How could one spice be included in the incense as two different species?"[24] Portaleone similarly censures Naḥmanides for suggesting that

knowledge of Greek in the Renaissance, see Moses A. Shulvass, "The Knowledge of Antiquity among the Italian Jews of the Renaissance," *Proceedings of the American Academy of Jewish Research* 18 (1948–9): 291–300.

22 *SG*, 87v: ובפירוש הסם הזה לא יכלנו לעמוד על אמתת מהותו מדברי המפרשים כי רש"י ז"ל בפירוש התורה כתב קידה היא שרש עשב בלשון חכמים קציעה See also Appendix I.

23 Portaleone refers to Nathan ben Yeḥiel, who lived in Rome in the eleventh century. A 1555 edition of the *Arukh* was edited by Portaleone's fellow Mantuan Moses Provenzali. On the latter, see Shlomo Simonsohn, *History of the Jews in the Duchy of Mantua* (Jerusalem: Kiryath Sepher, 1977), 729–30; and Robert Bonfil, "I responsi rabbinici come fonte storica," *Materia Giudaica* 9:1–2 (2004): 103–8.

24 *SG*, 87v: והנה גם בעל הערוך והמתרגמן לאטינו לעניות דעתי לא באו על אמתת משמעות הקציעה כי הקלופה היא הקאסיאה ואיך יכנס בקטרת שני פעמים גם יחד סם אחד *Arukh* (Pesaro: Soncino, 1517), 150a; see also *Arukh* (Venice: Bragadin, 1552), 142v. As was the custom among Italian Jews of the Renaissance, Portaleone uses the phrase "Latin translator" to refer to Jerome's translation of the Bible, commonly known as the Vulgate. For example, Abraham Farissol uses a nearly identical expression in his critical essay on the Vulgate; see his *Magen Avraham*, chap. 29. In the Vulgate, Exodus 30:24 reads "cassiae autem quingentos siclos in pondere sanctuarii olei de olivetis mensuram hin"; *qidah* is translated by Jerome as *cassia*, a rendering that persists in modern translations and may be found in the Jewish Publication Society's translation of the same verse.

since *qetzi'ah* is written in the plural (*qetzi'ot*) in Psalms 45:9, as are several other spices grouped in the category of *qosht*, it must mean that a double portion of spices in the group *qosht* is to be included in the final mixture. After responding that such a gloss lacks any textual support, Portaleone demurs and notes "nevertheless the Torah only commands that we take the choicest of each species; why would the Torah differentiate between *qosht* and the other spices?"[25] In the end Portaleone, left with no good options, has to guess. His recourse, not surprisingly, is to Greek: "Therefore my heart tells me that *qetzi'ah* is the spice called *agollochon* or *xyloaloe* in Greek. It is a very fragrant spice – there is none better than it among the other spices in the incense."[26]

One rabbi on whom Portaleone does consistently rely is Simeon ben Gamliel. In his chapter on *tzori*, or myrrh, Portaleone notes that the rabbis misidentified the spice. However, he reminds his readers that Simeon ben Gamliel, the second-century CE Palestinian rabbi, proposed the correct interpretation but that his views were rejected by other rabbis.[27] After reviewing ancient scientific work on myrrh and concluding that all scholars besides Theophrastus concur that myrrh is sap, rather than a fruit or a tree, Portaleone reflects that "one must therefore be mystified as to why our rabbi [Maimonides], of blessed memory, did not decide in favor of Rabbi Simeon ben Gamliel, who said that '*tzori* is nothing but sap that drips from balsam trees.'"[28] Portaleone goes on to relate how in the Babylonian Talmud's discussion of *tzori*, the rabbis ruled that the spice was originally taken from the tree itself and not from its sap. The import of this analysis is clear: Simeon ben Gamliel was, knowingly or not, in agreement with most ancient Greek and Roman scholars about the olfactory properties of the balsam tree and the proper part of the tree from which to extract its essential odor. Other Talmudic rabbis could not match their colleague's botanical expertise. At the chapter's

[25] *SG*, 88r: ועם כל זה התורה לא צותה אלא שנקח המובחר שבמיניהם ולמה תשים התורה הפרש בין הקושט ובין שאר הסממנים

[26] *SG*, 88r: על כן לבי אומר לי כי הקציעה היא הסם הנקרא בלשון יון אגאלוקון או גסילאלואי. והוא סם ריחני מאד אין טוב ממנו בכל שאר סממני הקטרת

[27] See BT Keritot 6a.

[28] *SG*, 83r: על כן יש לתמוה עד מאד על רבינו ז"ל מדוע לא פסק כרבן שמעון בן גמליאל דאמר הצרי אינו אלא שרף הנוטף מעצי הקטף Portaleone is referring to Maimonides, *Hilḥot Kelei HaMiqdash* 2:4, where he suggests that *tzori* means the balsam tree itself and not its sap. Maimonides' opinion and Simeon ben Gamliel's gloss are discussed in Naḥmanides' commentary to Exodus 30:34.

conclusion, Portaleone defends his allegiance to Simeon ben Gamliel. Portaleone writes, "I have not deviated from his exact intention in this matter, heaven forbid, because of what the gentile sages wrote. Instead, I have relied exclusively upon the exceedingly awesome and divine man, Rabbi Simeon ben Gamliel."[29] Simeon ben Gamliel, known to have had complete command of Greek, was famed as a natural scientist and leading member of the Sanhedrin, or rabbinic council of seventy that adjudicated Jewish disputes in first- and second-century Palestine, and his scholarship was highly valued by Portaleone.[30]

It is indicative of Portaleone's intellectual disposition that, as he moves forward in his chapters on incense, he mentions the rabbis less and less, preferring to structure his comments around ancient and medieval medical writings and contemporary botanical works. The rabbis do not fade from view entirely, but they play a conspicuously more minor role in later chapters. By my count there are twelve mentions of rabbinic literature in chapter 78, including Talmudic and Midrashic passages, against the same number of citations in chapter 88, which is more than twice as long. One explanation for this may simply be Portaleone's discursive style.[31] As topics veer farther and farther from his stated purpose, it makes sense that he would lose track of foundational Jewish texts. Another possibility may be that Portaleone felt there was little relevant in rabbinic writings as his discussion proceeded. Whereas earlier chapters dealt with the four types of spice explicitly mentioned in the Pentateuch (stacte, onycha, galbanum, and frankincense), the latter chapters identify and describe the remaining eleven that are never specified in the Bible. As Portaleone is forced to depart from canonical Jewish texts, it makes sense that he would look for information from other sources.

[29] *SG*, 83v: שלא נטיתי מכונתו זאת ח"ו בעבור מה שכתבו המחברים שלא מבני עמנו אלא על איש האלהים נורא מאד רבן שמעון בן גמליאל בלבד נשענתי

[30] Talmudic literature testifies to Simeon ben Gamliel's Hellenic qualifications and his botanical expertise. He is reputed to have said that the Torah may be correctly translated only into Greek (see Jerusalem Talmud Megillah 1:9). For examples attesting to his proficiency in natural sciences, see BT Pesaḥim 53a, where he differentiates various species of fruit-bearing trees.

[31] Peter Miller has recently flagged this aspect of *Shiltei HaGibborim*. See his "Lost and Found," 504, where he observes that, "like all good early modern encyclopedists, Portaleone is prone to digression."

GEOGRAPHY AND GREEK

Of all the fields of knowledge in which Portaleone was well versed, two were conspicuously helpful to him in his efforts to identify the elements of biblical incense: Greek philology and classical geography. In the seventy-eighth chapter of *Shiltei HaGibborim*, Portaleone identifies the element *tzori* (balsam).[32] After a few brief quotations from Talmudic literature, Portaleone reviews the comments of non-Jewish authorities, including Dioscorides, Galen, Avicenna, and Theophrastus, before turning to post-classical rabbinic literature to evaluate Jewish knowledge of the balsam plant. Isaac Abravanel (1437–1508) is his first object of scorn.[33] The fifteenth-century statesman and sage, in his commentary on Exodus, cites Rashi, who remarks that *nataf* (stacte) is balsam (*tzori*) and then goes on to state that "[the sap] drips from balsam trees. In the vernacular it is referred to as *gomma*."[34] Displeased with this gloss, Portaleone writes: "I am bewildered that he, who was an expert in the vernacular and in Latin, did not see that Rashi, of blessed memory, was not an expert in these languages. [Rashi] defined a specific spice with a general term for all resins that come from sap. For any kind of spice that derives from sap is called *gomma* in the vernacular."[35] Portaleone's criticism of Abravanel is based on the fact that the latter failed to highlight the inadequacy of Rashi's knowledge of Romance languages and, by extension, accurate botanical nomenclature. Abravanel, however, quickly moves beyond Rashi's gloss and defines balsam as *mastix*. Portaleone protests, insisting that

> what this sage said – "the correct [interpretation] is that it is *mastix*" – is also not true. For the *lentisco* [tree] that produces good *mastix* exists only on one of the Greek islands, called Chios in their language. In fact, this tree does grow in other places besides this one island. Furthermore, in

[32] *SG*, 83r.

[33] The literature on Abravanel is formidable. Benzion Netanyahu's *Don Isaac Abravanel, Statesman and Philosopher* (Philadelphia: Jewish Publication Society of America, 1953) remains a good introduction. More recently, see Eric Lawee, *Isaac Abravanel's Stance towards Tradition: Defense, Dissent and Dialogue* (Albany, NY: SUNY Press, 2001) and the essays collected by Menahem Kellner and Abraham Melamed in *Jewish History* 23:3 (September 2009).

[34] Rashi on Exodus 30:34, quoted in *SG*, 83r: והוא נוטף מעצי הקטף ובלעז קורין אותו גומא

[35] *SG*, 83r: ותמה אני מאד ממנו שהיה בקי בלשון לועז ולאטינו ולא ראה שרש"י ז"ל שלא היה בקי בלשונות האלה פירש שם סם אחד פרטי בשם אחד כולל לכל השרפים כי כל שרף יהיה מה שיהיה יקרא גומי בלשון לעז

> the Land of Israel the *lentisco* does not produce ideal *mastix* like it does on Chios. Therefore one cannot consider it among the "best fruits of the land," since our holy patriarch said "take of the best fruits of the land" (Genesis 43:11).[36]

Portaleone argues against Abravanel with a combination of superior botanical knowledge, geographic expertise, and scriptural sensitivity. The only specific criticism Portaleone articulates is that Abravanel should have had a better sense about the character of balsam because of his familiarity with Romance languages. Clearly, however, more is at stake here for Portaleone. His geographic knowledge, culled from Pliny and Strabo, and his botanical knowledge, gathered from Dioscorides and Theophrastus, put him at an advantage over Abravanel. Portaleone's medical education, which exposed him to works by all four of these ancient writers, positioned him to understand ancient incense in a more nuanced manner than Abravanel.[37] Finally, Portaleone would have had plenty of opportunities to see and handle various types of balsam. Attaining firsthand, practical knowledge of plants was praised in sixteenth-century botany. For example, Prospero Alpino, one of Portaleone's contemporaries, states in his work on balsam that it was "imported into many places in Italy" from Egypt and Syria but that "our physicians refuse to acknowledge it."[38]

[36] Ibid., 83r: ואינו גם כן נכון מה שאמר החכם הזה "והנכון שהוא מסטיצי" כי הלינטיסקו היוצא ממנו המסטיצי הטוב הוא בלבד באי אחת מהיונים הנקראת בלשונם קיאו עם כי האילן הזה הוא גדל גם כן במקומות אחרים חוץ מהאי הזאת וגם בארץ ישראל הלינטיסקו לא יעשה המאסטיקו השלם כמו בקיאו ולא יקרא אם כן מזמרת הארץ כמו שאמר אבינו הקודש "קחו מזמרת הארץ" אלא זמרת הארץ היתה באמת הבאלסאמו כי לא היה ממנו אז במקום אחר כי אם בארץ ישראל בלבד The verse from Genesis (43:11), which Portaleone does not cite in full, reads "And their father Israel said to them, 'if it must be so now, do this: take of the best fruits in the land in your utensils, and carry down a present to the man, a little balm, and a little honey, spices, and myrrh, nuts and almonds.'" Jewish Publication Society translation.

[37] For more on sixteenth-century medical education, see Richard J. Durling, "Girolamo Mercuriale's *de modo studendi*," *Osiris*, 2nd ser., 6 (1990): 181–95.

[38] Prospero Alpino (b. 1553) was a Venetian physician, student of Melchior Guilandinus (see Chapter 2), and scholar of Near Eastern botany. This quotation is from his *De balsamo dialogus*, bound with *De plantis Aegypti liber* (Venice: apud Franciscum de Franciscis Senensem, 1592), 60r: "cum et si in multa Italiae loca ex Aegypto, ac Syria huiusce plantae succus, fructus, lignaque; nunc vere comportentur, haec tamen agnoscere nostri medici renuant." On Alpino, see Giuseppe Ongaro, "Contributi alla biografia di Prospero Alpini," *Acta medicae historiae patavina* 8–9 (1961–2/1962–3): 79–168; Nancy Siraisi, "In Search of the Origins of Medicine: Egyptian Wisdom and Some Renaissance Physicians," in Valeria Finucci and Kevin Brownlee, eds., *Generation and Degeneration: Tropes of Reproduction in Literature and History from Antiquity through Early Modern Europe* (Durham, NC:

One chapter in *Shiltei HaGibborim* puzzles out the identification of *shechelet*, an element in the incense mixture made from the *operculum*, or closing flap, of snails.[39] The chapter provides an opportunity for Portaleone to censure Abravanel yet again. The thrust of Portaleone's criticism in this chapter is not so much that rabbis misidentified a component of incense but that they incompletely identified it, supplying only a Hebrew equivalent and neglecting to explore its scientific identity. Commiserating with his coreligionists by admitting that the identification of *shechelet* is exceedingly difficult, Portaleone concedes that he "had not seen in any of the commentaries one who wrote precisely what it [*shechelet*] is, other than as one who trifles."[40] Abravanel, at least, tried to equate the substance with a botanical term, remarking that "in the Roman language it is called *byzanzio*."[41] In his commentary on Exodus (30:34), Abravanel stops there and does not supplement his identification with any form of analysis; but Portaleone goes on to describe the origins of that name and the maritime context for the growth of *byzanzion*. Portaleone also remarks that in Greek this organism is called *blatta*, which has two meanings, both of which escaped Abravanel.[42] Not surprisingly, Abravanel, along with his rabbinic interlocutors, is found to be wanting in both geographic knowledge and botanical expertise. Indeed, the chapter includes Portaleone's criticism of several other rabbis' failure to accurately identify *shechelet*. For example, he derides Naḥmanides' view that *shechelet* should be identified with *tzipporen*, which, although potentially true, is an unsatisfactory interpretation.[43] "I am surprised," writes Portaleone, that Naḥmanides, "who was a great scholar of Torah and also a scholar of non-Jewish sciences, and fluent in Arabic, revealed a tiny bit and concealed so much more, especially

Duke University Press, 2001), 235–61, 237 n. 3; Nancy Siraisi, *History, Medicine and the Traditions of Renaissance Learning* (Ann Arbor: University of Michigan Press, 2007), 344–5, n. 33.

39 For *shechelet* in classical Jewish sources, see BT Keritot 6b.

40 *SG*, 83v: והנה קשה לי מאד כי לא ראיתי במפרשים מי שכתב בפירוש מה היא אלא כמתעתע

41 *SG*, 83v: בלשון רומי ביזאנציאו

42 In Latin, Portaleone informs us, *blatta* means a creature that chews through garments – i.e., a moth – and in Greek it refers to a creature of the sea otherwise known as *porpora*. *SG*, 83v.

43 Standard dictionaries of biblical and rabbinic Hebrew equate these two terms as well. See Marcus Jastrow, *A Dictionary of the Targumim, the Talmud Babli and Yerushalmi, and the Midrashic Literature*, 2 vols. in 1 (New York, 1996), s.v. שחלת, p. 1548.

since he had read what our rabbi [Maimonides] wrote on this issue."[44] Maimonides, Portaleone goes on to explain, completely identified and described the nature of *tzipporen*, while Naḥmanides was content to stop short of fuller description. After giving the Arabic equivalent of *shechelet* originally cited in Maimonides, Portaleone proposes that in Greek it might be *onyx euodes*, or possibly *blatta*, as the medieval physician Paul of Aegina suggested.[45] Appropriately, the chapter concludes with yet another slight on Abravanel, one that underscores his lack of Greek. "There are those among the Greeks," Portaleone writes, "who call it *blatta byzanzion* in order to clarify that it is not *porpora*. This, as I have noted, is perhaps what Don Abravanel, of blessed memory, wished to say, but omitted."[46] Portaleone's tone here is ironic: pointing out Abravanel's omission, while accompanying his name with not one but two honorifics, is a way of emphasizing the inadequacy of his remarks on *shechelet*.

Abravanel is by no means the only Jewish sage whom Portaleone ridicules for attempting serious botanical research without knowledge of Greek. The Mantuan physician excoriates the author of the *Arukh* for mangling a Greek word and confusing two plants: "The author of the *Arukh*, of blessed memory, wrote '*mor* … in Greek is *mosco*.' Until this day I have never known that the scented *mosco* is so-called in Greek."[47] Portaleone proceeds to note that *byron* is something that looks like white wool and has a sweet smell; on the tree the Greeks call this *peuke*, and in Latin it is called *picea*, in Arabic *artz*. Once again, owing

44 *SG*, 83v: ותמה אני עליו שהיה חכם גדול בתורה וגם היה חכם בחכמות החצוניות וידע בשלמות הלשון ערבי למה גלה טפח וכסה טפחיים בפרט אחרי שקרא מה שכתב רבינו בו See Naḥmanides to Exodus 30:34 and Maimonides, *Perush al Masechet Ohalot* 3:3; Maimonides, *Hilḥot Kelei Bet HaMiqdash* 2:1, 2, 4.

45 I have not been able to ascertain Portaleone's source. *Pauli Aeginetae opus de re medica* (Paris: apud Simonem Colinaeum, 1532), contains no mention of onyx euodes. Book 7, p. 50, discusses "onyches, conchulae indicae," a type of mollusc Portaleone may have had in mind: "Onyches conchyliorum Indicorum opercula sunt, quae suffitu strangulatione vuluarum concidentes foeminas excitant, item comitialeis: potae aluum turbant." Paul of Aegina's discussion of *blatta* concerns insects that are found in mills, rather than sea creatures. See ibid., book 7, p. 59.

46 *SG*, 83v: יש מהיונים שקוראים אותה בלאטה ביזאנציאון לפרש שאינה הפורפורא והוא מה שבאולי רצה והשמיט השר אברבאנילו ז"ל כאשר אמרתי

47 *SG*, 86r: ובעל הערוך ז"ל כתב ... מור וקציעה מור ואהלות בלשון יון מוסקו. ואני עד היום לא ידעתי שהמוסקו הריחני יקרא כן בלשון יון See *Arukh* (Pesaro: Soncino, 1517), 93v. See also *Arukh* (Venice: Bragadin, 1552), 94r–95v.

to his refined botanical knowledge, as well as his greater familiarity with Greek, Portaleone demonstrates his advantage over his rabbinic predecessors. Castigating not only Abravanel but also other postclassical rabbis, Portaleone exclaims, "It completely escapes me why they did not seek to know the truth of this matter from King Solomon, may peace be upon him."[48] Portaleone goes on to quote the book of Kings, where the Queen of Sheba is reported to have brought *mor* and other spices to King Solomon "from her own land," and also the Song of Songs, in which King Solomon, the supposed author of Song of Songs, states, "I shall go to the mountain of myrrh."[49] Portaleone describes how King Solomon learned to grow myrrh from the Queen of Sheba, and raised it on mountaintops, or at least on high mountain plains. An avid reader of Mattioli's commentary on Dioscorides' *De materia medica*, Portaleone read passages in which Mattioli cited Pliny (*Natural History* 12:15) discussing myrrh's origin among the Sabeans, a people known for cultivating myrrh and frankincense,[50] and whom Renaissance readers identified as the Queen of Sheba's subjects. Additionally, Portaleone was familiar with Theophrastus's discourse on myrrh (*De plantarum historia* 9:4), also quoted at length by Mattioli, which speaks of myrrh growing on high, snowy mountains.[51] Portaleone never proves the identification of *mor* as myrrh on precise philological or botanical grounds; he simply assumes its identification and uses classical literature to confirm cryptic statements in the Bible regarding myrrh's provenance.

Portaleone does not deviate from rabbinic teachings in a casual manner. On the contrary, when he disagrees with his rabbinic forbears, a sense of regret and even despair is palpable in his writing. Often, before he launches into an explanation at odds with rabbinic tradition, he struggles to come to terms with the theological implications of his words. For example, Portaleone begins a chapter on *kefat ha-Yarden* (Jordan

48 *SG*, 86v: כי נעלם ממני איך לא בקשו לדעת אמתות הדבר הזה משלמה המלך ע"ה

49 Song of Songs 4:6.

50 Pliny, *Natural History* 12:32, quoted in Mattioli, *Opera quae extant omnia* (Frankfurt: ex officina typographica N. Bassaei, 1598), book I, chap. 67, p. 88: "convehitur et ex sylvis laudata, petuntque eam etiam à Troglodytis Sabaei transitu maris."

51 Ibid., 88: "Gignitur thus et myrrha regione Arabum media circa Saba ... et exeunt thuris, myrrhaeque arbores aliae super montem, aliae in pede montis culturis propriis quamobrem aliae coluntur, aliae vitam agunt incultae. Montem istum praealtum affirmant, et ningi solitum."

amber) by lamenting the fact that Jewish sages have not contributed more to identifying Jordan amber:

> We shall pursue, if we are able, the scholars of our generation in order to learn from them the identity of *kefat ha-Yarden*, which is included in the incense. For this matter is exceedingly difficult for me, and I am not embarrassed to reveal my shame. Walking and wandering for many days now in the field of foolishness and confusion I do not know where I will turn for help. I found no water to quench my thirst, and my tongue cleaved to my cheek (Psalm 137:6). I have no words with which to convey to you even a clear hint (Job 26:14) of what I have heard when I ponder the matter within me. My heart is dismayed (Psalm 143:4) when I realize that my mind is ill at ease and cannot grasp what the great minds of the ages have written, such as Rashi, the author of the *Arukh*, *Kolbo*, and all the rest of them, of blessed memory. And I have not come, heaven forbid, to oppose my masters, for I will always seek Torah from their mouths, and if there is an oral tradition, I shall cheerfully accept all of its particulars, as is obligatory for anyone designated an Israelite. However, should permission be granted to refute at times the words of the sages, such that truth might emanate from disagreement, I will speak up (Job 32:17), and perhaps from within my foolishness their wisdom will shine like the light of the sun.[52]

Clearly, Portaleone has reservations about overturning the rulings of the sages. Just the same, he is confident that one result of his efforts will be the glorification and confirmation of their words. In his discomfort with correcting ancient scholars, Portaleone had partners in the world of sixteenth-century European botany. Giovanni Odorico Melchiori, in a laudatory letter published at the beginning of a 1568 edition of Mattioli's commentary on Dioscorides, describes the act of correcting the ancients as a "paradox," musing that "there are quite a few who say that it is something of a paradox for one to wish to go against the opinions of our ancient scholars. The common opinion, which you express, holds

[52] *SG*, 92v: ונרדפה אחרי חכמי דורנו לדעת מהם אם נוכל מה היא כפת הירדן הבאה בקטרת כי הנה קשה עלי מאד הדבר הזה ולא אבוש לגלות את חרפתי כי הנני הולך ותועה זה ימים רבים בשדה הסכלות והמבוכה ולא ידעתי אנה אפנה לעזרה כי לא מצאתי מים לרוות את צמאי דבקה לשוני לחכי ואין מלה בלשוני להגיד לכם שמץ דבר ברור ששמעתי בהגם בתוכי ישתומם לבי בזכרי כי אין דעתי מתישבת עלי לעמוד במה שכתבו גאוני עולם עליה כמו שהם רש"י בעל הערוך והכל בו וזולתם ז"ל. ואני לא באתי ח"ו לחלוק על רבותי כי תורה לעולם אבקש מפיהם ואם קבלה היא אקבל כל דבריה בסבר פנים יפות כמוטל על כל אשר בשם ישראל יכונה. אמנם אם הרשות נתונה להשיב לפעמים על דברי חכמים עד שמתוך הויכוח יתברר האמת אענה אף אני חלקי ואולי מתוך סכלותי כאור שמש יזרח חכמתם

that some of the basic and most important simples of the pharmacists, such as acoro, cinnamon, and aromatic calamo, and others besides these are not the true ones."[53] Melchiori's remarks illuminate the anxiety felt by some early modern botanists who deigned to correct the words of ancient authorities. At the same time, they indicate the broad diffusion of Portaleone's ideas and signal the professional culture that helped generate them.

CRITICISM OF ANCIENT GREEK AND LATIN SOURCES

Closely related to Portaleone's departure from rabbinic texts is his gradual disengagement from ancient Greek botanical literature. That disengagement from ancient botanical sources is, I suggest, rooted in the practice of sixteenth-century natural philosophy. Finding fault with and subsequently emending ancient scientific works was common practice in the second half of the sixteenth century.[54] As Portaleone's work commences, Dioscorides and, to a lesser extent, Theophrastus are cited as the ultimate arbiters of botanical accuracy. However, as the chapters proceed, Portaleone favors the accounts of Spanish and Portuguese travelers, local spice dealers, and pharmacists in Mantua, as well as his own experience. In the end, ancient and medieval sources of all kinds – Greek, Roman, and Jewish – take a backseat to contemporary works on pharmacology, medicine, and natural history. Portaleone's work may lend credence to an established trend in historical scholarship, that the discovery and study of the New World did in fact do much to displace the authority of ancient texts.[55]

[53] Giovanni Odorico Melchiori, dedicatory letter "allo eccellentissimo dottore M. Pietro Andrea Matthioli medico sanese, mio signore," in Pietro Andrea Mattioli, *I discorsi di M. Pietro Andrea Mattioli nelli sei libri di Pedacio Dioscoride Anazarbeo della Materia Medicinale* (Venice: Vincenzo Valgrisi, 1568), sig. ***3v- sig. ***4r at sig. ***4r: "nè mancano alcuni di dire, che sia quasi un paradosso il voler tenere contra l'opinione de' nostri vecchi e il commune uso, come fate voi, che alcuni de' primi e più importanti semplici delle speciarie, come l'Acoro, il Cinnamomo, il Calamo aromatico e altri, non sieno i veri." Dated "di Padova alli xx. di Ottobre, 1549."

[54] See Ogilvie, *The Science of Describing*, esp. 49–51.

[55] John Elliott, *The Old World and the New, 1492–1650* (Cambridge: Cambridge University Press, 1970). Cf. Anthony Grafton, *New Worlds, Ancient Texts: The Power of Tradition and the Shock of Discovery* (Cambridge, MA: Belknap Press of Harvard University Press, 1992).

One characteristic of Portaleone's censure of scientific texts from antiquity is his insistence that one ancient commentator rarely provides a complete description of any plant. On the topic of Dioscorides' description of myrrh, Portaleone states that, "since Dioscorides left out matters relevant to us about myrrh, it is important that we seek additional details. In this chapter I will translate for you what Pliny and Theophrastus said about myrrh." To mitigate the impact of relying so heavily on gentile commentators, Portaleone tells his readers to "learn from the words of these men who speak truthfully that King Solomon, may peace be upon him, knew quite well the identity of myrrh and its provenance many hundreds of years before them [Pliny and Theophrastus]."[56] The proof that Portaleone adduces is the familiar verse from Song of Songs: "I will go up to the mountain of myrrh." Compared to Dioscorides', Pliny's, and Theophrastus's detailed descriptions of this spice, Solomon's simple geographic observation is much less helpful for identifying the plant. Although Portaleone does explain the significance of Solomon's identification of myrrh as a plant that grows in high altitudes, next to Dioscorides' and Theophrastus's descriptions of myrrh, this praise of Solomon reads like a conciliatory gesture directed at his more traditionally minded coreligionists. Even so, several of Portaleone's peers in the sixteenth century praise King Solomon's botanical expertise while leaving out the specificities of his achievements; Caspar Bauhin, for example, does the same. In the first dedicatory epistle that opens the 1598 Latin version of Mattioli's work on Dioscorides, Bauhin writes to the Holy Roman emperor, to whom the book is dedicated:

> O Most Illustrious and Merciful Lord: among so many and so great a number [of tales], remarkable is this tale of Solomon, wisest of kings, namely, that, as part of the affairs of his rule, he desired to write a complete account of all plants, from the cedars of Lebanon to the Hyssop of the walls [of Jerusalem] so that he might proclaim the wisdom of the best

56 *SG*, 87r: ומדברי האנשים האלו המשיחים לפי תומם תלמדו ששלמה המלך ע"ה מאות רבות בשנים קודם להם ידע על נכון מה הוא המור ומקומו On Jewish apologetics in the Renaissance, see Arthur Lesley, "Il richiamo agli 'antichi.'" See also Lesley, "Jewish Adaptation of Humanist Concepts in Fifteenth- and Sixteenth-Century Italy," in Maryanne Cline Horowitz et al., eds., *Renaissance Rereadings: Intertext and Context* (Urbana: University of Illinois Press, 1988), 51–66.

> and greatest God. This history was destroyed (alas, we long for it) to the great detriment of humanity.[57]

Solomon's scientific prowess enchanted both Christian and Jewish scholars of Portaleone's time.

Perhaps the most trenchant and consistent of Portaleone's criticisms of the ancients is that, as opposed to traveling widely in order to discover and describe plants, they preferred to work from limited samples at their convenient disposal. In a section in which he praises the energetic efforts of various modern explorers and roving botanists, Portaleone remarks that they "walked and wandered to nearly all corners of the earth and saw what the ancients, sitting at ease in their tents, hastily recording their own hallucinations and vanities (Ecclesiastes 5:6), did not see."[58] This remark indicates Portaleone's preference for experience over convenience, travel over armchair antiquarianism, empiricism over speculation.[59]

According to Portaleone, sedentary scholarship engenders derivative scholarship. He complained that "all the ancient authors spoke at length about this spice, and they rambled on about *qinnamon* as a separate spice. All of the scholars copied repeatedly from one another – all lies! Each [copied] from his fellow [scholar] like a dog returning to its vomit (Proverbs 26:11)."[60] The origin of the misinformation, according to Portaleone, was Dioscorides, who identified the best type of *qinnamon*

[57] Mattioli, *Opera quae extant omnia* (Frankfurt: ex officina typographica N. Bassaei, 1598), unnumbered pages just before sig *2r: "memorabile est Illustrissime ac Clementissime Dux, regum illud sapientissimi Salomonis exemplum quod is inter tot tantaque imperii sui negotia, omnium Plantarum, quo Dei Opt. Max. sapientiam admirandam praedicaret, a Cedro inquam Libani usque ad Hyssosium murorum, Historiam texere voluerit, quae (heu optata!) non sine magno mortalium damno interiit."

[58] *SG*, 89v: אשר הלכו ושטו כמעט בכל חלקי העולם וראו מה שלא ראו הקדמונים היושבים תחת אהליהם במנוחה וכותבים חלומות והבלים בחפזה

[59] On the increasing emphasis upon empiricism in sixteenth-century intellectual life, see the essays collected in Gianna Pomata and Nancy G. Siraisi, eds., *Historia: Empiricism and Erudition in Early Modern Europe* (Cambridge, MA: MIT Press, 2005). See also Alessandro Guetta, "Can Fundamentalism Be Modern? The Case of Avraham Portaleone (1542–1612)," in David N. Myers et al., eds., *Acculturation and Its Discontents: The Italian Jewish Experience between Exclusion and Integration* (Toronto: University of Toronto Press, 2008), 99–115, where he points to two passages in Portaleone's *De auro dialoghi tres* (Venice: apud Io. Baptistam à Porta, 1584), 20, 140, that display the Mantuan physician's devotion to empiricism.

[60] *SG*, 89v: וממנה דברו כל המחברים הקדמונים בארוכה והרבו דברים על הקנמון כמו סם נפרד ממנה והעתיקו זה מזה ושבו כלם על דברי כזב ושקר האחד על חבירו ככלב שב על קיאו

as *mosilitico*. Among those who copied Dioscorides were Serapion "the Arab," Theophrastus, Galen, Strabo, and Avicenna. Portaleone has choice words for this group: "These worthless and reckless men (Judges 9:4) devised [much] in their own hearts (1 Kings 12:33), and all of them failed to see the light of truth. For they walked in such darkness that I am embarrassed and ashamed even to copy down their words – complete drivel. They are bereft of understanding (Obadiah 1:7)."[61] Portaleone's unusually strong denunciation of these authors, all of whom were respected medical authorities in the sixteenth century, and all of whom were taught in the standard medical curricula at Padua and other Italian universities, may best be understood as a form of humanist polemic. The physicians who "did not see the light of truth" and "walked in darkness" were ancient and medieval authorities, some of whom had fallen out of favor in the late sixteenth century. Immediately after castigating this group of pagan and Muslim writers, Portaleone calls upon the work of contemporary scholars whose practices were far more commendable in Portaleone's eyes. "Therefore," Portaleone writes, "I decided to return to the current authors[62] of our time such as Clusius."[63] It is to the "new authors" whom Portaleone relies upon that we now turn our attention.

Generally, Portaleone has only positive things to say about the contemporary scholars he discusses in his chapters on incense. The Spanish and Portuguese, in particular, are praised for their wanderlust and for their rigorous exploration of medicinal plants and herbs, and his Italian brethren are singled out for the proficiency of their medical learning. Portaleone's discussion of contemporary botanical and medical discoveries sheds light on his relationship to modern geographic discoveries and the importance of empiricism over book learning.

Early in Portaleone's work on incense, in his chapter on *mor* (myrrh), Portaleone informs his sons that "in recent years the Spanish have brought

[61] *SG*, 89v: ומה שבדו מלבם אנשים ריקים ופוחזים וכל האנשים האלה לא ראו אור האמת ובחשכה התהלכו עד כי בושתי וגם נכלמתי להעתיק דבריהם דברי הבאי אין תבונה בהם

[62] The expression המחברים החדשים is probably best understood as a Hebraicized version of *recentiores*.

[63] *SG*, 89v: לכן אמרתי לחזר אחרי המחברים החדשים שבזמננו כמו שהם הקלוסיאו On Clusius, see Florike Egmond, Paul Hoftijzer, and Robert P. W. Visser, eds., *Carolus Clusius: Towards a Cultural History of a Renaissance Naturalist* (Amsterdam: Royal Netherlands Academy of Arts and Sciences, 2007). Besides Clusius, in these lines Portaleone mentions Francisco López de Gómara (1510–60), André Thevet (1502–92), and others. See Miletto, *Glauben und Wissen*, 232–4.

from India, which is in the west [i.e., the West Indies], the sap of a certain tree which they call balsam. It is noble and quite fragrant, resembling in its features and very nearly in its form and essence the sap of fine *tzori*, which existed in our Holy Land."[64] Portaleone cites a portion of Nicolás Monardes' testimony of this plant: "As Niccolo Monardes, the Spaniard, wrote, [this plant] grows in the land they call 'New Spain,' and the Indians call this tree in their language *xilo*, and this tree is large, slightly smaller than our pomegranate trees, and its leaves resemble the leaves of the grass called in Greek *galeopsis*."[65] Portaleone goes on to provide equivalent terms for this plant in Arabic, Latin, and Italian and launches into a lengthy description of its flowers, branches, and shoots. Portaleone quotes Monardes a second time: "Niccolo Monardes also wrote that from the four portions of the world (these being Europe, Asia, Africa, and America) the Spaniards have brought back to Spain a certain resin that resembles our good *tzori*, and it comes from the tree in clusters, and is made from shells."[66] Compared to his treatment of both rabbinic sources and ancient Greek writings, Portaleone is rather credulous in accepting Monardes' reports; he does not critically evaluate them.

As much as Portaleone took from Monardes, he took even more from Mattioli. While discussing the incense component *qillufah* and the *agollochon* tree, from which it may derive, Portaleone remarks:

> As the Portuguese attested, who traveled by ship through the high southern seas (Proverbs 30:19), eastward toward the Orient, this tree grows on an island called *Taprobana*, and also in some adjacent lands. Thence these men transported to our realms whole shoots and branches, which not only emit a pleasant and wonderful aroma when burnt, but even when merely handled give off their fragrance and their scent.[67]

64 *SG*, 83r: דעו בני כי מעט הם השנים שהספרדים הביאו מהודו שבמערב שרף עץ אחד שקורין אותו באלסאמו והוא נכבד ומבושם מאד דומה בפעולותיו וכמעט בצורתו ועצמותו לשרף הצרי הטוב שהיה בארצנו הקדושה

65 Portaleone's source was very likely Mattioli, *Opera quae extant omnia* I:18, which quotes Monardes: "ex occidentali India in Hispaniam adfertur, liquor est arboris Indis Xilo dictae." Ibid., 62. He very well could have read Monardes directly. See the following note.

66 Nicolás Monardes (1512–88) was the coauthor with Carolus Clusius of *De simplicibus medicamentis ex occidentali India delatis, quorum in medicina usus est* (Antwerp: Plantin, 1574). There were several subsequent editions. On Monardes, see José Pardo Tomás, *Oviedo, Monardes, Hernández: el tesoro natural de América: colonialismo y ciencia en el siglo XVI* (Madrid: Nivola, 2002).

67 *SG*, 88r: והנה כאשר העידו אנשי פורטוגאלו ההולכים בספינות בלב ים הדרום קדמת ארץ המזרח העץ הזה הוא צומח באי אחת נקראת טאפרובאנה וגם בקצת ארצות הסמוכות לה. והאנשים האלה הם אשר נושאים משם בגלילותינו גזעי

This discussion of the origin and destination of the *agollochon* tree also indicates Portaleone's interest in and knowledge of Indian geography. He notes, for example, that it is a mere three days' journey from Seifico to Alcomiro. Mattioli was Portaleone's principle source for most botanical data, and Portaleone assimilated much from this world-renowned figure.[68]

For Portaleone, contemporary scholars helped to identify the elements of incense more than ancient authorities did. Portaleone's particular fondness for Garcia de Orta is a case in point; Portaleone gushes, "Among all of these I have chosen the words of Garcia de Orta, for they are clear to those who understand (Prov. 8:9)." For example, Portaleone quotes de Orta extensively on the spice *qinnamon*.[69] Portaleone shows that Garcia proves that *Cassia lignea, qinnamon*, and "our" *cannella* are the same spice.[70] Garcia de Orta provides Portaleone's strongest support for the claim that the spice he knew of in his time as cassia lignea was the same as *qillufah*.

HOLY PHARMACOLOGY: PORTALEONE'S RECONSTRUCTION OF BIBLICAL INCENSE

As Portaleone moves from describing elements of the incense mixture to assembling a portion of it, his methods as well as his sources of knowledge change. Having identified the ingredients of the incense mixture, the final chapter of Portaleone's work is more technical and practical than the others. It specifies how to construct the anointing oil. In order to do that, Portaleone had to employ his vast knowledge of classical and rabbinic literature. But it was also necessary for him to seek guidance and instruction from humbler informants. The final chapters of *Shiltei HaGibborim* that address the topic of incense invoke conversations with and lessons learned from glass makers, coopers, and spice grinders. This dimension of Portaleone's working method has never been explored.

וענפי האילן הזה שלמים כאשר הם שלא בלבד כשיודלקו יוצא הריח הטוב והמופלא מהם אלא גם במשמוש הידים עליהם יתנו את ריחם המבושם

68 Miletto, *Glauben und Wissen*, 286.

69 Carolus Clusius and Garcia de Orta, *Aromatum et simplicium aliquot medicamentorum apud Indos nascentium historia* (Antwerp: Plantin, 1567), chap. 15. De Orta's *Coloquios dos simples e drogas* was first published in Portuguese (Goa: Por Ioannes de Endem, 1563).

70 *SG*, 90r.

But it merits exploration, since the conspicuous presence of artisanal knowledge in a sprawling, deeply learned work of natural philosophy establishes connections between popular and learned practices.[71] It also clarifies the role of empirical skill in assisting Portaleone's endeavor to reconstruct a biblical product.

Recent scholarship has emphasized how closely connected artisans and scholars were in early modern Europe.[72] Most of this work, however, is concerned with Northern Europe.[73] Very little historiography addresses similar realities in Southern Europe, and even less attends to northern Italy.[74] Furthermore, many studies of the relationships between scholars and craftsmen in the sixteenth and seventeenth centuries are chiefly concerned with the question of the origins of the scientific revolution or, at the very least, how the New Philosophy of the seventeenth century depended on the entry of artisans into the knowledge-making process. Portaleone's receptiveness to nonbookish sources of learning constitutes another side to this story, one that underscores how an Italian Jewish physician assimilated both textual and manual learning.[75]

[71] Pamela O. Long, *Openness, Secrecy, Authorship: Technical Arts and the Culture of Knowledge from Antiquity to the Renaissance* (Baltimore: Johns Hopkins University Press, 2001), 176, 208.

[72] Pamela H. Smith, *The Body of the Artisan: Art and Experience in the Scientific Revolution* (Chicago: University of Chicago Press, 2004); Deborah Harkness, *Jewel House: Elizabethan London and the Scientific Revolution* (New Haven: Yale University Press, 2007).

[73] In addition to the two works just cited, I also have in mind the early seventeenth-century Leiden circle of physicians, pharmacists, and botanists that coalesced around Christiaen Porret (1554–1627), described by Claudia Swan in her "Making Sense of Medical Collections in Early Modern Holland: The Uses of Wonder," in Pamela H. Smith and Benjamin Schmidt, eds., *Making Knowledge in Early Modern Europe: Practices, Objects, and Texts, 1400–1800* (Chicago: University of Chicago Press, 2007), 199–213. See also Ole Peter Grell, "In Search of True Knowledge: Ole Worm (1588–1654) and the New Philosophy," in ibid., 214–32, which lists the Danish physician's modes of acquiring knowledge as "travel, books, face-to-face discussions, correspondence, collecting rare objects, and finally empiricism and experiment, all of them closely interrelated and interdependent." Ibid., 215.

[74] See, for example, Antonio Barrera Osorio, *Experiencing Nature: The Spanish American Empire and the Early Scientific Revolution* (Austin: University of Texas Press, 2006).

[75] Of all the studies mentioned in the previous three notes, only Grell's is especially concerned with a physician: Ole Worm. Harkness argues for the central role vernacular learning played in the coming of the Scientific Revolution, and William Eamon assumes that only charlatans, empirics, or medical outsiders were devoted to experimentation and concrete proof. See his "'With the Rules of Life and an Enema': Leonardo Fioravanti's Medical Primitivism," in J. V. Field and Frank A. J. L. James, eds., *Renaissance and Revolution: Humanists, Scholars, Craftsmen and Natural Philosophers in Early Modern Europe* (Cambridge: Cambridge University Press, 1993), 29–44.

Early modern authorities were aware of how important the manual trades were to scholarly advancement, and several urged their readers not to neglect manual laborers as potential sources of knowledge. Juan Luis Vives, in his *De tradendis disciplines*, writes that the cultured man "must not be ashamed to enter into the workshops and into the factories" and suggests that they ask questions of artisans, "trying to become cognizant of the details of their work."[76] In the same vein, Andreas Vesalius remarked in the preface to his *De humani corporis fabrica* that the decline of medicine in the medieval world may be attributed to "fashionable doctors despising the work of the hand." Those doctors, according to Vesalius, "assigned the manual treatments, which they considered necessary for their patients, to commoners and limited themselves to supervising."[77] Just as that neglect of manual practice damaged learned medicine, shunning artisans in early modern Europe could hamper a scholar's ability to understand the world around him.

Portaleone, like other natural philosophers of his time, operated under the Aristotelian assumption that nothing in the world ever disappears once it has been created, so long as the world itself endures. To that assumption he added a pious gloss by emphasizing that God is responsible for the permanence of creation: "Trees, plants, and creatures survive for all time according to His will." In Portaleone's mind, the elements that were used in the ancient incense mixture are still available for discovery and use in the contemporary world.[78] Some of those elements were retrievable only in remote corners of the Middle East, while others could be found in northern Italy's botanical gardens. Some were even available in Mantua's pharmacies. Portaleone is explicit about how

[76] Cited in Paolo Rossi, *Philosophy, Technology and the Arts in the Early Modern Era*, trans. Salvator Attanasio (New York: Harper & Row, 1970), 6.

[77] Cited in ibid., 7. I have modified Attanasio's translation slightly. For the Latin original, which Rossi does not provide, see Vesalius, *De humani corporis fabrica libri septem* (Basel: Johannes Oporinus, 1555 [1543]), sig. a2r: "Medicina eousque lacerari coeperit, quod primarium eius instrumentum, manus operam in curando adhibens, ita neglectum sit, ut ad plebeios ac disciplinis medicae arti subservientibus neutiquam instructos id quasi videatur esse demandatum." See also ibid., sig. a2v: "verum maxime post Gotthorum vastationem, quando omnes scientiae, antea pulcherrime florentes utque decebat exercitae, pessum iuere, lautiores medici primum in Italia, ad veterum Romanorum imitationem, manus operam fastidientes, quae in aegris manu facienda ducerent, servis praescribere, ac illis tantum architectorum modo astare, coeperunt."

[78] *SG*, 95v: כל מה שהוציאה הארץ במצות ה" בששת ימי בראשית מהאלנות והעשבים והבעלי חיים הם קיימים ברצונו תמיד

pharmacists helped him accomplish his work, and expresses his hope that his labor "will not be repulsive and loathsome (1 Samuel 15:9) in your eyes, for I have written it according to the specifications of the spice grinders."[79] Aware that he was writing about a religiously sensitive topic with unlettered artisans as his guides, Portaleone had humble hopes for his work's reception; he merely wished that it not be "hated and despised."

But Portaleone's exculpatory remarks should perhaps be taken rhetorically, since pharmacists may not have been condescended to by Europe's learned elite.[80] In fact, the role of the pharmacist in early modern culture is still understudied.[81] Unfortunately, few pharmacists left behind extensive records of their collections. Some state archives in Italy – for example, the one in Portaleone's birthplace, Mantua – contain records for ministries of *spezzieria*, or spice dealers. However, the documents preserved in Mantua's state archive deal exclusively with the ruling Gonzaga family's orders to one or two specially appointed "spice dealers of the duke" and tell scholars disappointingly little about the activities of other spice dealers working for clients besides the duke.[82] Even so, evidence from the later part of the sixteenth century attests that pharmacists were held in high esteem. Tomaso Garzoni, in his *Piazza universale di tutte le professioni del mondo* (Venice, 1585), writes concerning pharmacists that, "compared to other professions, they typically enjoy a very high rank, whether for the honor of the art itself, bearing a certain similarity to science ... or for the practitioners, who maintain their reputation with the seriousness befitting their profession."[83]

79 *SG*, 94r: עם כל זה לא תהיה המלאכה הזאת נמבזה ונמס בעיניכם כי כתבתי אותה כפי תנאי הרקחים Cf. 1 Samuel 15:9.

80 Several physicians, including Guillaume Rondolet in Toulouse and Francisco Sanches in Montpelier, lectured to pharmacists. At the University of Montpelier in the sixteenth century, pharmacists were given a rigorous education, including thorough training in Latin. See Jean-Pierre Bénézet, *Pharmacie et médicament en Méditerranée occidentale (XIIIe–XVIe siècles)* (Paris: Honoré Champion, 1999), 434.

81 See, however, Bénézet's *Pharmacie et médicament*.

82 See, for example, Archivio di Stato di Mantova, Magistrato ducale, busta IV: 1580–1689.

83 Tomaso Garzoni, *Piazza universale di tutte le professioni del mondo*, discorso LXXXIX: "De' speciari overo aromatari." I quote from Paolo Cherchi and Beatrice Collina's annotated edition (Turin: Einaudi, 1996), 2:1059: "fra gli altri professori ancora, tengono ordinariamente un luogo assai nobile, sí per l'arte in se stessa onorevole per aver una certa similitudine di scienza ... sí anco per se stesso, mantenendo la riputazione loro con la gravità condecente al lor mestieri."

Modern scholars, unfortunately, have not been as charitable as Garzoni. Peter Dilg has written on the role pharmacists and pharmacological systems of collecting played in shaping intellectual life in early modern Europe, and his work is a happy exception to this trend.[84] Dilg's scholarship ably demonstrates the centrality of pharmacology in sixteenth- to eighteenth-century Europe. He argues that apothecaries participated in more than just health-related sciences; they were intimately associated with natural history collections. He also notes how doctors and pharmacists often bonded, sometimes in learned interchange, other times during the course of routine visits, regarding their shared interests in zoology, mineralogy, and botany.[85]

In Portaleone's time, Mantua boasted a rich tradition of pharmacists and botanical gardens. Filipo Costa was one of the many figures in Portaleone's community who was involved not only in collecting – antiquities, specimens of plants, animals, fossils – but also in pharmacology. Costa's grandfather had been a spice dealer in Mantua at the beginning of the sixteenth century, and Costa's father as well as Costa himself served as "spice dealers to the 'King.'" Unlike many pharmacists, Costa left behind an impressive oeuvre, including the *Discorsi sopra le compositioni de gli Antidoti, & Medicamenti* (1576), his best-known work.[86] Indeed, numerous collectors and physicians cultivated gardens in and around Mantua, many of which, as the sixteenth century wore on, contained samples of plants from the New World.[87] Dwarfing them all, however, was the botanical garden of the Gonzaga family, which grew considerably in scope and fame during the reigns of Guglielmo (1550–87) and his successor Vincenzo I (1587–1612). In 1603 Zenobio Bocchi published a plan of the ducal garden entitled *Giardino de' Semplici in Mantova*.[88] In Mantua Portaleone was exposed to celebrated and well-stocked botanical gardens.

84 See Peter Dilg, "Apotheker als Sammler," in Andrea Grote, ed., *Macrocosmos in Microcosmo: Die Welt in der Stube: zur Geschichte des Sammelns 1450 bis 1800* (Opladen: Leske & Budrich, 1994), 453–74.

85 Ibid., 453–4.

86 For more on Costa, see Dario A. Franchini et al., *La scienza a corte: collezionismo eclettico, natura e immagine a Mantova fra Rinascimento e Manierismo* (Rome: Bulzoni, 1979), 41–4.

87 Ibid., 23.

88 Ibid., 130. Unfortunately, very few other plans or catalogs of botanical gardens survive from Mantua in this period. Ibid., 116.

At times Portaleone's treatment of technical matters such as volume and measurement is decidedly bookish. *Shiltei HaGibborim*'s final chapter, for example, deals with the weight of the various elements of the incense mixture. As he does so, we may observe his medical training, as well as his antiquarian sensibilities, most clearly.[89] Portaleone repeatedly refers to his profession's practices and even introduces a special "doctors' calculation" for the value of the *dinar*. Portaleone writes, "The dinar, in the opinion of all the doctors, is half a *scriptolo*." A few paragraphs later, Portaleone explains that the *drachma* consists of "twenty of our *unkiot*, as the doctors have said."[90] Portaleone was concerned with what a *dinar* is. Since it is clear that there are 368 *maneh* in the overall mixture, the only unresolved issue is the value of a *dinar*, since the *maneh* is, "according to everyone," equivalent to one hundred dinars. But with regard to dinars, Portaleone laments that, in a manner redolent of Cardano's comments on the *iugero*, "opinions are legion."[91] Portaleone makes no effort to hide his obvious professional pride: he even states that doctors know things that other people simply do not. For example, he notes that liquids such as honey, juice, water, and wine all have different capacities when put in the same vessel. This, Portaleone informs his reader, is knowledge that doctors are privy to.[92]

Occasionally Portaleone blends classical learning with real-world experience, as he does in his description of the process of grinding and drying out incense. He mentions how spice particles would enter and

89 Guiseppe Olmi has convincingly linked natural science and antiquarianism in sixteenth-century Europe. See his *L'inventario del mondo: catalogazione della natura e luoghi del sapere nella prima età moderna* (Bologna: Il Mulino, 1992), 256, 300. Nancy Siraisi has also developed this line of thinking in several articles, including "Anatomizing the Past: Physicians and History in Renaissance Culture," *Renaissance Quarterly* 53:1 (2000): 1–30, and "History, Antiquarianism, and Medicine: The Case of Girolamo Mercuriale," *Journal of the History of Ideas* 64:2 (2003): 231–51.

90 *SG*, 94r: לדעת כל הרופאים ... כאשר אמרו הרופאים

91 *SG*, 94r: והמנה לדברי הכל הם מאה דינרים לכל מנה אמנם במשקל הדינר רבו הדעות For Cardano's comment about the difficulty of calculating the *iugero*, see chap. 63 ("De mensuris superficierum") of his *Practica arithmetica* in *Hieronymi Cardani Mediolanensis, philosophi ac medici celeberrimi Opera Omnia* (Lyon: sumptibus Ioannis Antonii Huguetan et Marci Antonii Ravaud, 1663), 4:115, where, discussing Milanese, Paduan, and Roman units of measurement, he states that it is "impossible and tedious" to use multiple metrical standards: "impossibile enim est et taediosum ponerere diversitatem usus cunctarum nationum cum una regula cunctis satisfaciat."

92 *SG*, 94v: כאשר ידעו הרופאים

damage the spice grinder's throat, causing irritation and changing the quality of his voice. From his intimate knowledge of this practice, it is plausible that he either tried this or had at least been around enough spice dealers to know.[93] As a humanist, Portaleone included a classical reference and appropriately evoked the spirit in the temple, where voices would rise in unison, urging the head spice grinder to "grind the spice well." To make this image come alive to his readers, Portaleone compares this activity – for which there is no precise word in Hebrew – to the Latin noun *celeusma*. That term refers to the call that the head oarsman would shout out to his rowers to make them row in unison.[94] But Portaleone's description of drying incense betrays his most valued sources of knowledge: common practice in Mantua. For example, he uses the word *trocischi* to describe the piles of spices that Mantuan pharmacists lay out to dry in the sun: "They would assemble portions of roughly crushed spices and make of them *trocischi*, which are small, fine, squared piles [of spices] spread out in the open air until they are completely dry."[95] Then, Portaleone informs us, the process is repeated a second and third time.

Though it is hardly surprising that an active physician would display familiarity with the practices of contemporary pharmacology, it is noteworthy how Portaleone uses that knowledge to experiment with the particulars of the ancient temple service. Earlier in the sixteenth century, the Parisian physician Jean Fernel decried how much doctors depended on pharmacists; the relationship, Fernel maintained, should be inverted:

> The knowledge, collection, choice, culling, preservation, preparation, correction, and task of mixing of simples all pertain to pharmacists; yet it is especially necessary for the physician to be expert and skilled in these things. If, in fact, he wishes to maintain and safeguard his dignity and authority among the servants of the art, he should teach them these things.[96]

[93] *SG*, 95r: כי כשיודקו היטב תפרח ותעלה עפרורית הבשמים בגרונו של שוחק ותזיק בגרונו

[94] *SG*, 95r: היו מרימים קולם ואומרים הדק היטב נקראת הרמת הקול גם יחד בלשון לאטינו ציליאוסמה See Lewis and Short, *A Latin Dictionary* (Oxford: Oxford University Press, 1991 [1879]), 309, s.v. celeusma.

[95] *SG*, 95r: להעמיד יחד חלקי הסממנים הבלתי כתושים היטב והיו עושים מהם טרוציסקי והם חלקים קטנים דקים ומרובעים ושוטחים אותם לאויר עד שיבשו בשלמות

[96] Fernel, *Methodus medendi* (Basel, 1622), preface, quoted by Karen Meier Reeds, *Botany in Medieval and Renaissance Universities* (New York: Garland, 1991), 25–6. The Latin reads as follows: "simplicium cognitio, collectio, delectus, expurgatio, conservatio, praeparatio,

It is hard to tell how much Portaleone taught the spice grinders of Mantua. It is clear, however, that he learned much from them.

Another practice that connects the world of pharmacists to that of erudite natural philosophers is Portaleone's emphasis on visual proof, particularly the sort that comes from regularly handling botanical products. The habit of seeing and describing rare specimens encouraged not only precise identification of ancient plants but also criticism of ancient botanical authorities. Portaleone was hardly alone among early modern Italians in correcting classical descriptions of spices and incense. Portaleone gleefully reports that his contemporary Prospero Alpino, in his *De plantis aegyptis liber,* proved the "ancient physicians" were wrong about a specific type of myrrh.[97] Portaleone may have had in mind the fourteenth chapter of that work, entitled "On Balsam, which is called *Balassan* by the Egyptians." It opens as follows:

> The balsam plant grows throughout Egypt, does it not? ALPINO: Not at all: it flourishes in Arabia, where the Arabs attest the plant is much more robust than in Egypt. GUILANDINUS: Therefore Dioscorides, Theophrastus, Pliny, Justinus, to say nothing of other ancient writers, were wrong when they claimed that Balsam grew heartily in Egypt and Judaea? ALPINO: There is no doubt in my mind that those mistaken writers were not speaking of Balsam's place of origin, but were rather describing trees, sap, fruits and other things. Besides, it is to be doubted if they themselves ever even saw a living balsam tree.[98]

Alpino, like Portaleone, was a champion of firsthand experience. He wrote to Giovanni Mauroceno, the addressee of *De plantis aegyptiis,* that

correctio, et miscendi industria, seorsum, ad Pharmacopaeos referuntur ac pertinent, quorum tamen imprimis et Medicum gnarum peritumque esse oportet, siquidem apud artis ministros auctoritatem, dignitatem que suam retinere ac tueri velit, quos docere haec ipsas debet." For the Latin text, see Reeds, 184 n. 77. I have used Reeds's translation on pp. 25–6.

97 *SG*, 95v: כי שקר דברו הרופאים הקדמונים כאשר כתבו שהיה נטיעת הצרי עצמית וטבעית ליריחו ולמצרים

98 Prospero Alpino, *De plantis aegyptiis liber* (Venice: apud Franciscum de Franciscis Senensem, 1592), chap. 14, page 20r: "Nunquid balsami planta amplius in Aegypto vivit? ALPIN. Nequaquam, sed in Arabia foilici, quam Balsami feracem omnes tum Aegyptij, tum Arabes praedicant. GUILAND. Igitur Dioscorides, Theophrastus, Plinius, Iustinus atque alij ex antiquis scriptoribus permulti, qui Balsamum tantum in Aegypto et in Iudae olim vixisse prodiderunt, decepti sunt. ALPIN. Sine dubio illos non modo de loco Balsami patrio, sed etiam de arbore quoque, succo, fructibus atque aliis deceptos fuisse arbitror, ex quo etiam dubitandum esset ipsos balsami arborem viventem nusquam vidisse."

he "saw and observed these plants, in various places in Egypt."[99] After praising Alpino's work, Portaleone tells his sons that "should you want to know further comprehensive details about *tzori*, read his books,[100] which are in Latin. There you will find all that you seek, and you will see that even today we have this very sap that will never disappear from the world, with the grace of God, may His name be blessed, Amen."[101]

The emphasis on visual confirmation of botanical knowledge that Alpino stressed encouraged Portaleone's zeal in correcting ancient authorities. At several points in the course of his work on incense, Portaleone mentions having seen the plants and herbs he discusses. This stress on visual experience and material confirmation of textual authorities is something he shared with numerous scholars in sixteenth-century Europe. In her study of the legal culture of early modern England, Barbara Shapiro has shown that the meaning of the term "fact" changed from the mid-sixteenth to the mid-seventeenth century and came to indicate provable, observed action as opposed to rumor or report.[102] Botanists in later sixteenth-century Italy shared this belief in the importance of visual proof. In Mattioli's commentary on Dioscorides, for example, he frequently notes the availability of spices and herbs in his native Italy. While discussing balsam, Mattioli concedes that neither the sap nor the seeds nor the wood nor the bark of the balsam tree is imported into Italy unless by means of adulteration and impostures.[103] Nonetheless, Mattioli admits that he has seen versions of this plant, such as the one he observed in the Holy Roman

[99] Ibid., sig. a2r: " … de plantis, quas olim in locis Aegypti inspexi, ac observavi."

[100] Portaleone refers to Alpino's *De balsamo dialogus*, which was printed in the same 1592 edition of *De plantis aegyptiis liber*. See above, note 38.

[101] *SG*, 95v: ואם תרצו לדעת יתר פרטי הצרי בשלמות תקראו ספריו אלה שהם בלשון לאטינו כי שם תמצאו כל חפצכם ותראו שגם בזמננו יש לנו השרף הזה שלא יבצר ממנו לעולם בחסד ה' יתברך שמו אמן

[102] See Barbara Shapiro, *A Culture of Fact: England, 1550–1720* (Ithaca, NY: Cornell University Press, 2000). On the developing notion of fact in the early modern period, see also Lorraine Daston, "Marvelous Facts and Miraculous Evidence in Early Modern Europe," *Critical Inquiry* 18:1 (1991): 93–124, reprinted in James Chandler, Arnold I. Davidson, and Harry Harootunian, eds., *Questions of Evidence: Proof, Practice, and Persuasion across the Disciplines* (Chicago: University of Chicago Press, 1994): 243–74; Daston, "Baconian Facts, Academic Civility, and the Prehistory of Objectivity," *Annals of Scholarship* 8 (1991): 337–63, reprinted in Allan Megill, ed., *Rethinking Objectivity* (Durham, NC: Duke University Press, 1994), 37–64. Also, Simona Cerutti and Gianna Pomata have collected essays under the title *Fatti: storie dell'evidenza empirica*, in *Quaderni storici* 108:3 (December 2001).

[103] Mattioli, *Opera quae extant omnia*, book 1, chap. I: 18, page 59: "veruntamen diu est, quod in Italiam, ne in totam Europam, neque lachryma, neque semen, neque lignum, neque cortex importantur, nisi adulteriis, et imposturis vitiata."

emperor Ferdinand I's collection, which he had received as a gift from the Ottoman sultan Suleiman.[104] Mattioli also informs his readers that the Veronese collector and apothecary Francesco Calzolari, "exceedingly skilled in medical matters," brought him a sample of balsam while he was at Trent.[105] Just as Mattioli supplements his descriptions of plants with occasional anecdotes about having seen them, so did Portaleone point out his legitimate experience with the plants and herbs he discusses. For example, regarding the grape vine *lambrusca*, which flourished – and still flourishes – throughout the *mantovano*, Portaleone speaks from firsthand experience, commenting that "the plant of this flower resembles a desert vine, which we spoke about in the previous chapter. In Greek it is referred to as *oinanthe*, and in Italian *lambrusca*."[106] Using a combination of classical erudition, practical knowledge, and firsthand experience with the plants mentioned in the Bible and Talmud, Portaleone was able, as he thought, to establish the identity of most of the elements of the ancient incense mixture. This having been done, Portaleone set the stage for his assembly of the anointing oil, one of its chief ingredients.

MAKING BIBLICAL INCENSE: THE CONSTRUCTION OF A PROHIBITED PRODUCT

In premodern Jewish culture, replicating the ancient incense mixture was strictly proscribed. Portaleone was acutely aware of that proscription. The prohibition against making biblical incense originates in the Bible itself. The thirtieth chapter of Exodus describes the anointing oil and lists its contents: myrrh, cinnamon, calamus, cassia, and olive oil.[107]

104 Ibid., 60: "legitimum autem opobalsamum notis omnibus comprobatum, vidi tamen ego apud Imperatorem Ferdinandum Primum, Dominum meum clementissimum, a Solimano Turcarum imperatore dono missum, quibusdam con nonnullis aliis muneribus." Mattioli met Ferdinand when the Holy Roman emperor came to Trent in the early 1550s. Sara Ferri briefly discusses this episode in her essay "Profilo di Pietro Andrea Mattioli," in S. Ferri and E. Miraldi, eds., *I giardini dei semplici e gli orti botanici della Toscana* (Perugia: Quattroemme, 1993): 159–64, 161.

105 Mattioli, *Opera quae extant omnia*, 60: "cui simile omnino mihi visum est illud quod anno superiore detulit ad me Tridentum Franciscus Calceolarius Veronensis, rei medicae admodum peritus."

106 *SG*, 93r: ונטיעת הפרח הזה הוא דומה לנטיעת הכרם המדברית אשר אמרנו בפרק הקודם שנקראת בלשון יון אינאנטי או לאמברוסקה בלעז

107 Exodus 30:22–5.

A few verses later, scripture states that the oil "shall be a holy anointing oil to Me throughout your generations. Upon man's flesh shall it not be poured, nor shall you make any other like it, after its composition.... Whoever compounds any like it, or whoever puts any of it upon a stranger, shall be cut off from his people."[108] Talmudic authorities analyze this scriptural threat. The first chapter of the Babylonian Talmud tractate Keritot classifies "one who compounds the anointing oil" in the category of thirty-five other actions that may lead to forcible expulsion from the Jewish community.[109] Understandably, as Portaleone leaves behind his intellectual exercise of identification and description and moves toward a practical excursus on how to *make* a crucial element of that mixture, his first words are those of justification, caution, and self-defense.

He begins with a clever circumlocution, announcing that in this section he is merely "not concealing" information from his readers: "Therefore I shall not conceal from you the recipe for this fine and holy oil, that is the anointing oil."[110] Portaleone poses as one who merely refrains from concealment and also emphasizes the scriptural, and therefore unassailable, foundation of the assembly of this oil. Portaleone also acts as a supplicant before God, alluding to the Psalms and adopting liturgical themes from the Day of Atonement, writing "to God most high (Genesis 14:20), our King, and our God, I pour out my complaint (Psalm 142:3) with a heart cracked and crushed, and I plead (Deuteronomy 3:23) and pray to His holy dwelling (Psalm 68:6) in heaven."[111] Finally, the Mantuan physician legitimizes the construction of the oil of anointing, reminding his readers that, up until the time of King Josiah, the secrets of its proper mixture were known.[112]

To claim that the secrets of the anointing oil are latent in scripture, or that they were known far beyond the time of the Pentateuch, was not enough of a justification for flouting rabbinic law. He

[108] Exodus 30:31–3.

[109] See BT Keritot 2a.

[110] *SG*, 96r: ולמען לא אעלים מכם מרקחת השמן הטוב והקדוש הוא שמן המשחה

[111] *SG*, 96r: ולאל עליון מלכנו ואלהינו בלב נשבר ונדכה אשפוך שיחי ואתחנן ואתפלל אל מעון קדשו השמימה Cf. Psalms 51:19; 142:3.

[112] For more on King Josiah, see 2 Chronicles 34–5; 2 Kings 22–3; and BT Pesaḥim 56a for a list of his reforms.

needed a stronger one, and he found it through a selective reading of Maimonides' *Laws of the Temple Vessels*. Portaleone told his sons that "our rabbis, of blessed memory, permitted us to study the plain meaning [of scripture] in all matters ... you are studying in order to understand and instruct."[113] To his mind Portaleone's reconstruction of the incense mixture was undertaken "to understand and instruct." Portaleone also underscores Maimonides' ruling that "one who does this in order to study or transmit [the teaching] to the public is exempt [from punishment]."[114] Conveniently, Portaleone neglects to cite or mention the previous line of Maimonides' code, which is unambiguous about the illicit nature of Portaleone's project. Maimonides makes it plain that "one who compounds incense from these eleven spices according to these prescribed weights in order to smell it, even though he does not smell it, is condemned to a premature, divinely ordained death, provided that he does this intentionally. If, however, he did this inadvertently, without knowing it was prohibited, he must bring a fixed sin-offering."[115] It is almost certain that Portaleone was aware of this prohibition; nevertheless, he found his loophole in the law and exploited it fully.

Portaleone's exposition of how to create the ancient incense mixture is explicitly cast as an expansion of Maimonides' *Laws of the Temple Vessels* and implicitly formulated as an elaboration of Talmudic discussions about the proportions of the incense mixture. While rabbis in tractate Keritot do discuss the weight of the various elements of the incense mixture, the Talmudic text does not delve into technicalities. Instead, it contains such generalities as "Moses would boil the olive oil with the spices," and their "roots were first soaked in water, then removed from the water, then they poured oil over them."[116] Although there are some details about how much olive oil was used, and how much anointing oil emerged at the end of the process, the section lacks detail about the weight, quantity, and proportion of spices. Maimonides' treatment

[113] *SG*, 96r: רבותינו ז"ל התירו לנו הלמוד הפשוט בכל הדברים ... אבל אתה למד להבין ולהורות

[114] Maimonides, *Hilḥot Kelei HaMiqdash* 2:10: עשאה להתלמד בה או למסרה לצבור פטור Though Portaleone does not say so, the line comes from BT Keritot 5a.

[115] Maimonides, *Hilḥot Kelei HaMiqdash* 2:9: העושה קטרת מן אחד עשר סמנין אלו לפי משקלות אלו כדי להריח בה אף על פי שלא הריח חייב כרת על עשייתה אם עשה במזיד ובשוגג מביא חטאת קבועה

[116] BT Keritot 5a.

of this issue is fuller but not detailed enough to satisfy Portaleone. He announces to his readers, "I have decided to teach you the pharmacist's method of compounding the anointing oil. Listen and I will utter what the Lord places in my mouth (Numbers 22:38), since the Rav [Maimonides] in the first chapter, second section of the *Laws of the Temple Vessels* did not say enough about its pharmacology."[117] Framing his investigation as an elaboration of what Maimonides neglected to adequately treat, Portaleone grants his work legitimacy in the sphere of Jewish jurisprudence.

Jurisprudential justification was not the only type Portaleone sought; he provides a theological rationale for instructing his readers in the art of making the anointing oil, too.

> I adjure, by the Lord of Heaven and the Lord of Earth (Genesis 24:3), whoever reads this chapter of mine not to compound the oil after this [fashion] but rather [to make the oil] as God commands by the authority of the prophet. For we are in exile because of our sins, and we have contracted the ritual impurity imparted by a corpse. We are not able to purify ourselves properly through the process described in the written Torah, in the pericope *Ḥuqah* [Numbers 19:1ff.]. Since it is not unreasonable to think that an impure person might involve himself in this holy pharmacology, he should become pure exclusively by the instructions of God.[118]

Portaleone also cites verses attesting to God's mercy and his willingness to make the impure pure, and he adds as a closing:

> Praise is due to the Lord our God! For we have exerted ourselves and discovered, as far as I know, all that is necessary for the knowledge of the spices for incense: its preparation, weight, and manufacture – and also what is necessary for compounding the anointing oil, and the art by which it is done.[119]

117 *SG*, 97r: על כן יעדתי ללמד אתכם אופן רקוחו של שמן המשחה שמעו ואנכי אדבר כפי אשר ישים ה' בפי כי הרב בפרק הראשון של כלי המקדש פסקא שנית לא דבר ברקוחו כמספיק

118 *SG*, 100v: והנני משביע באלקי השמים ואלקי הארץ כל מי שיקרא פרקי זה שלא ירקח שמן כזה אלא במצות ה' על פי נביא בפרט כי אנו בגלותנו בגלל עונותינו טמאים אנחנו טומאת מת ולא נוכל לטהר את עצמנו על פי התורה הכתובה בפרשת חקת כדין וכשורה ואינו מן הראוי שהטמא יטפל עצמו ברקוח הקדוש הזה אלא כשיהיה טהור ובמצות ה' ביחוד

119 *SG*, 100v: והתהלה לה' אלהינו כי יגענו ומצאנו לפי דעתי כל הצריך בידיעת סממני הקטורת מכשיריה משקלה ופטומה וגם מה שצריך ברקוחו של שמן המשחה ומלאכתו

CONCLUSION

In applying the methods of Renaissance botany to the explication of Jewish texts Portaleone created new applications for the former and introduced a novel way of studying the latter. The Mantuan physician used the methodologies of learned medicine and natural philosophy to diversify his study of the Bible and postbiblical Jewish texts. One of the ways he did that was by preferring modern authors to ancient authorities. Another was by welcoming new forms of evidence, such as artisanal expertise, into his investigations. Like many early modern scholars, Portaleone did not cite all of the authorities he relied on. As a justification for that tendency, he professed, "I have not come to confuse the world with critiques and therefore I will omit them." To those words he added, in ecumenical fashion, "I seek the truth from whomever pronounces it."[120] The words of those who pronounced the truth were recorded in a variety of books: classical texts, rabbinic treatises, and Renaissance monographs. But, as we have seen, they were also uttered in the *piazze*, pharmacies, and workshops of late sixteenth- and early seventeenth-century Mantua.

[120] *SG*, 86r: ואני לא באתי לבלבל העולם בהשגות ולכן אשמיט אותם ואבקש האמת ממי שאמרו

Conclusion

Near the beginning of *Shiltei HaGibborim*, Abraham Portaleone's Hebrew encyclopedia, readers are greeted with an odd sight: the printed Greek alphabet, in both upper-case and lower-case fonts. The Mantuan physician claimed that he included Greek letters in his Hebrew book in order to clarify the comments of Jewish sages, some of whom spoke Greek and drew on its scientific traditions to understand the natural world around them.[1] But *Shiltei HaGibborim* is interlarded with more Greek words written by Dioscorides, Theophrastus, and their pagan peers than those spoken by Portaleone's Jewish forebears. Portaleone learned Greek as a medical student in order to study and practice medicine; he used it as an old, infirm man to elucidate his own Jewish tradition. Gianfrancesco Pico della Mirandola's observation in 1518, which appears at the beginning of this book, that "aspiring theologians" learn natural philosophy applies not only to Pico's Catholic contemporaries; it clearly applies as well to Pico's descendants, and Portaleone's contemporaries, in the world of learned Latinate culture.

In that culture, particularly its Italian variant of the later sixteenth century, natural philosophy had many applications and was enriched by a number of traditions. Just as natural philosophy helped Portaleone

[1] *SG*, 4r. On the Talmudic rabbis' knowledge and use of Greek for scientific purposes, see Saul Lieberman, *Greek in Jewish Palestine: Studies in the Life and Manners of Jewish Palestine in the II–IV Centuries C.E.* (New York: Jewish Theological Seminary, 1942), xx. In addition to the passage in *SG*, 4r, see also *SG*, 8r: הואיל כי בפרקי אלו בא פעמים רבות זכירת האלפא ביתא יונית אמרתי כי טוב הוא לכתוב לכם כאן צורתה משלם כדי שתבינו בנקלה מה שכתבתי בה מהמלות זרות עמה "Since the Greek alphabet is mentioned many times in these chapters of mine, I thought it best to write the alphabet here for you, in its complete form, so that with it you may easily understand the foreign words I have written in it [the Greek alphabet]."

write about his Jewish faith and history, Jewish texts helped his Catholic peers write about natural philosophy. In July 1587, for example, Orazio Augenio, then a professor of practical medicine at Turin, completed an epistolary treatise addressed to Serafino Olivieri, the dean of the Roman Rota, the highest ecclesiastical judicial tribunal.[2] Its subject was whether physical signs of virginity could be found in all women.[3] Augenio maintained that they could not, a position that Olivieri believed threatened canon law provisions for physical inspection in disputed matrimonial cases.[4] In support of his argument, he devoted a chapter of his treatise to "what the sign of virginity, which is mentioned in Deuteronomy, might be, both according to Jews and according to Christians."[5] Deuteronomy 22 presents the case of a bride whose virginity is disputed by her husband. Augenio cites the scriptural verse (Deuteronomy 22:17) that reads they shall "spread the clothing before the elders of the city," to determine if there are visible signs of her virginity on her gown, namely blood.[6] Augenio adds by way of clarification: "Rabbi Solomon [ben Isaac, or Rashi], among the Jews a very serious writer, and of a great reputation, says that these words should be understood metaphorically."[7] Beyond his mention of Rabbi

[2] For basic information on Augenio, see *DBI* 4:577–8. On his medical writings, see Nancy G. Siraisi, *Communities of Learned Experience: Epistolary Medicine in the Renaissance* (Baltimore: Johns Hopkins University Press, 2013), 62–84. For discussion of this treatise, see ibid., 75–6. Séraphin Olivier-Razali (1538–1609) became an auditor for Roman Rota in 1564 and held that position for forty years.

[3] Orazio Augenio, *Epistolarum et consultationum medicinalium prioris tomi libri XII [-alterius tomi libri XII]*, 2 vols. in 1 (Venice: apud Damianum Zenarium, 1592), 2:1r–8r. "Reverendissimo in Christo Patri Domino Domino Seraphino Olivario, Sanctissimi Domini Nostri Papae Capellano, eius Sacri Palatii Caussarum Auditori, Domino suo colendissimo. Ostenditur virgines foeminas eam non habere ex natura membranam, quam nonnulli interseptum, alii claustrum virginale, alii hymen vocant. Nullum certum, propriumque signum esse virginitatis. Et quod olim medicarum mulierum, quas hodie obstetrices vocant, ex Platone, et Galeno extiterit officium."

[4] Siraisi, *Communities of Learned Experience*, 76.

[5] Augenio, *Epistolae*, 2:7r–7v. "Quod signum sit virginitatis, cuius mentio fit in Deuteronomio, tum secundum Haebreos, tum secundum Christianos."

[6] Deuteronomy 22:17: "Expandent vestimentum coram senioribus civitatis."

[7] Augenio, *Epistolae*, 2:7r: "Rabi Salamon inter Haebreos scriptor gravissimus, et magni nominis, ea verba metaphorice intelligenda, cum praecipue dicat." Rashi's comment on Deuteronomy 22:17 reads הרי זה משל מחוורין הדברים כשמלה I have not been able to ascertain Augenio's precise source. He might have turned to Nicholas of Lyra's commentary on the Bible, or to Pietro Galatino's *Opus... de arcanis catholicae veritatis* (Ortona: per Hieronymum Suncinum, 1518), book 7, which concerns virginity. In book 7 of Galatino's work, however,

Solomon, or Rashi, Augenio drew additional support for his views from an unattributed "saying of the rabbis."[8] In his dispute with Olivieri, Augenio turned to the Bible and its Jewish expositors for confirmation of his views regarding the female anatomy.

The use of natural philosophy to explicate the Bible, and vice versa, was conspicuous in Italy from the middle of the sixteenth century to the beginning of the seventeenth. At that time and in that place, an interconfessional group of medical doctors pursued a unique form of scholarly writing that blended biblical and natural philosophic study. The eclectic works of Ulisse Aldrovandi, Andrea Bacci, Melchior Guilandinus, Amatus Lusitanus, David de' Pomi, and Abraham Portaleone belie easy classification or appellation. Jacques Le Goff once observed about twelfth-century literature that its "very nature ... is too subtle for the classificatory grids of present-day history."[9] The same may be said for the works examined in the foregoing pages. Rooted in the soil of Renaissance medical culture, they demonstrate a notable degree of intellectual agility. They display a tendency to approach ancient texts with more regard for their content, accuracy, and antiquity than for their sacrality. And they show how in the courts, universities, and colleges of physicians of northern Italy the classical canon was broadened to include not only newfound works from pagan antiquity but also the Bible.

The group of learned physicians this book has examined had intellectual cousins in Iberia and its dominions. Many Spanish and Portuguese physicians, however, skirted around the Bible rather than integrating it into their medical and philosophical writings. *Conversos* are a prime

Deuteronomy 22 is not mentioned. Nicholas of Lyra writes regarding cases of disputed virginity that "alii exponunt hebrei dicentes quod est locutio parabolica" and observes that "Scriptura sacra in pluribus locis habet talem modum loquendi metaphoricum." He does not mention Rashi. See *Biblie iampridem renovate pars prima [-sexta] complectens pentateuchum: una cum glosa ordinaria, et litterali moralique expositione Nicolai de Lyra, necnon additionibus Burgensis, ac replicis Thoringi, novisque distinctionibus et marginalibus summariisque annotationibus* (Basel: Froben, 1502), 356v.

8 Augenio, *Epistolae*, 2:7r: "ex iis unicuique constare potest, quid ex Rabinorum senentia de cruentato linteolo, ac certo signo virginitatis, sentire oporteat." Rabbinic statements on this issue may be found in *Sifrei*, §§ 236–8; Maimonides, *Mishneh Torah*, *Hilḥot Ishut*, chap. 11: §§ 9–12.

9 Jacques Le Goff, *The Birth of Purgatory*, trans. Arthur Goldhammer (Chicago: University of Chicago Press, 1984), 135.

example of this tendency.[10] Fearful of the Inquisition and its charges of Judaizing, they were understandably reluctant to address the Bible in any way that could reveal their heritage or expose imputed Jewish beliefs. In the 1550s, for example, the Spanish *converso* Andrés Laguna (1499–1559) composed a commentary on Dioscorides' *De materia medica* that bears some similarities to that of Amatus Lusitanus.[11] Where Amatus thought it proper to discuss King David's language, Laguna does not mention the Bible at all.[12] Nor do chapters on Balsam or Bitumen present opportunities for the Spanish physician to discuss their presence in biblical texts.[13] Similarly, in his work on meteorology, one book of which concerns its medical applications, Stephanus Rodericus a Castro (1559–1627) seldom mentions the Bible.[14] In one revealing instance, a Castro lists several mineralogical products with curative properties, including hyacinth and the horn of the *monocerote* – both commonly believed in the sixteenth century to be equivalents of biblical realia. But he does not cite the Bible at all.[15]

The most conspicuous work of natural philosophy from this period composed in Iberia that does address the Bible directly was not written by a *converso* but rather by Francisco Vallés (1524–92), physician to Phillip II. First published at Lyon in 1587, *De iis quae scripta sunt physice in*

[10] On the popularity of the medical profession among New Christians, see Yosef Hayim Yerushalmi, *From Spanish Court to Italian Ghetto: Isaac Cardoso: A Study in Seventeenth-Century Marranism and Jewish Apologetics* (New York: Columbia University Press, 1971), 70–2. On the same phenomenon elsewhere in the Sephardic diaspora, see Yosef Kaplan, "The Sephardim in North-Western Europe and the New World," in Haim Beinart, ed., *Moreshet Sepharad/The Sephardic Legacy* (Jerusalem: Magnes Press, 1992), 2:240–87, 280–1.

[11] Andrés Laguna, *Annotationes in Dioscoridem Anazarbeum* (Lyon: apud Gulielmum Rouillium, 1554). On Laguna and his *converso* background, see Harry Friedenwald, *The Jews and Medicine,* 2 vols. (Baltimore: Johns Hopkins University Press, 1944), 2:419–29; and James Nelson Novoa, "Andrés Laguna in Papal Rome: The Documents of the Mozoncillo Ecclesiastical Benefice," *Minvera* 25 (2012): 211–32 and works cited there. I thank Dr. Novoa for sharing his work with me.

[12] Laguna, *Annotationes,* "De myrrha," 36–7.

[13] Ibid., "De balsamo," 19–20; "De bitumine," 43–4. "Bitumen," or pitch, was the Vulgate rendering of one of the two adhesives used to seal Moses' cradle (Exodus 2:3).

[14] Stephanus Rodericus a Castro, *De meteoris microcosmi libri quatuor* (Florence: apud Iunctas, 1621). An exception is book 4, chap. 6, "De sanguinis menstrui veneno," 170–4, 173, which concerns Moses and the plagues he wrought on Egypt.

[15] Ibid., book 4, chap. 2, "Alexipharmaca unde habeant suam facultatem," 154–8, esp. 155–6.

libris sacris, sive de sacra philosophia (On those things that are written regarding physics in the Holy Scriptures; or, On sacred philosophy) is, at first glance, similar in tone and scope to the works composed by the Italian protagonists examined in this book. Biblical quotations lie aside references to ancient and medieval medical works. To glorify the Bible, Vallés applied his formidable scientific acumen and medical erudition to its scrutiny. But Vallés's exegetical imagination differs substantially from that of his Italian peers, in ways that underscore the uniqueness of Aldrovandi, de' Pomi, and Portaleone. Perhaps Vallés's exegetical imagination was limited by a network of correspondents that was smaller and less international than that enjoyed by his colleagues elsewhere in Europe.[16] Perhaps Iberian naturalists' disinterest in collecting objects and forming *Kunst- und Wunderkammern* induced a relationship to material culture that was abstract rather than concrete.[17] Perhaps they were wary of ecclesiastical and inquisitorial structures that were more rigid than those in Italy.

Whatever the reasons, *De iis quae scripta sunt* is the product of a very different mind and culture. In Vallés's book, the Bible is always the point of departure. It remains the touchstone for every topic discussed, and all of Vallés's learning serves to clarify scripture's meaning and justify its content with reference to ancient and contemporary scientific thought. Whereas the Spanish physician skips over Exodus 2 and its mention of the material form in which Moses' crib was constructed, which, as we have seen, engaged Guilandinus and Aldrovandi, he had much to say about chapter 15 of that book and its narrative of Moses turning bitter water into sweet.[18] This miracle cried out for scientific elucidation. The Italian writers analyzed in this book chose independent topics for analysis and integrated scrutiny of the Bible into them. The molds into which they poured their learning were shaped to produce knowledge about natural philosophical problems, linguistic puzzles, or antiquarian products – not biblical interpretation.

[16] Laurent Pinon, *Livres de zoologie de la Renaissance: une anthologie 1450–1700* (Paris: Klincksieck, 1995), 15.

[17] Brian Ogilvie, *The Science of Describing: Natural History in Renaissance Europe* (Chicago: University of Chicago Press, 2006), 62.

[18] Francisco Vallés, *De iis quae scripta sunt physice in libris sacris, sive de sacra philosophia* (Lyon: apud Franciscum Fabrum, 1595 [1587]), chap. 15, 108–10.

Vallés's relationship to the clergy is also very different from that of Aldrovandi. The Spaniard piously asserted that human intelligence is weak and fallible while the church remains strong and infallible.[19] To his mind intellectuals grappling with the Bible needed to fall back upon the authority and guidance of the church. Aldrovandi's experience inverts this formulation: the church needed him as much as he needed the church. After all, it was Cardinal Gabriele Paleotti and his brother Camillo who persuaded him to devote years of his life to an investigation of the Bible's natural history. In at least one important and populous diocese of northern Italy – Bologna – leading church officials not only welcomed the involvement of naturalists in biblical interpretation but actively sought it out.

Another revealing discrepancy between Vallés's work and that of the Italians featured in this book is Vallés's relative indifference to the Bible's original languages and his related tendency to accept scripture's claims at face value. Vallés appears to have had complete faith in his biblical text: he never questions the terminology of the Vulgate, and rarely calls upon other languages (such as Hebrew or Greek) to clarify obscure vocabulary.[20] Psalm 45 with its detailed botanical terminology fails to engage Vallés's attention; Psalm 77, with its description of "the doors of heaven" opening in order to rain down manna, does, and merits a chapter.[21] In his other published writings, such as his work on Hippocrates, attentiveness to language figures prominently.[22] But Vallés could not, or would not, apply the methods he used in medical research to those he employed in biblical study. As we have seen, the Italian protagonists of this book most certainly did.

Related to this faith in the solidity of the biblical text is a credulity with regard to the Bible's scientific inerrancy. In the preface to *De iis quae scripta sunt*, Vallés wrote "since some natural questions are woven into the line of discussion, I believe that they are all very true, since they

[19] Ibid., 6: "testor ante omnia, nihil me in hoc, aut ullo alio meorum operum asserere, nisi quatenus probetur a sancta Romana Ecclesia, penes quam veritas est et sapientia."

[20] One exception is ibid., chap. 1, p. 26, where Vallés notes that the Hebrew verb in the verse "et spiritus Domini ferebatur super aquas" (Genesis 1:2) is multivalent and can mean both "moved" and "lay upon."

[21] Ibid., chap. 57, 324–7.

[22] Craig Martin, "Printed Medical Commentaries and Authenticity: The Case of *De Alimento*," *Journal of the Washington Academy of Sciences* 90:4 (2004): 17–28, 21–2.

are dictated by the spirit of God."[23] In a similar vein, Vallés claimed that the Bible "contained a whole other doctrine – that is, a natural one."[24] Portaleone, Aldrovandi, and de' Pomi also believed in the Bible's truth. The assumption of scriptural veracity, at least doctrinally and juridically, may have been the same on the Iberian and Italian peninsulas. However, the way those learned communities engaged scripture's sacrality was markedly different. Vallés explains and ultimately justifies the Bible on scientific grounds to show that its ritual and narrative components stand up to scrutiny. He deployed his erudition to validate scripture. His Italian peers employed a greater range of intellectual commitments: imaginative, experiential, mechanical. They aspired, above all else, to animate scripture and showed that it could be resuscitated all around them. Portaleone's efforts to find new information to enliven one of Exodus's drier portions, Aldrovandi's receipt of wood understood to duplicate that mentioned in Ezekiel from the botanist Luca Ghini, and Aldrovandi's botanical romps in the Dolomite foothills with leading church officials in order to find manna, indicate a belief that the Bible's natural world could not be ignored or left in the charge of those officially appointed to interpret it; it had to be brought to life.

The legacy of Aldrovandi, de' Pomi, and Portaleone had a short afterlife. Fifty years after Guilandinus and Aldrovandi used the Bible to confirm their views on ancient cultivation of papyrus, Fernando Cardoso, the physician and apologist for Judaism who later took the name Isaac, made creative and historical use of the Old Testament in his scientific and antiquarian treatise on water. Shortly before departing his native Spain for Italy, where he would spend more than half his life, he wrote:

> Already in Alexander's time people would put ice in their drinks, since in his histories Cares of Mitilene wrote that Alexander decreed that, in the city of Petra, in India, thirty graves, or large pits, be built. He filled them with snow and laid oak branches over them so that the snow would be better preserved. But let us discover [this practice's] origin, which is of much greater antiquity: from the time of Solomon one may deduce that it

[23] Vallés, *De iis quae scripta sunt*, 5: "tamen cum quaedam in ipso sermonum ductu texantur naturalia, ea omnia verissima esse existimo, utpote quae, a summe vero Dei spiritu dictata sint."

[24] Ibid., 6: "ego mihi persuadeo atque omnibus persuasum volo, ut omnem aliam doctrinam, quae vera sit, ita naturalem, in his divinis libris contineri."

> [snow] had been used: "As the cold of snow in the time of harvest, so is a faithful messenger to them that send him: for he refresheth the soul of his masters." The wise one [Solomon] ... uses a simile, saying that [the messenger] pleases him as the coolness of the snow in the summer. This, then, is a clear signal that [snow] was used, since otherwise the comparison would be inappropriate.[25]

Cardoso used a verse from Proverbs to establish the antiquity of an alimentary practice. His Spanish predecessor Vallés also flagged this verse, but for a much different purpose: to exonerate alimentary practices in scripture – namely, the consumption of cold beverages.[26] Cardoso was not interested in vindicating scripture's dietetic statements; for him, as for Guilandinus and Aldrovandi before, the Bible served as a source for the history of the ancient world.

Even though their working methods may be discerned in later books, such as Cardoso's study of water and snow, the protagonists of this book did not attract students, devise a methodology, or inspire a movement. Their work is not an early manifestation of biblical criticism, nor should it be seen as an attempt to secularize sacred literature. Still, there were unintended outcomes of their work: inadvertently, these natural philosophers encouraged future students of the biblical past to study sacred history the same way they studied pagan history. Indeed, in Bologna during Aldrovandi's lifetime, scholars were doing just that: his friend Carlo Sigonio wrote his work on the Hebrew republic not as a polemicist or a theologian but as a historian.[27] Aldrovandi elided

[25] Fernando Cardoso, *Utilidades del agua i de la nieve, del bever frio i caliente* (Madrid: Alonso Martin, 1637), 55v–56r: "ya en tiempos de Alexandro se usava el bever con nieve, pues en sus historias que escrivio Cares Mitileneo, se refiere, que mandò en la ciudad de Petra en la India hazer treinta fosas, o cavas grandes, y llenarlas de nieve, echandole encima ramas de roble, que deste modo se conservava mejor. Mas de mayor antiguedad descubramos su principio, porque de tiempo de Salomon se colige averse usado, 'sicut frigus nivis in die messis, ita legatus fidelis ei, qui misit illum, animam ipsius requiescere facit.' ... Manifiesta el Sabio como queda descansado el animo del quien remite un fiel criado, quien con toda fidelidad se asegura que complirà con sus obligaciones: y usa da una similitud, diziendo que assi le recrea como el frio de la nieve en el estio; luego es clara señal que entonces se usava, pues de otro modo la comparacion fuera impropria." By "Cares Mitileneo" Cardoso refers to Cares of Mitilene's *Historias de Alejandro*. Cardoso quotes the Vulgate's translation of Proverbs 25:13. On Cardoso, see Yerushalmi, *From Spanish Court to Italian Ghetto*.

[26] Vallés, *De iis quae scripta sunt* [1595 ed.], chap. 61, 339–41.

[27] Carlo Sigonio, *De republica hebraeorum libri VII* (Frankfurt: apud haeredes Andreae Wecheli, 1583); B. Roussel, "Connaissance et interprétation du Judaism antique: des biblistes

differences between the Bible and other types of ancient literature by excerpting passages from both, juxtaposing them, and assigning them equal evidentiary value – as did de' Pomi and Portaleone. Commonplace books, a staple of sixteenth-century intellectual life that helped generate the sorts of treatises considered in this book, assessed facts – whether recent or ancient, bookish or empirical – as equivalent to each other.[28] By comparing the Bible's depictions of the natural world to those in pagan scientific writings, sixteenth-century natural philosophers unintentionally demoted the Bible from its exalted position in the canon of sacred literature. To their minds, they were promoting scripture, not demoting it; any literate person who read their works would understand the precise meaning of the Bible and thereby improve his knowledge of it.

Sixteenth-century naturalists could not predict that in the eighteenth century their works would be stripped of their spiritual message and anthologized in lavish encyclopedias such as Blasio Ugolini's *Thesaurus antiquitatum sacrarum* (Thesaurus of sacred antiquities).[29] Ugolini's antiquarian tomes presented the sacred past much the same way as contemporary works portrayed the Greek, Roman, Egyptian, and Etruscan

chrétiens de la seconde moitié du XVIe siècle," in Chantal Grell and François Laplanche, eds., *La République des lettres et l'histoire du Judaïsme antique XVIe–XVIIIe siècles* (Paris: Presses de l'Université Paris-Sorbonne, 1992), 21–50, 42; Paolo Prodi, "Vecchi appunti e nuove reflessioni su Carlo Sigonio," in Massimo Firpo, ed., *Nunc alia tempora, alii mores: storici e storia in età postridentina* (Florence: L. S. Olschki, 2005), 291–310, which sketches out connections between Sigonio, Paleotti, and Aldrovandi; Giudo Bartolucci, *La repubblica ebraica di Carlo Sigonio. Modelli politici dell'età moderna* (Florence: L. S. Olschki, 2007); William McCuaig, *Carlo Sigonio: The Changing World of the Late Renaissance* (Princeton: Princeton University Press, 1989); Kalman Neuman, "The Literature of the Respublica Judaica: Descriptions of the Ancient Israelite Polity in the Antiquarian Writing of the Sixteenth and Seventeenth Centuries" (Hebrew) (PhD diss., Hebrew University, 2002), iv.

28 Ann Blair, "Humanist Methods in Natural Philosophy: The Commonplace Book," *Journal of the History of Ideas* 53:4 (1992): 541–51, 545.

29 Blasio Ugolini, *Thesaurus antiquitatum sacrarum*, 34 vols. (Venice: J. G. Herthz, 1744–69). For example, Ugolini includes the Hebrew original and a Latin translation of portions of Abraham Portaleone's *SG*. See Ugolini, *Thesaurus*, vol. 11, cclvii–dxlviii. Discussing *SG*, Ugolini praises its erudition and says nothing about the work's clear spiritual and apologetic content: "in quo tanta sese ubique offert rerum praestantia et eruditio, ut merito ceteris, qui hoc argumentum illustrarunt, praeferendus esse videatur." Vol. 9, unnumbered pages before index.

past.[30] Unknowingly, sixteenth-century naturalists helped forge the tools with which eighteenth-century antiquarians and encyclopedists drained the Bible of its sacrality.

Of course, neither Portaleone nor Aldrovandi could see into the future or predict such a fate for their work or that of their peers. On the contrary, both emphasized the pious nature of their research. In 1611 Portaleone was an elderly hemiplegic, and he wrote his encyclopedia in a spirit of expiatory contrition:

> When God wanted to chasten me, I fell ill. Two years ago the whole left side of my body became as if dead, and I could no longer touch my hand to my breast nor walk in the street, even leaning on a cane, because of the loss of feeling and ability to move my limbs. I searched my behavior and saw (but only after Him who sees all) that in addition to my sins, which were more numerous than the hairs on my head, [I had] neglected the Torah. For I had dealings with the children of Greek wisdom, and I sought to reach the heights through philosophy and medicine, which lured me with their honeyed words to seek salvation in the ways of darkness, and thus prevented me from devoting myself to the heritage of the community of Jacob, as I should have.[31]

Portaleone's *Shiltei HaGibborim* displays ample evidence of "dealings with the children of Greek wisdom." Contrary to what Portaleone claimed, those dealings did not prevent him from enriching the "heritage of the community of Jacob." In fact, they enabled him to.

Unlike Portaleone, Aldrovandi did not struggle to reconcile his study of the Bible with his pursuit of natural philosophy; they were consonant endeavors for him. Some time after 1579, Aldrovandi reflected that "one of the greatest desires of my life has been to see Jerusalem and Mount Lebanon for devotion and also to know the great variety of

[30] See the introduction to Grell and Laplanche, eds., *La République des lettres et l'histoire du Judaïsme antique*. On antiquarianism in the eighteenth century, see Arnaldo Momigliano, "Ancient History and the Antiquarian," *Journal of the Warburg and Courtauld Institutes* 13 (1950): 285–315; Peter Miller, ed., *Momigliano and Antiquarianism: Foundations of the Modern Cultural Sciences* (Toronto: University of Toronto Press, 2007).

[31] Portaleone, *SG*, 2v. For discussion, see Alessandro Guetta, "Avraham Portaleone, le scientifique repenti," in Gad Freudenthal, Jean-Pierre Rothschild, and Gilbert Dahan, eds., *Torah et science: perspectives historiques et théoriques. Études offertes à Charles Touati* (Leuven: Peeters, 2001), 213–27.

plants set there by God."[32] Articulating the symbiosis between piety and knowledge of nature, Aldrovandi was speaking not only for himself but for a group of Italian naturalists – both Jewish and Christian – whose impact on biblical studies and religious culture in sixteenth-century Italy and beyond deserves to be better understood.

[32] BUB Ms. Aldrovandi 51, *De cruce*, 2 vols., 1:111r: "Io nell'età mia frà i maggiori desiderii che ho'havuto di vedere parte del mondo è stata Gierosolima, e questo monte Libano sì per devotione, sì anco per conoscere tanta varietà di piante generate dal grand' Iddio."

Appendix I

The Ancient Israelite Incense Mixture

BIBLICAL TEXT

Exodus 30:34–38

ויאמר יהוה אל משה קח לך סמים נטף ושחלת וחלבנה סמים ולבונה זכה בד בבד יהיה. ועשית אתה קטרת רקח מעשה רוקח ממולח טהור קדש. ושחקת ממנה הדק ונתתה ממנה לפני העדת באהל מועד אשר אועד לך שמה קדש קדשים תהיה לכם. והקטרת אשר תעשה במתכנתה לא תעשה לכם קדש תהיה לך ליהוה. איש אשר יעשה כמוה להריח בה ונכרת מעמיו

Jewish Publication Society Translation

And the Lord said to Moses, Take to you sweet spices, storax, and onycha, and galbanum; these sweet spices with pure frankincense; of each shall there be a like weight: And you shall make it a perfume, a confection according to the art of the apothecary, mixed together, pure and holy; And you shall beat some of it very small, and put of it before the Testimony in the Tent of Meeting, where I will meet with you; it shall be to you most holy. And as for the perfume which you shall make, you shall not make for yourselves according to its composition; it shall be to you holy for the Lord. Whoever shall make it like that, to partake of its scent, shall even be cut off from his people.

BABYLONIAN TALMUD KERITOT 6A

ת"ר: פיטום הקטרת הצרי והצפורן והחלבנה והלבונה משקל שבעים של שבעים מנה מור וקציעה שיבולת נרד וכרכום משקל ששה עשר של ששה עשר מנה הקושט שנים עשר קילופה שלשה וקנמון תשעה בורית כרשינה תשעה קבין יין קפריסין סאין תלתא קבין תלתא אם אין לו

יין קפריסין מביא חמר חיוריין עתיק מלח סדומית רובע מעלה עשן כל שהוא. ר' נתן אומר: אף כיפת הירדן כל שהוא. ואם נתן בה דבש פסלה. חיסר אחת מכל סממניה חייב מיתה

Soncino Translation

Our Rabbis have taught: the compound of incense consisted of balm, onycha, galbanum and frankincense, each in the quantity of seventy Maneh; of myrrh, cassia, spikenard and saffron, sixteen Maneh by weight; of costus twelve, of aromatic rind three, and of cinnamon nine Maneh; of lye obtained from leek, nine Kab; of Cyprus wine three Se'ah and three Kab, though if Cyprus wine is not available, old white wine may be used instead; of salt of Sodom the fourth of a Kab, and of Ma'aleh 'ashan a minute quantity. R. Nathan says: Also of Jordan resin a minute quantity. If, however, honey is added, the incense is rendered unfit; while if one omits one of the ingredients, he is liable to the penalty of death.

Appendix II

Ulisse Aldrovandi and Hebrew

The following manuscripts by Ulisse Aldrovandi display significant engagement with the Hebrew language. All of them may be found in Bologna's Biblioteca universitaria.

1. *Bibliologia* Ms. Aldrovandi 83 (2 vols.). Begun in 1580.
2. *De cruce* Ms. Aldrovandi 51 (2 vols.). Completed in 1597.
3. *Miscellanea de animalibus et plantis* Ms. Aldrovandi 97. Written over an extended period, mostly between 1581 and 1586.
4. *Lettere e discorsi* Ms. Aldrovandi 6 (3 vols.), especially vols. 2 and 3. Written over an extended period, mostly between 1578 and 1582.
5. *Ulyssi Aldrovandi et amicorum Dictionarium Latino-Syro-Chaldaicum* Ms. Aldrovandi 21 (3 vols.) Undated.
6. *De lucentibus* Ms. Aldrovandi 91. Completed in 1577.
7. *Theatrum biblicum naturale* Ms. Aldrovandi 54 (2 vols.). Begun in 1585.

Appendix III

The Index to Portaleone's *Responsorum et consultationum medicinalium liber* (1607)

Abraham Portaleone's *Responsorum et consultationum medicinalium liber* contains *responsa* and *consultationes* that Portaleone wrote to and received from more than forty correspondents. The men with whom Portaleone corresponded were of extremely variable fame. Illustrious physicians such as Girolamo Mercuriale, as well as nearly the entirety of the University of Padua's medical faculty at the turn of the seventeenth century, are prominently listed in this index. At the same time, obscure men, such as Jacobus Saravallus (Jacobo Saravallo) and Samuelis Limae (Samuele da Lima), grace its pages. I have not been able to identify every contributor. What follows after these brief remarks is a partial annotation of the index. When possible, I have listed the vernacular names of Portaleone's correspondents. When appropriate, I have given their institutional affiliation and noted their major works.

Portaleone corresponded with Jews as well as Christians. In this index Portaleone's son, David, lists the names of nearly all Christian correspondents his father wrote to or received letters from. However, in a clear act of obfuscation, he omitted from the index letters to or from Jews. For example, Portaleone wrote (in Latin) to Abraham Provenzali, a Jewish educator from Mantua and Portaleone's own teacher, on the topic of epilepsy and hysteria. See "Consilium Excellentissimi Patris de Histerica passim pro mulierum hebrea. Excellentissimo Legum Artiumque Doctori Domino Abrahae Provinciali Hebreo," 293r–298v. The letter is signed and dated "Abraham e Portaleonis Mantuanus Medicus hebraeus ita consulebat pridie nones Novembris anno ab origine mundi 5329" (12 November 1569). In the index to this collection the *consilium* is referred to only as "De Hysterica passione Excellentissimi Patris." In another *consilium*, Portaleone describes Provenzali as "l'excellentisimo dottore e non mai lodato a pieno Nostro Signor Abramo Provenzali, fedelissimo mio singolare Precettore." See 464r, "Epistola de suffusione occulorum Excellentissimi Patris." Curiously, Portaleone dates this letter according to the Jewish calendar and in Hebrew characters: שמ"א, or 1581. More examples of correspondence with Jews could be given. A *consilium* on hypochondriacal melancholy was composed "per donna Rachella do Foa Regensi Hebrea," 513v. A treatise on ancient deafness was written "pro Juvens da Foa Hebreo," 130v. Finally, a *consilium* on ulceration of the liver was sent to "D. Raffaello de Carminis Hebreo," 232r. The addressees of these final three examples are not listed in the index to *Responsorum et consultationum medicinalium liber*.

Index Consultationum Medicinalium quae in hoc libro continentur

[1] Giulio Cesare Claudino (ca. 1550–1618) was the author of *De ingressu ad infirmos libri duo* (Venice: apud Donatum Pasquardum agentem P. P. Tozzii, 1628). He also authored a book of medical letters: *Responsionum et consultationum medicinalium tomus unicus; in duas sectiones partitus, in quarum prima Responsiones; in altera Consultationes continentur* (Frankfurt: sumptibus Lazari Zetzneri, 1607).

[2] Eustachio Rudio (1551–1611) was the author of a number of works on pulse, the heart, the soul, and ulcers. On him, see Nancy G. Siraisi, *Avicenna in Renaissance Italy: The Canon and Medical Teaching in Italian Universities after 1500* (Princeton: Princeton University Press, 1987), 114, 115, 117, and 277.

[3] Alessandro Vigonza was the second professor extraordinarius of practica at the University of Padua. See Siraisi, *Avicenna in Renaissance Italy*, 116, 118.

[4] Girolamo Fabrizi d'Acquapendente (1533–1619) taught at the University of Padua from 1565. Duke Guglielmo called him to Mantua to pronounce a medical opinion on the suspected virginity of his son's bride Margherita Farnese; d'Acquapendente's opinion helped annul the marriage. For more on this episode, see Adalberto Pazzini, "La Medicina alla corte dei Gonzaga a Mantova," 291–351, in *Mantova e i Gonzaga nella Civiltà del Rinascimento. Atti del convegno dall'Accademia Nazionale dei Lincei e dall'Accademia Virgiliana con la collaborazione della città di Mantova sotto l'alto patronato del Presidente della Repubblica Italiana Giovanni Leone, Mantova 6–8 ottobre 1974* (Mantua: Accademia Virgiliana, 1977), 339, 324. For more on Fabrizi, see Nancy G. Siraisi, *History, Medicine, and the Traditions of Renaissance Learning* (Ann Arbor: University of Michigan Press, 2007), 65; Gianna Pomata, "*Praxis Historialis*: The Uses of *Historia* in Early Modern Medicine," in

Gianna Pomata and Nancy G. Siraisi, eds., *Historia: Empricism and Erudition in Early Modern Europe* (Cambridge, MA: MIT Press, 2005, 105–46, 116–18.

[5] Girolamo Mercuriale (1530–1606). See Chapter 4, note 2. His best-known work was an antiquarian treatise on gymnastics, *Hieronymi Mercvrialis Foroliviensis de arte gymnastica libri sex* (Venice: apud Juntas, 1569).

[6] Giovanni Tomasso Minadoi (1545–1615) was professor ordinarius at the University of Padua. In addition to his medical teaching and writing he composed a *Historia della guerra fra Turchi et Persiani ... cominciando dall'anno MDLXXVII* (Venice: Andrea Muschio, & Barezzo Barezzi, 1588). See Siraisi, *Avicenna in Renaissance Italy*, 114 n. 110.

[7] See Chapter 4.

[8] Emilio Campilongo (1550–1604) was professor ordinarius of practica at the University of Padua. His *De arthritide liber unus* (Venice, apud Paulum Meietum, 1586) was published in several editions. Ercole Sassonia (1551–1607) was professor of anatomy and surgery at the University of Padua. He published extensively on venereal disease, melancholy, pulses, fevers, and practical medicine. See Siraisi, *Avicenna in Renaissance Italy*, 114 n. 110.

[9] Stefano Pampuri of Cassalmagiore.

[10] Filippo Cavriani (1536–1606) lived in Mantua and wrote several *discorsi* about Tacitus (Florence: Giunti 1597, 1600). See Bruno Spigarolo, *Filippo Cavriana: mantovano del XVI secolo, letterato tacitista, storico e politico* (Mantua: Sometti, 1999). Scipione Aquiliani was the author of *De placitis philosophorum, qui ante Aristotelis tempora floruerunt* (Venice: apud Ioannem Guerilium, 1620).

11 Perhaps Giovanni Battista Codronchi (1547–1628), author of *De annis climactericis: nec non De ratione vitandi eorum pericula, itemque De modis vitam producendi … commentarius* (Cologne: Matthaei Smitz, 1623).

[12] Ioannes Iacobus Bottattius, or Giovanni Iacopo Bottazzo, of Montecastello. His *Dialogi maritimi* were published at Mantua in 1547 by Iacopo Ruffinelli. He was one of the founders of the Accademia degli Argonauti. See *DBI* 13:422–3.

[13] Andreas Schato (1539–1603), German mathematician and physician. Professor of mathematics at the University of Wittenberg and, after 1592, professor ordinarius of medicine at that university.

[14] Alessandro Massaria (1510–98) was appointed to the first ordinarius chair in practica at the University of Padua in 1587.

[15] Orazio Augenio (ca. 1527–1603) was the second professor ordinarius of theoria. He published two volumes of *epistolae* and *consultationes*. See *Horatii Augenii a monte sancto medici, et philosophi praestantissimi ... Epistolarum et consultationum medicinalium Libri XII* (Venice: apud Damianum Zenarium 1592 [1579]). See also my discussion at the beginning of the Conclusion.

[16] Guglielmo I (1538–87) was Duke of Mantua from 1550 to 1587. He was succeeded by Vincenzo Gonzaga (1562–1612), who ruled the duchies of Mantua and Montferrat from 1587 until his death in 1612.

17 Johanna of Austria was the daughter of Emperor Ferdinand I. She married Francesco of Tuscany in 1565.

18 Giovanni Zecchi hailed from Bologna. He wrote books about fever, Hippocratic aphorisms, and urine. He also published a collection of *consultationes*. See *Ioannes Zecchii liber primus consultationum medicinalium* (Rome: apud Gulielmum Facciottum, ad instantiam Ioannis Martinelli, 1599).

19 See note 16.

20 Girolamo Capivaccio (1523–89) published a number of works including a *Nova methodus medendi* (Frankfurt: apud Joannem Feyrabendium, 1593). Some of his medical letters were included in a late sixteenth-century collection: *Consiliorum medicinalium, conscriptorum*

a praestantissimis atque exercitatissimis nostrorum temporum medicis, liber singularis (Frankfurt: apud Andreae Wecheli haeredes, Claudium Marnium et Joannes Aubrium, 1598).

21 Samuel of Lima did not leave behind any medical writings. He was a Jewish physician who wrote to Portaleone about a case of possible leprosy involving an unnamed Venetian Jew. See *Consilium Excellentisimi Doctor Samuelis di Lima di Lepra pro Nobili Hebreo Veneto*, which begins "Domino Abrahamo e Portaleonis Medico Excellentissimo Mantuano, Doctor Lima Medicus hebreus S.P.D." *Responsorum et consultationum medicinalium liber*, 234r. Samuel of Lima signed his letter according to the Jewish calendar: "Venetiis die 9 nisan 5350," ibid., 235v. In Portaleone's response, he does the same: 22 Nisan 5350 (5350 corresponds to 1590).

22 Giovanni Battista Pona (1565–1630) was a Veronese apothecary and botanist whose most well-known work was *Monte Baldo descritto da Giovanni Pona veronese, in cui si figurano, & descrivono molte rare piante de gli antichi, da' moderni fin' hora non conosciute* (Venice: Roberto Meietti, 1617). Monte Baldo, west of Verona, was prized as a lush site for the study of plants. Pona also owned a museum in Verona. See his *Index multarum rerum quae repositorio suo [Johannis Ponae] adservantur* (Verona, 1601), as cited in Paula Findlen, *Possessing Nature: Museums, Collecting, and Scientific Culture in Early Modern Italy* (Berkeley: University of California Press, 1994), 180.

23 Giulio Alessandrini (1506–90) was a physician and one of the authors of *Salubrium sive de sanitate tuenda, libri triginta tres* (Cologne: apud Geruinum Calenium & haeredes Quentelios, 1575).

[24] Cristoforo Guarinoni Fontani (d. 1602) was a Veronese physician. His work was included in a volume of *sententiae* on Aristotle's *De anima* (Frankfurt: imprimebat Ioannes Saurius sumptibus Nicolai Steinii Bibliopolae & Notarii, 1601); he also published medical *consilia*. See his *Consilia medicinalia in quibus universa praxis medica exacte pertractatur* (Venice: Baglionus, 1610).

[25] This *discursus* was written in November 1592 to Vincenzo Gonzaga, the Duke of Mantua.

[26] This *discursus* was also written in November 1592 to Vincenzo Gonzaga, the Duke of Mantua. Discursus Excellentisimi Patris de Lapido Bezahar dieto ad instantiam signorissimo D. Ducis Mantuae ecc[elentissimo]. 23 November 1592.

[27] Giovanni Battista Baccanelli (1508/9–1571) was from Reggio Emilia. He was the author of *De consensu medicorum in curandis morbis: libri quatuor* (Lyon: Honoratus, 1572).

[28] Elsewhere in this collection Portaleone wrote a case history for Guglielmo Cattaneo. See "Brevis Historia Massimi Gulielmi Cattanei conscripta ab Excellentissimo papi," 112r. I have

De melancholia Hippochondriaca Auricalchi pro eodem	Cap: 140 fol: 414
De Hydrope timpanitica Ex.mi Bertutii[29]	Cap: 141 fol: 416
Responsio Ex.mi Patris ad eundem	Cap: 142 fol: 418
De tumore Lienis palpitatione in sinistra gena, et parte ipsius Nasi, Ex.mi Corregii ad Ex.mum Patrem	Cap: 143 fol: 427
Responsio Ex.mi Patris ad eundem	Cap: 144 fol: 429
De vino Calybeato utrum i[dem] competat in schyrro lienis non exq[ui]sito Ex.mi Pagani ad Ex.mum Patrem	Cap: 145 fol: 432
Responsio Ex.mi Patris ad eundem	Cap: 146 fol: 433
De Gutturis Hernia Ex.mi Patris	Cap: 147 fol: 436
De Gutturis Hernia innominati medici	Cap: 148 fol: 447
De Gutturis Hernia innominati medici	Cap: 149 fol: 449
De Gutturis Hernia Ex.mi Achati Fer[rariensis][30]	Cap: 150 fol: 450
De Retentione Urinae Medici Casalensis	Cap: 151 fol: 451
Responsio Ex.mi Patris de Retentione Urinae	Cap: 152 fol: 452
De scirrho Meseraei Ex.mi Patris	Cap: 153 fol: 457
Responsio Ex.mi Cassolae de scirrho Meseraei[31]	Cap: 154 fol: 460
De numero et differentia Panum, et quid sit Panis lotus et aquaticus Ex.mi Patris	Cap: 155 fol: 462
Epistola de suffusione occulorum Ex.mi Patris	Cap: 156 fol: 464
Responsio praedictae epistolae	Cap: 157 fol: 464

not been able to identify Guglielmo Cattaneo. A certain Alphonsus Cataneus Ferrariensis gave morning lectures on *medicina theorica* at La Sapienza in Rome in 1587. See Emanuele Conte, *I maestri della sapienza di Roma dal 1514 al 1787: i rotuli e altre fonti* (Rome: Nella sede dell'Istituto Palazzo Borromini, 1991), 1:126.

29 Alfonso Bertocci was best known as the author of a *Methodus generalis et compendiaria ex Hippocratis, Galeni, et Avicennae placitis deprompta ac in ordinem redacta* (Lyon: apud Gabrielem Coterium, 1558).

30 I cannot precisely identify this figure, but a certain "Achates" composed an Italian prose prologue to a sixteenth-century miscellany in the possession of Berlin's Kupferstichkabinett, Ms. 79 D5. See Paul Oskar Kristeller, *Iter Italicum* (London: Warburg Institute, 1963–97), 3:468b.

31 Scipio Cassola, along with Giovanni Francesco Boccalini, published a work entitled *Scipionis Cassolae cum Joanne Francisco Boccalino medico Asulano disceptatio an epithematum usus antiquis medicis fuerit cognitus* (Parma: apud Seth Viottum, 1565).

[32] The Longius who was the recipient of this *responsio* was perhaps the philologist Joseph Lang[e] (1570–1615), rather than Johann Lange, the longtime court physician at the court of the Elector Palatine in Heidelberg, who wrote unkindly about Jewish physicians and was unlikely to have corresponded with one. See Chapter 4, note 28 for more on Lang[e]. Finally, it is possible Portaleone corresponded with Antonius Longus, who gave a funeral oration at the University of Padua upon the death of Nicolao Pontio in 1585. See Antonio Riccoboni, *De gymnasio patavino … commentariorum libri sex* (Padua: apud Bolzetam, 1598), 129r.

[33] Caretto is a small village in Liguria about eighty kilometers west of Genoa. It is not known who the village's marquis was at the time Portaleone wrote.

Bibliography

Manuscripts

Belluno, Biblioteca Civica

Lollino, Aloysio, Vite di Francesco Piccolomini, Jacopo Zabarella, Tommaso Peregrino, Melchior Guillandino, Antonio Riccobono, Girolamo Mercuriali, Guido Pancirola, Faustino Sommo, Giuseppe Molezio, Bastesiano Monticolo, Professori nell'Univ. di Padova. Ms. 505

Bologna, Archivio Isolani

Ms. F. 30 (30/1–2–3)

Ms. F. 60 /134, CN 88

Bologna, Biblioteca dell'Archiginnasio

Pomi, David de'. *Discorso maraviglioso sopra la guerra promossa da Selim Imperator di Turchi*. Ms. A 428.

Bologna, Biblioteca universitaria

Aldrovandi, Ulisse. *Bibliologia*. 2 vols. Ms. Aldrovandi 83

De cruce. 2 vols. Ms. Aldrovandi 51

Discorso naturale. Ms. Aldrovandi 91

Lexicon latino-hebraico et syro-chaldaicum rerum quae in Sacris Bibliis leguntur. 3 vols. Ms. Aldrovandi 21

Methodus theatri biblici naturalis. Ms. Aldrovandi 48

Miscellaneous. Ms. Aldrovandi 66

Miscellaneous. 6 vols. Ms. Aldrovandi 124

Miscellaneous. Ms. Aldrovandi 97

Pandechion epistemonicon. 83 vols. Ms. Aldrovandi 105

Theatrum biblicum naturale. 2 vols. Ms. Aldrovandi 54

Cambridge, University Library

Bertinoro, Ovadiah, Untitled Ms. Add. 395

London, British Library

Anonymous, *Sodot Avanim uMaragliot*, Ms. Oriental 2396

Mantua, Archivio di Stato

Spezeria. Magistrato ducale, busta IV: 1580–1689.

New York, Jewish Theological Seminary

Cases, Moses ben Samuel. *Bi'ur al Masechet Middot*, Ms. Rab. 23

Oxford, Bodleian Library
Yagel, Abraham. *Beit Ya'ar HaLevanon*, Ms. Reggio 10
Paris, Bibliothèque nationale
Portaleone, Abraham. *Abrahami Portaleonis Medici Mantuani Hebrei Responsorum et consultationum medicinalium liber*, Ms. Latin 13004

Printed Books Before 1800

a Castro, Rodericus. *Roderici à Castro. Medicus Politicus, sive de officiis medico-politicis tractatus*. Hamburg: ex bibliopolio Frobeniano, 1614.

a Castro, Stephanus Rodericus. *De meteoris microcosmi libri quatuor.* Florence: apud Iunctas, 1621.

Alessandrini, Giulio. *Salubrium sive de sanitate tuenda, libri triginta tres.* Cologne: apud Geruinum Calenium & haeredes Quentelios, 1575.

Almosnino, Moses ben Baruch. *Tefilah le-Moshe.* Salonika, 1563.

Yedei Moshe. Salonika, 1582.

Alpino, Prospero. *Prosperi Alpini de plantis aegypti liber: in quo non pauci, qui circa herbarum materiam irrepserunt, errores, deprehenduntur, qourum causa hactenus multa medicamenta ad usum medicine admodum.* Venice: Franciscum de Franciscis, 1592.

Aquiliani, Scipione. *De placitis philosophorum, qui ante Aristotelis tempora floruerunt.* Venice: apud Ioannem Guerilium, 1620.

Arias Montano, Benedict. *Antiquitatum iudaicarum libri IX.* Lyon: apud F. Raphelengium, 1593.

Biblia sacra. Antwerp: Christophorus Plantinus, 1572.

Phaleg: sive de gentivm sedibvs primis, orbisque terrae situ liber. Antwerp: Plantin, 1572.

Arnaldus de Villa Nova. *Arnaldi Villanovani Opera Omnia.* Basil: ex Officina Pernea per Conradvm Waldkirch, 1585.

Augenio, Orazio. *Epistolarum et consultationum medicinalium prioris tomi libri XII.* Venice: apud Damianum Zenarium, 1602 [1592].

Avicenna. *Avicennae principis et philosophi sapientissimi libri in re medica omnes qui hactenus ad nos pervenere. Id est libri canonis quinque, de viribus cordis, de removendis nocumentis in regimine.* Venice: apud Vincentium Valgrisium, 1564.

Baccanelli, Giovanni Battista. *De consensu medicorum in curandis morbis: libri quatuor.* Lyon: Honoratus, 1572.

Bacci, Andrea. *Andreae Baccii Elipidiani philosophi, medici et civis romani, de gemmis et lapidibus pretiosis, eorumque viribus et usu tractatus, italica lingua conscriptus: nunc vero non solum in latinum sermonem conversus verum etiam utilissimis annotationibus & observationibus auctior redditus.* Frankfurt: Matthias Becker, 1603.

De naturali vinorum historia. Rome: ex typographia Nicolai Mutii, 1596.

L'Alicorno. Discorso dell' eccellente medico, et filosofo M. Andrea Bacci nel quale si tratta della natura dell' Alicorno, & delle sue virtù eccellentissime. Florence: Giorgio Marescotti, 1573.

Le XII Pietre Preciose, le quali adornavano i vestimenti del sommo sacerdote: discorso dell' Alicorno et delle sue virtù: et della gran bestia detta Alce da gli antichi. Rome, 1587.
Bauhin, Caspar. *Pinax theatrum botanicum*. Basel: Impensis Johannis Regis, 1671.
Belon, Pierre. *De admirabili operum antiquorum et rerum suspiciendarum praestantia liber primus. De medicato funere, seu cadavere condito, et lugubri defunctorum eiulatione liber secundus. De medicamentis nonnullis, servandi cadaveris vim obtinentibus liber tertius*. Paris: Guglielmo Cavellat, 1553.
Berchoir, Pierre. *Dictionarii seu repertorii moralis Petri Berchorii Pictaviensis ordinis divi benedicti pars prima*. Venice: apud Haeredem Hieronymi Scoti, 1574.
Bertocci, Alfronso. *Methodus generalis et compendiaria ex Hippocratis, Galeni, et Avicennae placitis deprompta ac in ordinem redacta*. Lyon: apud Gabrielem Coterium, 1558.
Bibliander, Theodorus. *De ratione communi omnium linguarum et literarum commentarius*. Zurich: Christoph Frosch, 1548.
Bochart, Samuel. *Hierozoicon sive bipertitum opus de animalibus s. scripturae*. Frankfurt: Zunner, 1675.
Bono, Giacomo Antonio. *Del terremoto dialogo*. Modena: P. Gadaldini & fratelli, 1571.
Bottazzo, Giovanni Iacopo. *Dialogi maritime*. Mantua: Iacopo Ruffinelli, 1547.
Bozzola, Giovanni Battista. *Universum sacrosanctum concilium tridentinum*. Brescia: J. B. Bozola, 1563.
Calepino, Ambrogio. *Ambrosii Calepini dictionarium linguarum septem: iam demum accurata emendatione, atque infinitorum locorum augmentatione, collectis ex bonorum authorum monumentis, omnium vocum significationibus*. Basil: Petri, 1575.
Camillo, Leonardo. *Speculum lapidum clarissimi artium et medicine doctoris Camilli Leonardi Pisaurensis*. Venice: Melchior Sessas & Petrus de Ravanis sociis, 1516.
Campilongo, Emilio. *De arthritide liber unus*. Venice: apud Paulum Meietum, 1586.
Cangiamila, Francesco Emanuello. *Embriologia sacra, ovvero dell'uffizio de' sacerdoti, medici, e superiori, circa l'eterna saluta de' bambini racchiusi nell'utero, libri quattro*. Milan: Giuseppe Cairoli, 1751.
Capivaccio, Girolamo. *Nova methodus medendi*. Frankfurt: apud Joannem Feyrabendium, 1593.
Cardano, Girolamo. *De subtilitate libri XXI*. Lyon: Gulielmus Rovillium, 1550.
Caro, Isaac. *Toledot Yitzhak*. Constantinople, 1518.
Casaubon, Isaac. *De rebus sacris exercitationes XVI*. Geneva, 1655.
Cassola, Scipio, and Giovanni Francesco Boccalini. *Scipionis Cassolae cum Joanne Francisco Boccalino medico Asulano disceptatio an epithematum usus antiquis medicis fuerit cognitus*. Parma: apud Seth Viottum, 1565.
Castell, Edmund. *Lexicon heptaglotton, hebraicum, chaldaicum, syriacum, samaritanum, aethiopicum, arabicum, conjunctim; et persicum, separatim*. London: Thomas Roycroft, 1669.
Catalano, Abraham. *Olam Hafukh*. Edited by Cecil Roth. Vol. IV (14): *Kovetz Al Yad*. 1946 [orig. 1630].

Chevalier, Antoine Rodolphe. *Rudimenta hebraicae linguae*. Paris: Stephanus, 1567.

Claudino, Giulio Cesare. *De ingressu ad infirmos libri duo*. Venice: apud Donatum Pasquardum agentem P. P. Tozzii, 1628.

Clusius, Carolus, and Garcia de Orta. *Aromatum et simplicium aliquot medicamentorum apud Indos nascentium historia*. Antwerp: Plantin, 1567.

Codronchi, Giovanni Battista. *De annis climactericis: nec non De ratione vitandi eorum pericula, itemque De modis vitam producendi … commentarius*. Cologne: Matthaei Smitz, 1623.

Cohen, Tobias. *Ma'aseh Tuviyyah*. Venice: Bragadin, 1705.

Colombo, Realdo. *Realdi Columbi de re anatomica: libri XV*. Paris: Wechel, 1562 [1559].

Costa, Filippo. *Discorsi di M. Filippo Costa Mantovano sopra le compositioni degli antidoti, & medicamenti, che piu si costumano di dar per bocca. Di nuovo dal medesimo in questa seconda impressione ricorretti*. Mantua: Francesco Osanna, 1586.

Daléchamps, Jacques. *C. Plinii Secundi historiae mundi*. Lyon: Bartholomeaus Honoratus, 1587.

de Laguna, Andrés. *Pedacio Dioscorides Anazarbeo: acerca de la materia medicinal, y de los venenos mortiferos*. Salamanca: Mathias Gast, 1563.

Dolce, Lodovico. *Trattato delle gemme che produce la natura*. Venice: G. Battista and G. Bernardo Sessa, 1565.

Donati, Marcello. *De medica historia mirabili libri sex*. Mantua: Franciscum Osanam, 1586.

du Chesne, Joseph. *Le richezze della riformata farmacopea*. Translated by Giacomo Ferrari. Venice: Giovanni Guerigli, 1619.

Durante, Castore. *Herbario novo*. Rome: Bartholomeo Bonfadino, & Tito Diani, 1585.

Il tesoro della sanità. Pisaro: Bartholomeo Cesani, 1565.

Epiphanius. *Sancti Patris Epiphanii episcopi Cypri ad Diodorum Tyri episcopum, de XII gemmis, quae erant in veste Aaronis, liber graecus, & e regione latinus, Iola Hierotarantino interprete: cum corollario Conradi Gesneri*. Zurich: Gesner, 1565.

Fabrici d'Aquapendente, Girolamo. *De formatu foetu*. Venice: Franciscus Bolzetta, 1606.

Falloppio, Gabriele. *Gabrielis Falloppii Mutinensis, physici ac chirurgici praeclarissmimi opera quae adhuc extant omnia*. Frankfurt: Andreas Wechels, 1584.

Ficino, Marsilio. *De vita libri tres*. Binghamton, NY: Medieval & Renaissance Texts & Studies in conjunction with the Renaissance Society of America, 1989.

Fioravanti, Leonardo. *Dello specchio di scientia universale*. Venice: Valentini, 1624.

Del regimento della peste. Venice: Andrea Revenoldo, 1565.

Il tesoro della vita humana. Venice: Gli Heredi di Melchior Sessa, 1582.

Fontani, Cristoforo Guarinoni. *Consilia medicinalia in quibus universa praxis medica exacte pertractatur*. Venice: Baglionus, 1610.

Sententiarum Aristotelis de anima seu mente humana interpretatio. Frankfurt: imprimebat Ioannes Saurius sumptibus Nicolai Steinii Bibliopolae & Notarii, 1601.

Fuchs, Leonhart. *De historia stirpium commentarii insignes*. Basel: in officina Isingriniana, 1542.

Galen. *Galeni omnia quae extant opera: in lat. sermonem conversa*. Venice: Giunta, 1565.

Galeni septima classis, artem morborum curatricem describit promptaque ad id opus remedia quem plurima subjungit, necnon quae ad deligationes, luxationes, & fracturas attinet, chirurgiam. Florence: Giunti, 1541.

Gesner, Conrad. *De omni rerum fossilium genere, gemmis, lapidibus, metallis, et huiusmodi libri aliquot, plerique nunc primum editi. Operâ Conradi Gesneri: quorum catalogum sequens folium continet*. Zurich: Iacobus Gesnerus, 1565.

Guilandinus, Melchior. *De stirpibus aliquot, epistolae V*. Padua: Gratiosus Perchacinus, 1558.

De stirpium aliquot nominibus vetustis ac novis. Basil: apud Nicolaum Episcopium juniorem, 1557.

Melchioris Guilandini Papyrus, hoc est, commentarius in tria C. Plinij Maioris de papyro capita: accessit Hieronymi Mercurialis repugnantia, qua pro Galeno strenuè pugnatur. Venice: apud M Antonium Ulmum, 1572.

Hippocrates. *Magni Hippocratis medicorum omnium facile principis: opera omnia quae extant, in VIII sectiones ex erotiani mente distributa*. Frankfurt: Wechels, 1596.

Ibn Yahia, Gedaliah. *Shalshelet Ha-Kabbalah*. Venice: Zuan di Gara, 1586.

Jiménez de Cisneros, Francisco. *Biblia polyglotta*. Alcalá de Henares: Arnaldi Guillelmi de Brocario, 1514.

Josephus, Flavius. *Flavii Iosephi opera, in sermonem latinum iam olim conversa*. Basel: Froben, 1567.

Iosippus de bello iudaico. Basil: Henrichus Petrus, 1559.

Kimḥi, David. *Sefer Ha-Shorashim thesaurus linguae sanctae sive dictionarium hebreum*. Venice: Giustiniani, 1547.

Laguna, Andrés. *Annotationes in Dioscoridem Anazarbeum*. Lyon: apud Gulielmum Rouillium, 1554.

Lampronti, Isaac. *Paḥad Yiẓhak*. Lyck, 1874 [1750–].

Langius, Joseph. *Adagia sive sententiae proverbiales graecae, latinae, germanicae ex praecipuis autoribus collectae*. Strasbourg: Rihel, 1596.

Epigrammaton libri XV. Strasbourg: Zetzner, 1595.

Index omnium vocabulorum quae in omnibus M. Val. Martialis poematum libris reperiuntur. Strasbourg: Zetzner, 1595.

Leoniceno, Niccolò. *Nicolai Leoniceni Vincentini de Plinii, & plurium aliorum medicorum in medicina erroribus opus primum Angelo Politiano dedicatum*. Ferrara: Joannes Maciochius, 1509.

Nicolai Leoniceni Vicentini, philosophi et medici clarissimi, opuscula. Basel: Cratandrum, 1532.

Lipsius, Justus. *Opera omnia*. Antwerp: Moretus, 1637.

López de Gómara, Francisco. *Historia general de las Indias*. Medina del Campo: por Guillermo de Millis, 1553.

Lusitanus, Amatus. *Curationum medicinalium centuria sexta*. Venice: apud Vincentium Valgrisium, 1556.

In Dioscorides Anazarbei de materia medica libros quinque enerrationes. Lyon: apud viduam Balthazari Arnoletti, 1558.
Manardi, Giovanni. *Epistolarum medicinalium libri duodeviginti*. Basel, 1535.
Marini, Marco. *Annotationes literales in Psalmos*. Bologna, 1748.
Arca Noe thesaurus linguae sanctae novus. Venice: apud Ioannem Degaram, 1593.
Massa, Nicolo. *Epistolarum medicinalium tomus alter*. Venice: ex officinal Stellae Jordani Zilleti, 1558.
Mattioli, Pietro Andrea. *Epistolarum medicinalium libri quinque*. Lyon: apud Cesarem Farinam, 1564.
I discorsi di M. Pietro Andrea Matthioli. Nelli sei libri di Pedacio Dioscoride Anazarbeo della materia medicinale. Venice: Vincenzo Valgrisi, 1568.
Petri Andreæ Matthioli medici cæsarei et Ferdinandi Archiducis Austriæ, opera quæ extant omnia: hoc est, commentarij in VI libros Pedacij Dioscoridis Anazarbei de medica materia. Frankfurt: ex officina typographica Nicolai Bassæi, 1598.
Mercuriale, Girolamo. *Hieronymi Mercurialis Foroliviensis responsorum, et consultationum medicinalium tomus primus*. Venice: apud Iolitos, 1587.
Hieronymi Mercurialis Foroliviensis responsorum, et consultationum medicinalium tomus tertius. Venice: Franciscum de Franciscis Senensem, 1597–1604.
Hieronymi Mercurialis Foroliviensis responsorum, et consultationum medicinalium tomus quartus. Venice: apud Iuntas, 1604.
Hieronymi Mercurialis Foroliviensis de arte gymnastica libri sex. Venice: apud Juntas, 1569.
Minadoi, Giovanni Tomass. *Historia della guerra fra Turchi et Persiani … cominciando dall'anno 1577*. Venice: Andrea Muschio, & Barezzo Barezzi, 1588.
Moscato, Judah. *Nefutzot Yehudah*. Venice: Juan de Gara, 1589.
Modena, Leon. *Ari Nohem*. Leipzig: K. Tauchnitz, 1840 [orig. 1639].
Galut Yehudah. Venice: Giacomo Sarzina, 1602.
Münster, Sebastian. *Shilush leshonot dictionarium trilingue*. Basel: Henricus Petrus, 1530.
Veteris instrumenti tomus secundus, prophetarum oracula atque hagiographa continens. Basel, 1535.
Pagnini, Sante. *Biblia: habes in hoc libro prudens lector utriusque instrumenti nouam translationem æditum*. Lyon: Antonius du Ry, 1528.
Psalterium nuper translatum ex hebraeo, chaldaeo, et graeco. Rome: n.pr., 1521.
Thesauri hebraicae linguae, olim a Sante Pagnino Lucensi conscripti, epitome. Antwerp: Plantin, 1572.
Thesaurus linguae sanctae. Paris: Stephanus, 1548.
Pansa, Mutio. *Della libraria vaticana, ragionamenti di Mutio Pansa divisi in quattro parti*. Rome: G. Martinelli, 1590.
Paul of Aegina. *Pauli Aeginetae opus de re medica*. Paris: apud Simonem Colinaeum, 1532.
Plinius Secundus, Gaius. *C. Plinii Secundi naturalis historiae pars*. Venice: in aedibus haeredum Aldi et Andreae Asulani soceri, 1535–6.
Pomi, David de'. *Brevi discorsi et efficacissimi ricordi per liberare ogni citta oppressa dal mal contagioso da David de Pomis*. Venice: appresso G. Perchacino, 1577.

De medico hebraeo enarratio apologica apposita sunt non paucorum amplissimorum principum, quam multa decreta, in hebraeorum favorem constituta annectuntur quinetiam in tractatus calce, nonnulla aurea dicta; ex priscorum hebraeorum monumentis excerpta; nunc primum, latinitate donata, & in lucem edita. Venice: apud Joannem Variscum, 1588.

Discorso intorno a l'humana miseria, e sopr'al modo di fuggirla. Venice: Appresso Giordano Ziletti e compagni, 1572.

Dittionario novo hebraico/Tsemah David, molto copioso: dechiarato in tre lingue. Venice: apud Ioannem de Garo, 1587.

Enarratio brevis de senum affectibus praecavendis, atque curandis: rationali methodo decorata, aeque atque praestantissimis, arcanisque auxiliis, in quibusdam profligandis morbis, insignita in qua. Venice: apud Joannem Variscum, 1588.

Pona, Giovanni Battista. *Monte Baldo descritto da Giovanni Pona veronese, in cui si figurano, & descrivono molte rare piante de gli antichi, da' moderni fin' hora non conosciute.* Venice: Roberto Meietti, 1617.

Portaleone, Abraham. *Shiltei Ha-Gibborim.* Mantua, 1612.

Postel, Guillaume. *De etruriae regionis, quae prima in orbe europaeo habitata est, originibus, institutis, religione, & moribus & imprimis de aurei saeculi doctrina & vita praestantissima quae in divinationis sacrae usu posita est ... commentatio.* Florence: Torrentini, 1551.

Riccoboni, Antonius. *De gymnasio patavino Antonii Riccoboni commentariorum libri sex.* Padua: Bolzeta, 1598.

Rocca, Angelo. *Bibliotheca apostolica vaticana a Sixto V. Pont. Max. in splendidiorem commodioremque locum translata et a fratre Angelo Roccha ... commentario.* Rome: ex typographia apostolica Vaticana, 1591.

Rueff, Jakob. *De conceptu et generatione hominis, et iis quae circa haec potissimum considerantur, libri sex.* Zurich: Christophorus Froschoverus, 1554.

Scaliger, Joseph. *Opuscula varia ante hac non edita omnium catalogum post praefationem lector inveniet.* Paris: apud Drouard, 1610.

Scaligerana, ou bons mots, rencontres agreables, et remarques judicieuses & Sçavantes De J. Scaliger. Amsterdam, n.p. 1695.

Schenck, Johann. *Hortus patavinus, cui accessere M. Guilandini conjectanea synonymica plantarum.* Frankfurt: Johann Theodor de Bry, 1608.

Sforno, Obadiah. *Kitve Rabi 'Ovadyah Sforno: perush le-sifre Yonah, Ḥavakuk u-Zekharyah, Shir Ha-Shirim, Kohelet, Iyov u-Tehilim: Pirkei Avot, Or 'Amim, igrot, derashot, she'elot u-teshuvot.* Jerusalem: Mosad ha-Rav Kuk, 1983.

Sigonio, Carlo. *De republica hebraeorum libri VII.* Frankfurt: apud haeredes Andreae Wecheli, 1583.

Sommo, Judah. *Ẓaḥut bediḥuta de-kiddushin.* Edited by J. Schirmann. Jerusalem: Sifre Tarshish, 1965 [orig. c. 1550].

Steuchus, Augustinus. *Veteris testamenti ad hebraicam veritatem recognitio.* Lyon: Gryphius, 1529.

Ugolinus, Blasius. *Thesaurus antiquitatum sacrarum.* Venice: J.G. Herthz, 1744–69.

Vallés, Francisco. *De iis quae scripta sunt physice in libris sacris sive de sacra philosophia liber singularis.* Lyon, 1595.

Various authors. *Consiliorum medicinalium, conscriptorum a praestantissimis atque exercitatissimis nostrorum temporum medicis, liber singularis*. Frankfurt: apud Andreae Wecheli haeredes, Claudium Marnium et Joannes Aubrium, 1598.

Medicæ artis principes, post Hippocratem et Galenum. Græci latinitate donati [ab Iunio Paulo Crasso aliisque]. Aretaeus, Ruffus Ephesius, Oribasius, Paulus Aegineta, Aëtius, Alex. Trallianus. Paris: Henricus Stephanus, 1567.

Vesalius, Andreas. *Andreae Vesalii de humani corporis fabrica libri septem*. Basel: Johannes Oporinus, 1555.

Vielmi, Girolamo. *De sex diebus conditi orbis liber*. Venice: Giunta, 1575.

Weidner, Paul. *Mishnah Pirke Abot sententiae hebraicae ad vitae institutionem perutiles breviter explicatae et praeclarissimis dictis tam Sacram quam aliarum Scripturarum illustratae a Paulo Weidnero*. Vienna: Michaël Zimmerman, 1563.

Yagel, Abraham ben Hananiah. *Moshia Ḥosim*. Venice: Zuan di Gara, 1587.

Zecchi, Giovanni. *Ioannes Zecchii liber primus consultationum medicinalium*. Rome: apud Gulielmum Facciottum, ad instantiam Ioannis Martinelli, 1599.

Printed Books since 1800

Abramson, Shraga. "The 'Arukh' of Rabbi Nathan Ben Yehiel of Rome." *Sinai* 95:1–2 (1984): 27–42.

Albala, Ken. *Eating Right in the Renaissance*. Berkeley: University of California Press, 2002.

Allen, Don Cameron. *The Legend of Noah: Renaissance Rationalism in Art, Science, and Letters*. Urbana: University of Illinois Press, 1949.

Ankori, Zvi. *Yahadut ve-Yavanut Notsrit: Mifgash ve-'Imut bi-Meruzat ha-Dorot*. Tel Aviv: University of Tel Aviv, 1984.

Anonymous. *Book of Secrets of Precious Stones*. Jerusalem: Yerid ha-sefarim, 2004.

Antin, Paul, ed. *Saint Jérome sur Jonas*. Paris: Sources Chrétiennes, 1956.

Aranoff, Deena. "Elijah Levita: A Jewish Hebraist." *Jewish History* 23 (2009): 17–40.

Arbel, Benjamin. "Jews in International Trade: The Emergence of the Levantines and Ponentines." In *The Jews of Early Modern Venice*, edited by R. C. Davis and B. Ravid, 73–96. Baltimore: Johns Hopkins University Press, 2001.

Asad, Talal. *Formations of the Secular: Christianity, Islam, Modernity*. Stanford: Stanford University Press, 2003.

Asaf, Simḥa. *Meḳorot le-toldot ha-ḥinukh be-Yiśra'el*. New York: Bet Ha-Midrash le-rabanim ba-Amerika, 2001–9 [orig. Jerusalem, 1925–9].

Askenazi, E., ed. *Divrei ḥakhamim*. Metz, 1849.

Asksamija, Nadja. "Architecture and Poetry in the Making of a Christian Cicero: Giovanni Battista Campeggi's Tuscolano and the Literary Culture of the Villa in Counter-Reformation Bologna." *I Tatti Studies* 13 (2010): 127–91.

Bacchi, Maria Cristina. "Ulisse Aldrovandi e i Suoi Libri." *L'Archiginassio* 100 (2005): 255–366.

Baldini, Ugo. "Cardano e Aldrovandi nelle Lettere del Sant'uffizio Romano all'inquisitore di Bologna (1571–1573)." *Bruniana e Campanelliana* 6 (2000): 145–63.

Baldini, Ugo, and Leen Spruit. *Catholic Church and Modern Science: Documents from the Archives of the Roman Congregations of the Holy Office and the Index*. Rome: Libreria editrice vaticana, 2009.

Banchi, Franco. *Il pranzo di S. Giovanni: racconti da tavola del rinascimento fiorentino*. Florence: LoGisma, 1997.

Barkai, Ron. *A History of Jewish Gynaecological Texts in the Middle Ages*. Leiden: Brill, 1998.

Les infortunes de Dinah: le livre de la génération: la gynécologie juive au moyen age. Paris: Cerf, 1991.

Baron, Salo. "Azariah de' Rossi's Historical Method." In *History and Jewish Historians: Essays and Addresses*, edited by Arthur Hertzberg and Leon A. Feldman, 205–39. Philadelphia: Jewish Publication Society of America, 1964.

Barón Fernández, José. *Andrés Vesalio: su vida y su obra*. Madrid: Consejo Superior de Investigaciones Científicas Instituto Arnaldo de Vilanova, 1970.

Barrera-Osorio, Antonio. *Experiencing Nature: The Spanish American Empire and the Early Scientific Revolution*. Austin: University of Texas Press, 2006.

Bartolucci, Guido. *La repubblica ebraica di Carlo Sigonio. Modelli politici dell'Età Moderna*. Florence: L. S. Olschki, 2007.

"Venezia nel pensiero politico ebraico rinascimentale: un testo ritrovato di David de' Pomis." *Rinascimento* 44 (2005): 225–47.

Baruchson, Shifra. *Sefarim ve-ḳor'im: tarbut ha-ḳeri'ah shel Yehude Iṭalyah be-shilhe ha-Renesans*. Ramat-Gan: Bar Ilan University Press, 1993.

Bates, A. W. *Emblematic Monsters: Unnatural Conceptions and Deformed Births in Early Modern Europe*. Clio Medica, vol. 77. Wellcome Series in the History of Medicine. Amsterdam: Rodopi, 2005.

Bedouelle, Guy. "Le débat catholique sur la traduction de la Bible en langue vulgaire." In *Théorie et pratique de l'exégèse: Actes du troisième colloque international sur l'histoire de l'exégèse biblique au XVIe siècle (Genève, 31 août–2 septembre 1988)*, edited by Irena Backus and Francis Higman, 39–59. Geneva: Librarie Droz S.A., 1990.

Bellonci, Maria. *Segreti dei Gonzaga*. Milan: A. Mondadori, 1966.

Ben-Menahem, N. "Towards a Bibliography of R. Moses Almosnino" (Hebrew). *Sefunot* 11 (1978): 135–85.

Bénézet, Jean-Pierre, and Jean Flahaut. *Pharmacie et médicament en méditerranée occidentale: (XIIIe–XVIe siècles)*. Genève: H. Champion Slatkine, 1999.

Bentley, Jerry H. *Humanists and Holy Writ: New Testament Scholarship in the Renaissance*. Princeton: Princeton University Press, 1983.

Biale, David, ed. *Cultures of the Jews: A New History*. New York: Schocken Books, 2002.

Blair, Ann. "The Collective Commentary as Reference Genre." In *Der Kommentar in der frühen Neuzeit*, edited by Ralph Häfner and Markus Völkel, 115–32. Tübingen: Max Niemeyer Verlag, 2006.

"Humanist Methods in Natural Philosophy: The Commonplace Book." *Journal of the History of Ideas* 53:4 (1992): 541–51.

"Mosaic Physics and the Search for a Pious Natural Philosophy in the Late Renaissance." *Isis* 91 (2000): 32–58.

Bland, Kalman P. "Issues in Sixteenth-Century Jewish Exegesis." In *The Bible in the Sixteenth Century*, edited by David Steinmetz, 50–67. Durham, NC: Duke University Press, 1990.

Blondheim, D. S. *Les parlers judéo-romans et la vetus latina: étude sur les rapports entre les traductions bibliques en langue romane des juifs au moyen age et les anciennes versions*. Paris: Librarie Ancienne Édouard Champion, 1925.

Boksenboim, Yaakov. *Iggrot Yehudei Italya*. Tel Aviv: Tel Aviv University Press, 1994.

Bonfil, R. "Aliens Within: The Jews and Antijudaism." In *Handbook of European History, 1400–1600: Late Middle Ages, Renaissance, and Reformation*, edited by Thomas Brady, Heiko Oberman, and James Tracey, 263–97. Leiden: Brill, 1994.

"Aspects of the Social and Spiritual Life of the Jews in the Venetian Territories at the Beginning of the Sixteenth Century." *Zion* 41 (1976): 68–96.

"Change in the Cultural Patterns of a Jewish Society in Crisis: Italian Jewry at the Close of the Sixteenth Century." *Jewish History* 3:2 (1988): 11–30.

"Il Rinascimento: la produzione esegetica di 'O. Servadio Sforno." In *La lettura ebraica delle scritture*, edited by Sergio S. Sierra, 261–77. Bologna: EDB, 1995.

Rabbis and Jewish Communities in Renaissance Italy. Translated by Jonathan Chipman. Oxford: Published for the Littman Library by Oxford University Press, 1990.

Bono, James J. "The Languages of Life: Jean Fernel (1497–1558) and Spiritus in Pre-Harveian Bio-medical Thought." PhD dissertation, Harvard University, 1981.

Borschbert, Peter. "The Euro-Asian Trade in Bezoar Stones (approx. 1500 to 1700)." In *Artistic and Cultural Exchanges between Europe and Asia, 1400–1900*, edited by Michael North, 29–43. Aldershot: Ashgate, 2010.

Bos, Gerrit. "The Creation and Innovation of Medieval Hebrew Medical Terminology: Shem Tov ben Isaac, 'Sefer ha-Shimmush.'" In *Islamic Thought in the Middle Ages: Studies in Text, Transmission and Translation, in Honour of Hans Daiber*, edited by Anna Akasoy and Wim Raven, 195–218. Leiden: Brill, 2008.

"Hayim Vital's 'Practical Kabbalah and Alchemy': A 17th Century Book of Secrets." *Journal of Jewish Thought and Philosophy* 4 (1994): 55–112.

"A Late Medieval Hebrew-French Glossary of Biblical Animal Names." *Romance Philology* 63 (2009): 71–94.

"The Literature of Hebrew Medical Synonyms: Romance and Latin Terms and their Identification." *Aleph: Historical Studies in Science and Judaism* 5 (2005): 169–211.

"Shem Tov ben Isaac, Glossary of Botanical Terms, Nos. 1–18." *Jewish Quarterly Review* 92:1–2 (July–October 2001): 21–40.

Brisson, Luc, Marie-Hélène Congourdeau, and Jean-Luc Solère. *L'embryon, formation et animation: antiquité greque et latine, traditions hébraïque, chrétienne, islamique*. Paris: Librarie Philosophique J. Vrin, 2008.

Buck, August. "Die Medizin im Verständnis des Renaissancehumanismus." In *Humanismus und Medizin*, edited by Rudolf Schmitz and Gundolf Keil, 181–98. Weinheim: Acta Humaniora, 1984.

Burke, Peter. *The Historical Anthropology of Early Modern Italy: Essays on Perception and Communication*. Cambridge: Cambridge University Press, 1987.

"A Survey of the Popularity of Ancient Historians, 1450–1700." *History and Theory* 5:2 (1966): 135–52.

Burmeister, Karl Heinz. *Sebastian Münster: Eine Bibliographie mit 22 Abhandlungen*. Weisbaden: G. Pressler, 1964.

Burnett, Stephen. "Christian Hebrew Printing in the Sixteenth Century: Printers, Humanism and the Impact of the Reformation." *Helmantica* 51:154 (2000): 13–42.

From Christian Hebraism to Jewish Studies: Johannes Buxtorf (1564–1629) and Hebrew Learning in the Seventeenth Century. Leiden: Brill, 1996.

"Reassessing the 'Basel-Wittenberg Conflict': Dimensions of the Reformation-Era Discussion of Hebrew Scholarship." In *Hebraica Veritas? Christian Hebraists and the Study of Judaism in Early Modern Europe*, edited by Alison Coudert and Jeffrey Shoulson, 181–201. Philadelphia: University of Pennsylvania Press, 2004.

Bylebyl, J. J. "The School of Padua: Humanistic Medicine in the Sixteenth Century." In *Health, Medicine and Morality in the Sixteenth Century*, edited by Charles Webster, 335–70. Cambridge: Cambridge University Press, 1979.

Campanini, Saverio. "Un intellettuale ebreo del rinascimento: 'Ovadyah Sforno a Bologna e i suoi rapporti con i cristiani." In *Verso l'epilogo di una convivenza: gli ebrei a Bologna nel XVI secolo*, edited by Maria Giuseppina Muzzarelli, 99–128. Bologna: Giuntina, 1996.

Capellmann, Carolus. *Pastoralmedizin*. Paderborn: Bonifacius, 1920.

Cardano, Girolamo. *De Subtilitate*. Milan: F. Angeli, 2004.

Carnevali, Luigi. *Il Ghetto di Mantova con appendice sui medici ebrei*. Mantua, 1884.

Carpi, Daniel. "Jewish Graduates of the University of Padua during the 16th Century." In Daniel Carpi, *Be-tarbut ha-Renesans u-ven ḥomot ha-geto: meḥkarim be-toldot ha-Yehudim be-Italyah ba-me'ot ha-14.-ha-17*, 96–130. Tel Aviv: University Publishing Project, 1989.

"Rabbi Judah Messer Leon and His Activity as a Doctor" (Hebrew). *Michael* 1 (1973): 277–301.

Carra, G., and A. Zanca. "Gli statuti del collegio dei medici di Mantova del 1559." *Atti e memorie dell'accademia virgiliana di Mantova, Classe di scienze fisiche e techniche* 2 (1977).

Cassuto, Umberto. *Gli ebrei a Firenze nell'età del Rinascimento*. Florence: Tipografia Galletti e Cocci, 1918.

Ceard, Jean. "Le 'De Originibus' de Postel et la linguistique de son temps." In *Postello, Venezia e il suo mondo, Atti del Ii Convegno Internazionale su Postel*, edited by M. L. Kuntz, 19–44. Florence: L. S. Olschki, 1988.

Celata, Giuseppe. "Gli ebrei in una società rurale e feudale: Pitigliano nella seconda metà del Cinquecento." *Archivio storico italiano* 138 (1980): 197–255.

Centi, Timoteo M. "L'attività letteraria di Santi Pagnini (1470–1536) nel campo delle scienze bibliche." *Archivum Fratrum Praedicatorum* 15 (1945): 5–51.

Cerutti, Simona, and Gianna Pomata, eds. *Fatti: storie dell'evidenza empirica. Quaderni storici* 108:3 (December 2001).

Chambers, David, ed. *Venice: A Documentary History, 1450–1630*. Toronto: Published by University of Toronto Press in association with the Renaissance Society of America, 2001.

Chomarat, Jacques. *Grammaire et rhétorique chez Érasme*. 2 vols. Paris: Belles Lettres, 1981.

Cigogna, Emmanuele. *Delle inscrizioni veneziane: raccolte ed illustrate*. Venice: Giuseppe Orlandelli, 1824.

Cochrane, Eric W. *Italy, 1530–1630*. London: Longman, 1988.

Considine, John. *Dictionaries in Early Modern Europe: Lexicography and the Making of Heritage*. Cambridge: Cambridge University Press, 2008.

Conte, E. *I maestri della sapienza di Roma dal 1514 al 1787: i rotuli e altre fonti*. Rome: Nella sede dell'Istituto Palazzo Borromini, 1991.

Coudert, A., and J. S. Shoulson. *Hebraica Veritas? Christian Hebraists and the Study of Judaism in Early Modern Europe*. Philadelphia: University of Pennsylvania Press, 2004.

Crisciani, Chiara. "Histories, Stories, Exempla, and Anecdotes: Michele Savonarola from Latin to Vernacular." In *Historia: Empiricism and Erudition in Early Modern Europe*, edited by Gianna Pomata and Nancy G. Siraisi, 297–324. Cambridge, MA: MIT University Press, 2005.

"L'individuale nella medicina tra medioevo e umanesimo: i 'Consilia.'" In *Umanesimo e medicina: il problema dell' "individuale,"* edited by Roberto Cardini and Mariangela Regoliosi, 1–32. Rome: Bulzoni, 1996.

Cuomo, Luisa Ferretti. "Dalle glosse giudeo-italiane dell''Arukh': accessori." In *Il mio cuore è a Oriente*, edited by Francesco Aspesi et al., 435–56. Milan: Cisalpino, 2008.

Dahan, G., ed. *Gersonide en son temps. Science et philosophie médiévales*. Louvain-Paris: E. Peeters, 1991.

Dallari, Umberto. *I rotuli dei lettori legisti e artisti dello studio bolognese dal 1384 al 1799*. Bologna: Regia tipografia dei Fratelli Merlani, 1888–1924.

Danieli, Natascia. "Sull'epistolografia ebraica in Italia nei secoli XVI–XVIII." *Annali di Ca' Foscari, serie orientale* 42:3 (2003): 29–56.

Daremberg, Charles. *Œuvres de Rufus D'Éphèse, texte collationné sur les manuscrits, traduit pour la première fois en français, avec une introduction. Publication commencée par C. Daremberg, Continuée*. Paris, 1879.

Daston, Lorraine. "Baconian Facts, Academic Civility, and the Prehistory of Objectivity." *Annals of Scholarship* 8 (1991): 337–63. Reprinted in Allan Megill, ed., *Rethinking Objectivity*, 37–64. Durham: Duke University Press, 1994.

"Marvelous Facts and Miraculous Evidence in Early Modern Europe." *Critical Inquiry* 18 (1991): 93–124. Reprinted in James Chandler, Arnold I. Davidson, and Harry Harootunian, eds., *Questions of Evidence. Proof, Practice, and Persuasion across the Disciplines*, 243–74.Chicago: University of Chicago Press, 1994.

Davies, Martin. *Aldus Manutius: Printer and Publisher of Renaissance Venice*. Tempe: Arizona Center for Medieval and Renaissance Studies, 1999.

Daxelmüller, Christoph. "Zwischen Kabbala und Martin Luther – Elijah Levita Bachur, eine Jude zwischen den Religionen." In *Wechselseitige Wahrnehmung der Religionen im Spätmittelalter und in der frühen Neuzeit*, edited by Ludger Grenzmann, Thomas Haye, Nikolaus Henkel, and Thomas Kaufmann, 231–50. Berlin: de Gruyter, 2009.

De Bellis, Ennio. "Cenni sulla dottrina della *demonstratio* nel pensiero di 'Avraham de Balmes." In *Gli ebrei nel Salento: secoli IX–XVI*, edited by Fabrizio Lelli, 285–99. Galatina: Congedo Editore, 2013.

DeJob, Charles. *De l'influence du concile de trente sur la littérature du siècle de Louis XIV*. Paris: Ernest Thorin, 1884.

De Jonge, H. J. "The Study of the New Testament in the Dutch Universities, 1575–1700." In *Leiden University in the Seventeenth Century*, edited by Th. H. Lunsing Scheurleer and G. H. M. Posthumus Meyjes, 65–110. Leiden: Brill, 1975.

De Lange, Nicholas. *Hebrew Scholarship and the Medieval World*. Cambridge: Cambridge University Press, 2001.

Delisle, Candice. "The Letter: Private Text or Public Place? The Mattioli-Gesner Controversy about the Aconitum Primum." *Gesnerus* 61:3–4 (2004): 161–76.

Delisle, Leopold. *Inventaire des manuscrits latins conserves a la bibliotheque nationale sous les numeros 8823–18613*. Paris: A. Durand et Pedone-Lauriel, 1863.

Delph, Ronald. "Italian Humanism in the Early Reformation: Agostino Steuco (1497–1548)." PhD dissertation, University of Michigan, 1987.

Del Riccio, Agostino. *Istoria delle pietre*. Turin: Umberto Allemandi, 1996.

de Toni, G. B. "Melchiorre Guilandinus." In *Gli scienziati italiani*, edited by A. Mieli, 73–76. Rome: Casa editrice Leonardo da Vinci, 1933.

Dian, G. *Alcuni ricordi della medicina al tempo della Repubblica veneta*. Venice: A. Pellizzato, 1909.

Dilg, Peter. "Apotheker als Sammler." In *Macrocosmos in Microcosmo: Die Welt in der Stube. Zur Geschichte des Sammelns 1450 bis 1800*, edited by Andreas Grote, 453–74. Opladen: Leske und Budrich, 1994.

"Die botanische Kommentarliteratur Italiens um 1500 und ihr Einfluss auf Deutschland." In *Kommentar in der Renaissance*, edited by August Buck and Otto Herding, 225–52. Boppard: Boldt, 1975.

Di Liscia, Daniel. *Method and Order in Renaissance Philosophy of Nature: The Aristotle Commentary Tradition*. Brookfield, VT: Ashgate, 1997.

Diller, Aubrey. *Bibliotheca graeca manuscripta cardinalis Dominici Grimani, 1461–1523*. Mariano del Friuli: Ed. della Laguna, 2003.

Dionisotti, A. C. "Greek Grammars and Dictionaries in Carolingian Europe." In *The Sacred Nectar of the Greeks: The Study of Greek in the West in the Early Middle Ages*, edited by Michael W. Herren and Shirley Ann Brown, 1–56. London: King's College London, 1988.

The Uses of Greek and Latin Historical Essays. London: Warburg Institute, University of London, 1988.

Dioscorides, Pedanius. *Der Wiener Dioskurides*. Graz: Akademische Druck und Verlagsanstalt, 1999.

Dotti, Franco, and Attilio Zanca. "Fatti e figure della medicina mantovana durante il tardo rinascimento." In *Mantova e i Gonzaga nella Civiltà del Rinascimento. Atti del convegno dall'Accademia Nazionale dei Lincei e dall'Accademia Virgiliana con la collaborazione della città di Mantova sotto l'alto patronato del Presidente della Repubblica Italiana Giovanni Leone, Mantova 6–8 ottobre 1974*, 393–97. Mantua: Accademia Virgiliana, 1977.

Duni, Matteo. *Tra religione e magia: storia del prete modenese Guglielmo Campana (1460?–1541)*. Florence: L. S. Olschki, 1999.

Under the Devil's Spell: Witches, Sorcerers, and the Inquisition in Renaissance Italy. Syracuse, NY: Syracuse University Press, 2007.

Dunkelgrün, Theodor. "The Hebrew Library of a Renaissance Humanist: Andreas Masius and the Bibliography to His *Iosuae Imperatoris Historia* (1574), with a Latin Edition and an Annotated English Translation." *Studia Rosenthaliana* 42–3 (2010–11): 197–252.

"The Multiplicity of Scripture: The Confluence of Textual Traditions in the Making of the Antwerp Polyglot Bible (1568–1573)." PhD dissertation, University of Chicago, 2012.

Durling, R. J. "Girolamo Mercuriale's De Modo Studendi." *Osiris* 6 (1990): 181–95.

Eamon, W. *Science and the Secrets of Nature: Books of Secrets in Medieval and Early Modern Culture*. Princeton: Princeton University Press, 1994.

"'With the Rules of Life and an Enema': Leonardo Fioravanti's Medical Primitivism." In *Renaissance and Revolution: Humanists, Scholars, Craftsmen and Natural Philosophers in Early Modern Europe*, edited by J. V. Field and Frank A. J. L. James, 29–44. Cambridge: Cambridge University Press, 1993.

Egmond, Florike, Paul Hoftijzer, and Robert P. W. Visser, eds. Carolus Clusius: *Towards a Cultural History of a Renaissance Naturalist*. Amsterdam: Royal Netherlands Academy of Arts and Sciences, 2007.

Elliot, John. *The Old World and the New: 1492–1650*. Cambridge: Cambridge University Press, 1974.

Ermini, Giuseppe. *Storia della università di Perugia*. Bologna: Nicola Zanichelli, 1947.

Farmer, Stephen Alan, ed. and trans. *Syncretism in the West: Pico's 900 Theses (1486); the Evolution of Traditional, Religious, and Philosophical Systems*. Tempe, AZ: Medieval and Renaissance Texts and Studies, 1998.

Fedalto, Giorgio. *Ricerche storiche sulla posizione giuridica ed ecclesiastica dei greci a Venezia nei secoli XV e XVI*. Florence: L. S. Olschki, 1967.

Fernández Álvarez, Manuel, ed. *La Universidad de Salamanca*. 3 vols. Salamanca: University of Salamanca, 1989.

Fernández Marcos, Natalio. *Introducción a las versiones griegas de la biblia. Textos y estudios Cardenal Cisneros*. Madrid: Consejo Superior de Investigaciones Cientificas, 1979.

Ferorelli, Nicola. *Gli ebrei nell'italia meridionale dall'età romana al secolo XVIII*. Bologna: Arnaldo Forni, 1980 [orig. 1915].

Ferrari, G. E. "Le opere a stampa del Guilandinus." In *Libri e stampatori in Padova*, edited by Giuseppe Bellini, 377–463. Padua: Tipografia Antoniana, 1959.

Ferrari, Giovanna. *L'esperienza del passato: Alessandro Benedetti filologo e medico umanista*. Florence: L. S. Olschki, 1996.

Ferrari, Marco. "I Secreti Medicinali." In *Cultura popolare nell'Emilia Romagna: medicina, erbe e magia*, edited by G. Adami and G. Tamagnini, 82–97. Milan: Silvana, 1981.

Ferri, Sara, ed. *Pietro Andrea Mattioli, Siena 1501–Trento 1570: la vita, le opere.* Perugia: Quattroemme, 1997.

"Profilo di Pietro Andrea Mattioli." In *I giardini dei semplici e gli orti botanici della Toscana*, edited by S. Ferri, and E. Miraldi, 159–64. Perugia: Quattroemme, 1993.

Field, Frederick. *Origenis Hexaplorum Quae Supersunt Sive Veterum Interpretum Graecorum in Totum Vetus Testamentum Fragmenta.* Hildesheim: G. Olms, 1964.

Fincati, Mariachiara. "Il restauro medievale dell'Esateuco ambrosiano a 147 Inf." BA thesis, Università Cattolica del Sacro Cuore, 2008.

"Per la storia dell'Esateuco ambrosiano a 147 Inf." *Aevum: rassegna di scienze storiche, linguistiche, filologiche* 83 (2009): 299–339.

Findlen, Paula. *Athanasius Kircher: The Last Man Who Knew Everything.* New York: Routledge, 2004.

"The Formation of a Scientific Community: Natural History in Sixteenth-Century Italy." In *Natural Particulars: Nature and the Disciplines in Renaissance Europe*, edited by Anthony Grafton and Nancy G. Siraisi, 369–400. Cambridge, MA: MIT Press, 1999.

"The Museum: Its Classical Etymology and Renaissance Genealogy." *Journal of the History of Collections* 1:1 (1989): 59–78.

Possessing Nature: Museums, Collecting, and Scientific Culture in Early Modern Italy. Berkeley: University of California Press, 1994.

"Possessing the Past: The Material World of the Italian Renaissance." *The American Historical Review* 103:1 (1998): 83–114.

Finkel, Ephraim. *R. Obadja Sforno als Exeget*. Breslau: Schatzky, 1896.

Firpo, Luigi. *Gastronomia del rinascimento*. Turin: Unione tipografico-editrice torinese, 1974.

Fragnito, Gigliola. "The Central and Peripheral Organization of Censorship." In *Church, Censorship, and Culture in Early Modern Italy*, edited by Gigliola Fragnito, 13–49. Cambridge: Cambridge University Press, 2001.

La Bibbia al rogo: la censura ecclesiastica e i volgarizzamenti della scrittura (1471–1605). Bologna: Il Mulino, 1997.

Proibito Capire: la chiesa e il volgare nella prima età moderna. Bologna: Il Mulino, 2005.

Franceschini, Adriano. "Privilegi dottorali concessi ad ebrei a Ferrara nel sec. XVI." *Atti e memorie della Deputazione provinciale ferrarese di storia patria* 3:19 (1975): 163–95.

Franchini, Dario. *La scienza a corte: collezionismo eclettico, natura e immagine a Mantova fra rinascimento e manierismo*. Rome: Bulzoni, 1979.

Frati, Lodovico. *Catalogo dei manoscritti di Ulisse Aldrovandi*. Bologna: N. Zanichelli, 1907.

Freudenthal, Gad. "Cosmogonie et physique chez Gersonide." *REJ* 145 (1986): 295–314.

"Gersonides: Levi Ben Gershom." In *History of Islamic Philosophy*, edited by Seyyed Hossein Nasr and Oliver Leaman, 739–54. London: Routledge, 2000.

ed. *Studies on Gersonides: A Fourteenth-Century Jewish Philosopher-Scientist.* Collection de travaux de l'Académie Internationale d'Histoire des Science, 36. Leiden: Brill, 1992.

Friedenwald, Harry. "Apologetic Work of Jewish Physicians." *JQR*, n.s., 32 (1941): 228–30, 407–8.

The Jews and Medicine. 2 vols. Baltimore: Johns Hopkins Press, 1944.

Funkenstein, Amos. *Theology and the Scientific Imagination: From the Middle Ages to the 17th Century.* Princeton: Princeton University Press, 1986.

Fürst, Julius. *Bibliotheca Judaica: Bibliographisches Handbuch der gesammten jüdischen Literatur mit Einschluss der Schriften über Juden und Judenthum und einer Geschichte der jüdischen Bibliographie.* 3 vols. Leipzig: W. Engelmann, 1849–63.

Garin, Eugenio. "L'umanesimo italiano e la cultura ebraica." In *Storia d'Italia, Annali, 11. Gli ebrei in Italia I: Dall'Alto Medioevo all'età dei ghetti*, edited by C. Vivanti, 361–83. Turin: Einaudi, 1996.

Garzoni, Tomaso. *La piazza universale di tutte le professioni del mondo.* Turin: G. Einaudi, 1996.

Gebhardt, Oscar, ed. *Graecus Venetus. Pentateuch Proverbiorum Ruth Cantici Ecclesiastae Threnorum Danielis Versio Graeca.* Leipzig: F.A. Brockhaus, 1875.

Geiger, Abraham. "Symmachus der Übersetzer der Bibel." *Jüdische Zeitschrift für Wissenschaft und Leben* 1 (1862): 39–64.

Gentilcore, David. *Healers and Healing in Early Modern Italy.* Manchester: Manchester University Press, 1998.

Medical Charlatanism in Early Modern Italy. Oxford: Oxford University Press, 2006.

Gillet, Philippe. *Par mets et par vins: voyages et gastronomies en Europe: Xve–Xviiie siècles.* Paris: Payot, 1985.

Ginsberg, Christian D., ed. and trans. *Jacob ben Chajim ibn Adonijah's Introduction to the Rabbinic Bible, Hebrew and English ... and the Massoreth ha-Massoreth of Elias Levita, being an exposition of the massoretic notes on the Hebrew Bible or the ancient critical apparatus of the Old Testament ...* London, 1867.

Glade, Winfried. *Die Taufe in den vorcanisianischen katholischen Katechismen des 16. Jahrhunderts im deutschen Sprachgebiet.* Nieuwkoop: B. de Graaf, 1979.

Gosselin, E.A. "A Listing of the Printed Editions of Nicholas de Lyra." *Traditio* 26 (1970): 399–426.

Grafton, Anthony. *Cardano's Cosmos: The Worlds and Works of a Renaissance Astrologer.* Cambridge, MA: Harvard University Press, 1999.

Defenders of the Text: The Traditions of Scholarship in an Age of Science, 1450–1800. Cambridge, MA: Harvard University Press, 1994.

"The Identities of History in Early Modern Europe: Prelude to a Study of the Artes Historicae." In *Historia: Empiricism and Erudition in Early Modern Europe*, edited by Gianna Pomata and Nancy Siraisi, 41–74. Cambridge, MA: MIT Press, 2005.

Joseph Scaliger: A Study in the History of Classical Scholarship. 2 vols. Oxford-Warburg Studies. Oxford: Oxford University Press, 1983–93.

New Worlds, Ancient Texts: The Power of Tradition and the Shock of Discovery. Cambridge, MA: Belknap Press of Harvard University Press, 1992.

"On the Scholarship of Politian and its Context." *Journal of the Warburg and Courtauld Institutes* 40 (1977): 150–88.

"Rhetoric, Philology and Egyptomania in the 1570s: J. J. Scaliger's Invective against M. Guilandinus's Papyrus." *Journal of the Warburg and Courtauld Institutes* 42 (1979): 167–94.

Grafton, Anthony, and Nancy G. Siraisi, eds. *Natural Particulars: Nature and the Disciplines in Renaissance Europe*. Cambridge, MA: MIT Press, 1999.

Grafton, Anthony, and Joanna Weinberg. *"I Have Always Loved the Holy Tongue": Isaac Casaubon, the Jews, and a Forgotten Chapter in Renaissance Scholarship*. Cambridge, MA: Harvard University Press, 2011.

Green, Jonathon. *Chasing the Sun: Dictionary Makers and the Dictionaries They Made*. New York: Henry Holt, 1996.

Grell, Chantal. *La République des lettres et l'histoire du Judaïsme antique: Xvie–Xviiie siècles*. Paris: Presses de l'Université Paris-Sorbonne, 1992.

Grell, Ole Peter. "In Search of True Knowledge: Ole Worm (1588–1654) and the New Philosophy." In *Making Knowledge in Early Modern Europe*, edited by Pamela Smith and Benjamin Schmidt, 214–32. Chicago: University of Chicago Press, 2007.

Grendler, Paul. "Italian Biblical Humanism and the Papacy." In *Biblical Humanism and Scholasticism in the Age of Erasmus*, edited by Erika Rummel, 227–76. Leiden: Brill, 2008.

The Universities of the Italian Renaissance. Baltimore: Johns Hopkins University Press, 2002.

Griffiths, Richard. *The Bible in the Renaissance: Essays on Biblical Commentary and Translation in the Fifteenth and Sixteenth Centuries*. Burlington, VT: Ashgate, 2001.

Griñó, Raimundo. "El Meturgeman de Elías Levita y el 'Arukh De Natán Ben Yehiel como fuentes de la lexicografía targúmica." *Biblica* 60:1 (1979): 110–17.

Güdemann, M. *Geschichte des Erziehungswesens und der Kultur der Juden in Italien während des Mittelalters*. Vienna: Alfred Hölder, 1884.

Guetta, Alessandro. "Abraham Portaleone from Science to Mysticism." In *Jewish Studies at the Turn of the Twentieth Century*, vol. 2: *Judaism from the Renaissance to Modern Times*, edited by Angel Sáenz-Badillos and Judit Targarona Borrás, 40–7. Leiden: Brill, 1999.

"Avraham Portaleone, le Scientifique Repenti." In *Torah et Science: Perspectives historiques et théoriques. Études offertes à Charles Touati*, edited by Gad Freudenthal, Jean-Pierre Rothschild, and Gilbert Dahan, 213–27. Leuven: Peeters, 2001.

Gutwirth, Eleazer. "Amatus Lusitanus and the Location of Sixteenth-Century Cultures." In *Cultural Intermediaries: Jewish Intellectuals in Early Modern*

Italy, edited by David Ruderman and Giuseppe Veltri, 216–34. Philadelphia: University of Pennsylvania Press, 2004.

"Jewish Bodies and Renaissance Melancholy: Culture and the City in Italy and the Ottoman Empire." In *The Jewish Body: Corporeality, Society, and Identity in the Renaissance and Early Modern Period*, edited by Maria Diemling and Giuseppe Veltri, 57–92. Leiden: Brill, 2009.

Habermann, Abraham. *Ha-madpis Zo'an di Garah u-reshimat sifre bet defuso, 324–370 (1564–1610)*. Lod: Mekhon Haberman, 1982.

"The Printer Israel ha-Zifroni and His Son Elishma, and the List of Books Which Were Printed by Them" [Hebrew]. In his *Studies in the History of Hebrew Printers and Books*, 215–92. Jerusalem: R. Mas, 1978.

Harkness, Deborah E. *The Jewel House: Elizabethan London and the Scientific Revolution*. New Haven: Yale University Press, 2007.

Harrán, Don. "Jewish Dramatists and Musicians in the Renaissance: Separate Activities, Common Aspirations." In *Musicologia Humana: Studies in Honor of Warren and Ursula Kirkendale*, edited by Siegried Gmeinwieser et al., 291–304. Florence: L. S. Olschki, 1994.

Harrison, Peter. *The Bible, Protestantism, and the Rise of Natural Science*. Cambridge: Cambridge University Press, 1998.

Harth, H., ed. *Lettere/ Poggio Bracciolini*. I: *Lettere a Niccolò Niccoli*. 3 vols. Florence: L. S. Olschki, 1984–7.

Harvey, Steven, ed. *The Medieval Hebrew Encyclopedias of Science and Philosophy*. Dordrecht: Kluwer Academic Publishers, 2000.

Haugen, Kristine Louise. "A French Jesuit's Lectures on Vergil, 1582–1583: Jacques Sirmond between Literature, History and Myth." *Sixteenth Century Journal* 30:4 (1999): 967–85.

Heide, Albert van der. "Created at Dusk: Abraham's Ram in Medieval Jewish Bible Exegesis." In *Jewish Studies in a New Europe: Proceedings of the Fifth Congress of Jewish Studies in Copenhagen 1994*, edited by Ulf Haxen, Hanne Trautner-Kromann, and Karen Lisa Goldschmidt Salamon, 365–71. Copenhagen: C.A. Reitzel A/S International Publishers, 1998.

Heller, J. L. "Notes on the Meaning of κολοκύντη." *Illinois Classical Studies* 10:1 (1985): 67–116.

Heller, Marvin. "Ambrosius Froben, Israel Zifroni and Hebrew Printing in Freiburg im Breisgau." *Gutenberg-Jahrbuch* 80 (2005): 137–48.

Holborn, Hajo, and Annemarie Holborn, eds. *Desiderius Erasmus Roterdamus Ausgewählte Werke*. Munich: C. H. Beck'sche Verlagsbuchhandlung, 1933.

Höpfl, Hildebrand. *Beiträge zur Geschichte der Sixto-Klementinischen Vulgata, nach gedruckten und ungedruckten Quellen von P. Hildebrand Höpfl*. Freiburg i. B.: Herder, 1913.

Horbury, William. *Hebrew Study from Ezra to Ben-Yehuda*. Edinburgh: T&T Clark, 1999.

Iakerson, Shimon. "An Autograph Manuscript by Elijah Levita in St Petersburg." In *Omnia in Eo: Studies on Jewish Books and Libraries in Honour of Adri Offenberg Celebrating the 125th Anniversary of the Bibliotheca Rosenthaliana in Amsterdam*. *Studia Rosenthaliana* 38–9 (2006): 178–85.

Idel, Moshe. *Language, Torah, and Hermeneutics in Abraham Abulafia*. Albany: State University of New York Press, 1988.

Rabbi Menachem Recanati Ha-Mekubal. Jerusalem: Shocken, 1998.

"The Study Program of R. Yoḥanan Alemanno." *Tarbiz* 48 (1979): 303–31.

Israel, Jonathan. *Diasporas within a Diaspora: Jews, Crypto-Jews, and the World of Maritime Empires (1540–1740)*. Boston: Brill, 2002.

Israëls, A. H. *Testamen Historico-Medicum, Exhibens Collectanea Gynaecologica, Quae Ex Talmude Babylonico Depromsit*. Groningen: P. van Zweeden, 1845.

Jacoby, David. "Jewish Doctors and Surgeons in Crete under Venetian Control." In *Tarbut Ve-Ḥevrah be-Toldot Yisrael Bi-Yeme-Ha-Benayim*, edited by Reuven Bonfil, Menahem Ben-Sasson, and Joseph Hacker, 431–44. Jerusalem, 1989.

Jacquart, Danielle. "Theory, Everyday Practice, and Three Fifteenth-Century Physicians." In *Renaissance Medical Learning: Evolution of a Tradition*, edited by Michael R. McVaugh and Nancy G. Siraisi, 140–60. Philadelphia: History of Science Society, 1991.

Jütte, Daniel. "Abramo Colorni, jüdischer Hofalchemist Herzog Friedrichs I., und die hebräische Handelskompanie des Maggino Gabrielli in Würtemberg am ende des 16. Jahrhunderts." *Aschkenaz-Zeitschrift für Geschichte und Kultur der Juden* 15 (2005): 435–98.

Kagan, Richard L. "Universities in Castile 1500–1700." *Past and Present* 49 (1970): 44–71.

Kaplan, Yosef. *An Alternative Path to Modernity: The Sephardi Diaspora in Western Europe*. Leiden: Brill, 2000.

"Wayward New Christians and Stubborn New Jews: The Shaping of a Jewish Identity." *Jewish History* 8:2 (1994): 27–41.

Kassell, Lauren. "'The Food of Angels': Simon Forman's Alchemical Medicine." In *Secrets of Nature: Astrology and Alchemy in Early Modern Europe*, edited by William R. Newman and Anthony Grafton, 345–84. Cambridge, MA: MIT Press.

Kaufmann, David. "Jewish Ethical Wills: Texts and Additions." *JQR*, o.s., 4:2 (1892): 333–41.

"Leone de' Sommi Portaleone (1527–92): Dramatist and Founder of a Synagogue at Mantua." *JQR* 1 (1898): 445–61.

Kelley, Donald. *Foundations of Modern Historical Scholarship: Language, Law, and History in the French Renaissance*. New York: Columbia University Press, 1970.

Kessler, Eckhard, and Ian Maclean, eds. *Res et verba in der Renaissance*. Wiesbaden: Harrassowitz in Kommission, 2002.

Kisch, Guido, ed. *Pseudo-Philo's Liber Antiquitatum Biblicum*. Notre Dame: University of Notre Dame, 1949.

Klepper, Deeana Copeland. *The Insight of Unbelievers: Nicholas of Lyra and Christian Reading of Jewish Text in the Later Middle Ages*. Philadelphia: University of Pennsylvania Press, 2007.

Klijn, Albertus Frederik Johannes. *Seth in Jewish, Christian and Gnostic Literature*. Leiden: Brill, 1977.

Kottek, Samuel S. "Jews between Profane and Sacred Science in Renaissance Italy: The Case of Abraham Portaleone." In *Religious Confessions and the Sciences in the Sixteenth Century*, edited by Jurgen Helm and Annette Winkelman, 108–18. Leiden: Brill, 2001.

Krey, Phillip D. W., and Lesley Smith, eds. *Nicholas of Lyra: The Senses of Scripture.* Leiden: Brill, 2000.

Kristeller, Paul Oskar. *Iter Italicum.* London: Warburg Institute, 1963–97.

Kristeller, Paul Oskar, et al. *Catalogus Translationum et Commentariorum: Mediaeval and Renaissance Latin Translations and Commentaries; Annotated Lists and Guides.* Washington, DC: Catholic University of America Press, 1960–.

Kudlien, F. "Zwei medizinische Polemiken am ende des XVI Jahrunderts." *Gesnerus* 22 (1965): 85–92.

Kümmel, Werner. "Melancholie und die Macht der Musik: Die Krankheit König Sauls in der historischen Diskussion," *Medizinhistorisches Journal* 3–4 (1968–69): 189–209.

Lain Entralgo, Pedro. *La Historia Clinica: Historia y teoria del relato patografico.* Madrid: Consejo Superior de Investigaciones cientificas, 1950.

LeBachelet, X.-M. *Bellarmin et la Bible Sixto-Clementine.* Paris: G. Beauchesne, 1911.

Laplanche, François. *L'écriture, le sacré et l'histoire: erudites et politiques protestants devant La Bible en France au XVIIe siècle.* Amsterdam: APA-Holland University Press, 1986.

Lawee, Eric. *Isaac Abravanel's Stance towards Tradition: Defense, Dissent and Dialogue.* Albany, NY: SUNY Press, 2001.

Lehoux, Françoise. *Le cadre de vie des médecins parisiens aux XVIe et XVIIe siècles.* Paris: A. et J. Picard, 1976.

Lelli, Fabrizio. "L'Educazione ebraica nella seconda metà del '400: poetica e scienze naturali nel Ḥay Ha-'Olamim di Yoḥanan Alemanno." *Rinascimento* 36 (1996): 75–136.

Lesley, Arthur. "Jewish Adaptation of Humanist Concepts in Fifteenth- and Sixteenth-Century Italy." In *Renaissance Rereadings: Intertext and Context*, edited by Maryanne Cline Horowitz, 52–64. Urbana: University of Illinois Press, 1988.

Lieberman, Saul. *Greek in Jewish Palestine: Studies in the Life and Manners of Jewish Palestine in the II–IV Centuries C.E.* New York: Jewish Theological Seminary of America, 1942.

Long, Pamela. *Openness, Secrecy, Authorship: Technical Arts and the Culture of Knowledge from Antiquity to the Renaissance.* Baltimore: Johns Hopkins University Press, 2001.

Lowry, Martin. *The World of Aldus Manutius: Business and Scholarship in Renaissance Venice.* Ithaca, NY: Cornell University Press, 1979.

Lüthy, Christoph. "What to Do with Seventeenth-Century Natural Philosophy? A Taxonomic Problem." *Perspectives on Science* 8:2 (2000): 164–95.

Luzzati, Michele. "Il medico ebreo e il contadino: un documento pisano del 1462." *La Rassegna mensile di Israel* 45 (1979): 385–92.

Maclean, Ian. *Logic, Signs, and Nature in the Renaissance: The Case of Learned Medicine.* Cambridge: Cambridge University Press, 2002.

"The Medical Republic of Letters before the Thirty Years War." *Intellectual History Review* 18:1 (2008): 15–30.

Maggiulli, Gigliola. *Nomenclatura micologica latina*. Genoa: Istituto di Filologia Classica e Medievale, 1977.

Manuel, Frank. *The Broken Staff: Judaism through Christian Eyes*. Cambridge, MA: Harvard University Press, 1992.

Margolin, Jean. *Pratiques et discours Alimentaires à la Renaissance: actes du colloque de Tours de Mars 1979, Centre d'Études Supérieures de la Renaissance*. Paris: G.-P. Maisonneuve et Larose, 1982.

Martin, Craig. "Printed Medical Commentaries and Authenticity: The Case of De Alimento." *Journal of the Washington Academy of Sciences* 90:4 (2004): 17–28.

Martin, John. *Venice's Hidden Enemies: Italian Heretics in a Renaissance City*. Berkeley: University of California Press, 1993.

McCuaig, William. *Carlo Sigonio: The Changing World of the Late Renaissance*. Princeton: Princeton University Press, 1989.

Mecchia, Angelo. "Cenni di geriatria in un'opera del medico umbro Davide de' Pomi (1525–1600)." *Pagine di Storia della medicina* 10 (1996): 58–62.

Migne, J. P. *Patrologiae cursus completus series latina*. 221 vols. Paris: J. P. Migne 1844–64.

Miletto, Gianfranco. *La biblioteca di Avraham ben David Portaleone secondo l'inventario della sua eredità*. Florence: L. S. Olschki, 2013.

"Die Zulassung der jüdischen Ärzte in Italien während der Gegenreform: der Fall Portaleone." *Biblische Notizen* 116 (2003): 48–55.

Glauben und Wissen im Zeitalter der Reformation: der salomonische Tempel bei Abraham Ben David Portaleone (1542–1612). Berlin: de Gruyter, 2004.

"The Teaching Program of David Ben Abraham and His Son Abraham Provenzali in Its Historical-Cultural Context." In *Cultural Intermediaries: Jewish Intellectuals in Early Modern Italy*, edited by David Ruderman and Giuseppe Veltri, 127–48. Philadelphia: University of Pennsylvania Press, 2004.

Miller, Peter N. "Lost and Found." *JQR*, n.s., 97:4 (2007): 502–7.

Momigliano and Antiquarianism: Foundations of the Modern Cultural Sciences. Toronto: University of Toronto Press, 2007.

Momigliano, Arnaldo. "Ancient History and the Antiquarian." *Journal of the Warburg and Courtauld Institutes* 13 (1950): 285–315.

Tra storia e storicismo. Pisa: Nistri-Lischi, 1985.

Morisi Guerra, Anna. "Incontri ebraico-cristiani. Il Salterio poliglotto di Santi Pagnini." In Morisi Guerra, *Itinerari ebraico-cristiani: società, cultura, mito*, 9–37. Fasano: Schena, 1987.

"Santi Pagnini traducteur de la Bible." In *Théorie et pratique de l'exégèse*, edited by I. Backus and F. Higman, 191–98. Geneva: Droz, 1990.

Mottana, A. "Le 'miracolose virtù delle pietre pretiose per salute del vivere humano' di Scipione Vasolo: un trattatello rinascimentale sulle gemme come mezzi per mantenersi in salute senza ricorrere a medicine." *Rendiconti Lincei* 16:1 (2005): 19–73.

Mugnai Carrara, Daniela. *La Biblioteca di Nicolò Leoniceno: tra Aristotele e Galeno, cultura e libri di un medico umanista*. Florence: L. S. Olschki, 1991.

"Profilo di Niccolò Leoniceno." *Interpres* 2 (1979): 169–212.

Münster, Ladislao. "L'*Enarratio brevis de senum affectibus*' [bref commentaire aux maladies des vieillards] de David de' Pomi, le plus grand médecin israélite au XVIe siècle." *Revue d'Histoire de la Médicine Hebraique* 20 (1954): 7–16, 125–36. Reprinted in *Mélanges d'histoire de la médicine hébraïque; études choisies de la "Revue d'histoire de la médicine hébraïque" (1948–1985)*, edited by Gad Freudenthal and Samuel Kottek, 161–81. Leiden: Brill, 2003.

Myers, David N., et al., eds. *Acculturation and Its Discontents: The Italian Jewish Experience between Exclusion and Integration.* Toronto: University of Toronto Press, 2008.

Nance, Brian. "Wondrous Experience as Text: Valleriola and the Observationes Medicinales." In *Textual Healing: Essays on Medieval and Early Modern Medicine*, edited by Elizabeth Lane Furdell, 101–18. Leiden: Brill, 2005.

Nauert, Charles. "Humanists, Scientists, and Pliny: Changing Approaches to a Classical Author." *American Historical Review* 84:1 (1979): 72–85.

Navarrini, Roberto. "Note sui medici ebrei attivi in Mantova nei secoli XV–XVIII." *Postumia: annali del museo d'arte moderna dell'Alto Mantovano* 6 (1995): 64–9.

Nelles, Paul. "Juste Lipse et Alexandrie: les origines antiquaires de l'histoire des Bibliothèques." In *Le pouvoir des bibliothèques. La mémoire des livres dans la culture occidentale*, edited by Marc Baratin and Christian Jacob, 224–42. Paris: Albin Michel, 1996.

"The Renaissance Ancient Library Tradition and Christian Antiquity." In *Humanists and their Libraries*, edited by R. de Smet, 157–71. Brussels: Peeters, 2002.

Netanyahu, B. *Don Isaac Abravanel, Statesman and Philosopher*. Philadelphia: Jewish Publication Society of America, 1953.

Neuman, Kalman. "The Literature of the Respublica Judaica: Descriptions of the Ancient Israelite Polity in the Antiquarian Writing of the Sixteenth and Seventeenth Centuries." PhD dissertation, Hebrew University, 2002.

Novoa, James Nelson. "Andrés Laguna in Papal Rome: The Documents of the Mozoncillo Ecclesiastical Benefice." *Minvera* 25 (2012): 211–32.

Nummedal, Tara. *Alchemy and Authority in the Holy Roman Empire*. Chicago: University of Chicago Press, 2007.

Nutton, Vivian. *Ancient Medicine*. London: Routledge, 2004.

"Greek Science in the Sixteenth-Century Renaissance." In *Renaissance and Revolution: Humanists, Scholars, Craftsmen and Natural Philosophers in Early Modern Europe*, edited by J. V. Field and Frank A. J. L. James, 15–28. Cambridge: Cambridge University Press, 1993.

"Hellenism Postponed: Some Aspects of Renaissance Medicine, 1490–1530." *Sudhoffs Archiv* 81 (1997): 158–70.

"John Caius and the Eton Galen: Medical Philology in the Renaissance." *Medizinhistorisches Journal* (1985): 227–52.

ed. *Medicine at the Courts of Europe, 1500–1837*. London: Routledge, 1990.

"'Prisci Dissectionum Professores:' Greek Texts and Renaissance Anatomists." In *The Uses of Latin and Greek: Historical Essays,* edited by A. C. Dionisotti, Anthony Grafton, and Jill Kraye, 111–26. London: Warburg Institute, 1988.

"The Rise of Medical Humanism: Ferrara, 1464–1555." *Renaissance Studies* 11:1 (1997): 2–19.

Oberman, Heiko A. *The Harvest of Medieval Theology: Gabriel Biel and Late Medieval Nominalism*. Cambridge, MA: Harvard University Press, 1963.

Oberman, Heiko A., and Frank A. James III, eds. *Via Augustini: Augustine in the Later Middle Ages, Renaissance, and Reformation: Essays in Honor of Damasus Trapp, O.S.A.* Leiden: Brill, 1991.

O'Connor, Michael. "A Neglected Facet of Cardinal Cajetan: Biblical Reform in High Renaissance Rome." In *The Bible in the Renaissance: Essays on Biblical Commentary and Translation in the Fifteenth and Sixteenth Centuries*, edited by Richard Griffiths, 71–94. London: Ashgate, 2001.

Offenbach, A. *Bibliography of the Works of Jacob Jehudah Leon (Templo)*. Studia Rosenthaliana 12:1–2 (1978): 111–32.

Ogilvie, Brian W. "Natural History, Ethics, and Physico-Theology." In *Historia: Empiricism and Erudition in Early Modern Europe*, edited by Nancy G. Siraisi and Gianna Pomata, 75–104. Cambridge, MA: MIT Press, 2005.

The Science of Describing: Natural History in Renaissance Europe. Chicago: University of Chicago Press, 2006.

Old, Hughes. *The Shaping of the Reformed Baptismal Rite in the Sixteenth Century*. Grand Rapids, MI: Eerdmans, 1992.

Olmi, Giuseppe. *Inventario del Mondo: catalogazione della natura e luoghi del sapere nella prima età moderna*. Milan: Il Mulino, 1992.

"'Molti Amici in Varij Luoghi': Studio della natura e rapporti epistolari nel secolo XVI." *Nuncius. Annali di Storia della Scienza* 1 (1991): 3–31.

Olmi, Giuseppe, and Paolo Prodi. "Art, Science, and Nature in Bologna c. 1600." In *The Age of Correggio and the Carracci: Emilian Painting of the Sixteenth and Seventeenth Centuries*, 213–36.Washington, DC: National Gallery of Art, 1986.

Ongaro, Giuseppe. "Contributi alla biografia di Prospero Alpino." *Acta medicae historiae patavina* 8–9 (1961): 79–168.

Pagel, Walter. "Religious Motives in the Medical Biology of the XVIIth Century." *Bulletin of the Institute of the History of Medicine* 3 (1935): 97–128, 213–31, 265–312.

Paladini, Alba. *Il De arcanis di Pietro Galatino: traditio giudaica e nuove istanze filologiche*. Galatina: Congedo, 2004.

Palmer, Richard. "Medical Botany in Northern Italy in the Renaissance." *Journal of the Royal Society of Medicine* 78 (1985): 149–57.

"Nicolò Massa, His Family and His Fortune." *Medical History* 25:4 (1981): 385–410.

Pani, Giancarlo. "Un centenaire a rappeler: l'edition sixtine de la septante." In *Théorie et pratique de l'exégèse: Actes du Troisième Colloque international sur l'histoire de l'exégèse biblique au XVIe siècle (Genève, 31 août–2 septembre 1988)*, edited by Irena Backus and Francis Higman, 413–28. Geneva: Droz, 1990.

Parente, Fausto. "La chiesa e il Talmud." In *Gli Ebrei in Italia*, edited by Corrado Vivanti, 521–643. Turin: G. Einaudi, 1996.

Park, Katharine. *Doctors and Medicine in Early Renaissance Florence*. Princeton: Princeton University Press, 1985.

"The Organic Soul." In *The Cambridge History of Renaissance Philosophy*, edited by Charles B. Schmitt and Quentin Skinner, 464–84. Cambridge: Cambridge University Press, 1988.

Park, Katharine, and L. Daston, eds. *The Cambridge History of Science*. Vol. 3: *Early Modern Science*. Cambridge: Cambridge University Press, 2003.

Wonders and the Order of Nature, 1150–1750. New York: Zone Books, 1998.

Park, Katharine, and John Henderson. "'The First Hospital among Christians': The Ospedale di Santa Maria Nuova in Early Sixteenth-Century Florence." *Medical History* 35 (1991): 164–88.

Paschini, Pio. "Un cardinale editore: Marcello Cervini." In Paschini, *Cinquecento romano e riforma cattolica*, 185–217. Rome: Facultas Theologica Pontificii Athenaei Lateranensis, 1958.

Pazzini, Adalberto. "La medicina alla corte dei Gonzaga a Mantova." In *Mantova e i Gonzaga nelle civiltà del rinascimento*, 291–351. Mantua: A. Mondadori, 1977.

Pazzini, Massimo. "Registrazione e definitione del lemma nel dizionario di Rabbi David De Pomis." *Liber Annuus* 43 (1993): 261–76.

Penkower, Jordan S. "The Chapter Divisions of the 1525 Rabbinic Bible." *Vetus Testamentum* 48:3 (1998): 350–74.

"Jacob ben Hayyim and the Rise of the Biblia Rabbinica." PhD dissertation, Hebrew University, 1982.

"S. D. Luzzatto, Vowels, and Accents and the Date of the Zohar." In *Samuel David Luzzatto*, edited by Robert Bonfil, Isaac Gotlieb, and Hannah Kasher, 79–130. Jerusalem: Magnes Press, 2004.

Perles, Joseph. *Beiträge zur Geschichte der hebräischen und aramäischen Studien*. Munich: Theodor Ackermann, 1884.

Peroni, Vincenzo. *Biblioteca bresciana di Brescia 1818–23*. Bologna: Forni, 1968.

Perrat, Charles. "Les humanistes amateurs de papyrus." *Bibliothèque de l'école des Chartes* 109 (1951): 173–92.

Pinon, Laurent. "Conrad Gesner and the Historical Depth of Renaissance Natural History." In *Historia: Empiricism and Erudition in Early Modern Europe*, edited by Gianna Pomata and Nancy G. Siraisi, 241–59. Cambridge, MA: MIT Press, 2005.

Livres de zoologie de la Renaissance: une anthologie 1450–1700. Paris: Klincksieck, 1995.

Pomata, Gianna. "Sharing Cases: The Observationes in Early Modern Medicine." *Early Science and Medicine* 15 (2010): 193–236.

Pomata, Gianna, and Nancy G. Siraisi, eds. *Historia: Empiricism and Erudition in Early Modern Europe*. Cambridge, MA: MIT Press, 2005.

Porfyriou, Heleni. "La diaspora greca in italia dopo la caduta di Constantinopoli: Ancona, Napoli, Livorno e Genova." In *I greci a venezia*, edited by Maria Francesca Tiepolo and Eurigio Tonetti, 151–84. Venice: Istituto Veneto di Scienze, Lettere, ed Arti, 2002.

Portuondo, Maria. "The Study of Nature, Philosophy, and the Royal Library of San Lorenzo of the Escorial." *Renaissance Quarterly* 63:4 (2010): 1106–50.

Pozzi, G. *Introduzione a Hermolai Barbari Castigationes Plinianae et in Pomponium Melam*. Padua: Antenore, 1972.

Premuda, Loris. "La medicina e l'organizzazione sanitaria." In *Storia Della Cultura Veneta: Il Seicento Vol. 4/Pt. 2*, edited by Girolamo Arnaldi and Manlio Pastore Stocchi, 115–50. Vicenza: N. Pozza, 1984.

Preto, Paolo. *Peste e società a Venezia nel 1576*. Vicenza: N. Pozza, 1978.

Preuss, Julius. *Biblical and Talmudic Medicine*. Translated by Fred Rosner. New York: Sanhedrin Press, 1978.

Prijs, Joseph. *Die Basler hebräischen Drucke, 1492–1866. Bearbeitet von J. Prijs. Ergänzt und herausgegeben von Bernhard Prijs*. Olten: Urs Graf-Verlag, 1964.

Prodi, Paolo. *Il Cardinale Gabriele Paleotti (1522–1597)*. Rome: Edizioni di Storia e Letteratura, 1959–67.

"Vecchi appunti e nuove reflessioni su Carlo Sigonio." In *Nunc alia tempora, alii mores: storici e storia in età postridentina*, edited by Massimo Firpo, 291–310. Florence: L. S. Olschki, 2005.

Raz-Krakotzkin, Amnon. *The Censor, the Editor, and the Text*. Translated by Jackie Feldman. Philadelphia: University of Pennsylvania Press, 2007.

Reeds, Karen. *Botany in Medieval and Renaissance Universities*. New York: Garland, 1991.

"Renaissance Humanism and Botany." *Annals of Science* 33 (1976): 519–42.

Reiner, Elchanan. "The Ashkenazi Élite at the Beginning of the Modern Era: Manuscript versus Printed Book." In *Jews in Early Modern Poland*, edited by Gershon Hundert, 85–98. Polin, vol. 10. Oxford: Basil Blackwell Institute for Polish-Jewish Studies, 1997.

"The Attitude of Ashkenazi Society to the New Science in the Sixteenth Century." *Science in Context* 10 (1997): 589–603.

"Transformations in the Polish and Ashkenazic Yeshivot during the Sixteenth and Seventeenth Centuries and the Dispute over Pilpul" (Hebrew). In *Ke-Minhag Ashkenaz ve-Polin: Sefer Yovel le-Chone Shmeruk*, edited by Israel Bartal, Chava Turnianksy, and Ezra Mendelsohn, 9–80. Jerusalem: Zalman Shazar, 1989.

Rhodes, Dennis E. *La vita e le opere di Castore Durante e della sua famiglia*. Viterbo: Agnesotti, 1968.

Rice, Eugene. *Saint Jerome in the Renaissance*. Baltimore: Johns Hopkins University Press, 1985.

Richardson, Brian. *Print Culture in Renaissance Italy: The Editor and the Vernacular Text, 1470–1600*. Cambridge: Cambridge University Press, 1994.

Rieger, Paul, and Hermann Vogelstein. *Geschichte der Juden in Rom*. Berlin: Mayer & Müller, 1895.

Roger, Jacques. *Les Sciences de la vie dans la pensée française du XVIIIe siècle: La génération des animaux de Descartes a l'encyclopédie*. Paris: Colin, 1963.

Rossi, Azariah de'. *The Light of the Eyes*. Translated and edited by Joanna Weinberg. New Haven: Yale University Press, 2001.

Rossi, Paolo. *Philosophy, Technology, and the Arts in the Early Modern Era*. Translated by Salvator Attanasio. New York: Harper & Row, 1970.

Roth, Cecil. *The Jewish Contribution to Civilization*. London: Macmillan, 1938.

The Jews in the Renaissance. Philadelphia: Jewish Publication Society of America, 1977 [1959].

Rothschild, J.-P. "Les listes de livres, reflet de la culture des juifs en Italie du nord au XVe et au XVIe siècle?" In *Manoscritti, frammenti e libri ebraici nell'Italia dei secoli XV–XVI*, edited by G. Tamani and A. Vivian, 163–93. Rome: Carucci, 1991.

Roussel, B. "Connaissance et Interprétation du Judaism Antique: des Biblistes Chrétiens de la Seconde Moitié du XVIe Siècle." In *La République des Lettres et l'histoire du Judaïsme antique XVIe–XVIIIe siècles*, edited by Chantal Grell and François Laplanche, 21–50. Paris: Presses de l'Université Paris-Sorbonne, 1992.

Ruderman, David. *Early Modern Jewry: A New Cultural History*. Princeton: Princeton University Press, 2010.

Essential Papers on Jewish Culture in Renaissance and Baroque Italy. New York: New York University Press, 1992.

"The Italian Renaissance and Jewish Thought." In *Renaissance Humanism: Foundations, Forms, and Legacy*, edited by Albert Rabil Jr., 1:382–433. Philadelphia: University of Pennsylvania Press, 1988.

Jewish Enlightenment in an English Key: Anglo-Jewry's Construction of Modern Jewish Thought. Princeton: Princeton University Press, 2000.

Jewish Thought and Scientific Discovery in Early Modern Europe. New Haven: Yale University Press, 1995.

Kabbalah, Magic, and Science: The Cultural Universe of a Sixteenth-Century Jewish Physician. Cambridge, MA: Harvard University Press, 1988.

"Unicorns, Great Beasts, and the Marvelous Variety of Things in Nature in the Thought of Abraham B. Hananiah Yagel." In *Jewish Thought in the Seventeenth Century*, edited by Isidore Twersky, and Bernard Septimus, 343–64. Cambridge, MA: Harvard University Press, 1987.

The World of a Renaissance Jew: The Life and Thought of Abraham Ben Mordecai Farissol. Cincinnati: Hebrew Union College Press, 1981.

Ruderman, David, and Giuseppe Veltri, eds. *Cultural Intermediaries: Jewish Intellectuals in Early Modern Italy*. Philadelphia: University of Pennsylvania Press, 2004.

Rutkin, H. Darrel. "Astrology." In *Cambridge History of Science*, vol. 3: *Early Modern Science*, edited by Katharine Park and Lorraine Daston, 541–61. Cambridge: Cambridge University Press, 2008.

Sacerdote, Gustave. "Deux index expurgatoires de livres Hebreux." *REJ* 30 (1896): 262–71.

Salvesen, Alison. *Symmachus in the Pentateuch*. Manchester: University of Manchester, 1991.

Sánchez Manzano, María Asunción. *Prefacios de Benito Arias Montano a La Biblia Regia de Felipe II*. Vol. 32: *Colección Humanistas Españoles*. Salamanca: Universidad de León, 2006.

Santoro, M. "La polemica pliniana fra Leoniceno e Collenuccio." *Filologia Romanza* 3 (1956): 162–205.

Sarton, George. *Introduction to the History of Science*. Washington, DC: Carnegie Institution, 1927.

Saxl, Fritz. "Veritas Filia Temporis." In *Philosophy and History: Essays Presented to Ernst Cassirer*, edited by R. Klibansky and H. J. Paton, 197–222. Oxford: Clarendon Press, 1936.

Scalvanti, Oscar. "Lauree in medicina di studenti israeliti a Perugia nel secolo XVI." *Annali della facoltà di Giurisprudenza di Perugia*, 3rd ser., 7 (1910): 91–129.
Schäfer, Daniel. *Geburt aus dem Tod. Der Kaiserschnitt an Verstorbenen in der abendländischen Kultur*. Hürtgenwald: Guido Pressler, 1999.
Schiller-Szinessy, Salomon. *Catalogue of the Hebrew Manuscripts Preserved in the University Library, Cambridge*. Cambridge, 1876.
Schmitt, Charles B. *Gianfrancesco Pico della Mirandola (1469–1533) and His Critique of Aristotle*. The Hague: Martinus Nijhoff, 1967.
"Philosophy and Science in Sixteenth-Century Italian Universities." In *The Renaissance: Essays in Interpretation*, edited by André Chastel et al., 297–336. London: Methuen, 1982.
Schmitz, Rudolf, and Gundolf Keil, eds. *Humanismus und Medizin*. Weinheim: Acta Humaniora, 1984.
Schulte, F., and A. L. Richter, eds. *Canones et decreta concilii Tridentini*. Leipzig, 1853.
Sella, Domenico. *Italy in the Seventeenth Century*. London: Longman, 1997.
Serassi, Pierantonio. *La vita di Torquato Tasso*. Rome: Pagliarini, 1785.
Sermoneta, Giuseppe. "Considerazioni frammentarie sul giudeo-italiano." *Italia: Studi e ricerche sulla cultura e sulla letteratura degli ebrei d'Italia* 1 (1976): 1–29; 2 (1978): 62–106.
Un volgarizzamento giudeo-italiano del Cantico dei Cantici. Florence: G. C. Sansoni, 1974.
Serrai, Alfredo. *Storia della Bibliografia*. Rome: Bulzoni, 1993.
Shalem, Shimon. *Rabi Mosheh Alshekh*. Jerusalem: Ben Zvi Institute, 1966.
Shalev, Zur. "Sacred Geography, Antiquarianism and Visual Erudition: Benito Arias Montano and the Maps in the Antwerp Polyglot Bible." *Imago Mundi: The International Journal for the History of Cartography* 55:1 (2003): 56–80.
Sacred Worlds and Words: Geography, Religion, and Scholarship, 1550–1700. Leiden: Brill, 2012.
Shapiro, Barbara. *A Culture of Fact: England, 1550–1720*. Ithaca, NY: Cornell University Press, 2000.
Shatzmiller, Joseph. *Shylock Reconsidered: Jews, Moneylending, and Medieval Society*. Berkeley: University of California Press, 1990.
Sheehan, Jonathan. *The Enlightenment Bible: Translation, Scholarship, Culture*. Princeton: Princeton University Press, 2005.
Shuger, Deborah. *The Renaissance Bible: Scholarship, Sacrifice, and Subjectivity*. Berkeley: University of California Press, 1994.
Shulvass, Moses. *The Jews in the World of the Renaissance*. Leiden: Brill, 1973.
"The Knowledge of Antiquity among the Italian Jews of the Renaissance." *Proceedings of the American Academy for Jewish Research* 18 (1949): 291–310.
Siegmund, Stefanie. *The Medici State and the Ghetto of Florence: The Construction of an Early Modern Jewish Community*. Stanford: Stanford University Press, 2006.
Simoncelli, Paolo. *La lingua di Adamo: Guillaume Postel tra accademici e fuoriusciti fiorentini*. Florence: L. S. Olschki, 1984.

Simonsohn, Shlomo. *History of the Jews in the Duchy of Mantua*. Jerusalem: Kiryath Sepher, 1977.

"Jewish Education in the Renaissance (until the 17th Century)" (Hebrew). In *Entsiklopedya Ḥinukhit*, 4:376–81. Jerusalem: Mosad Bialik, 1959–74.

Siraisi, Nancy G. "Anatomizing the Past: Physicians and History in Renaissance Culture." *Renaissance Quarterly* 53 (2000): 1–30.

Avicenna in Renaissance Italy: The Canon and Medical Teaching in Italian Universities after 1500. Princeton: Princeton University Press, 1987.

"Cardano and the History of Medicine." In *Girolamo Cardano. Le opere, le fonti, la vita*, edited by Marialuisa Baldi and Guido Canziani, 342–62. Milan: F. Angeli, 1999.

The Clock and the Mirror: Girolamo Cardano and Renaissance Medicine. Princeton: Princeton University Press, 1997.

"Giovanni Argenterio and Sixteenth-Century Medical Innovation: Between Princely Patronage and Academic Controversy." *Osiris* 6 (1990): 161–80.

"History, Antiquarianism, and Medicine: The Case of Girolamo Mercuriale." *Journal of the History of Ideas* 64 (2003): 231–51.

History, Medicine, and the Traditions of Renaissance Learning. Ann Arbor: University of Michigan Press, 2007.

"In Search of the Origins of Medicine: Egyptian Wisdom and Some Renaissance Physicians." In *Generation and Degeneration: Tropes of Reproduction in Literature and History from Antiquity through Early Modern Europe*, edited by Valeria Finucci and Kevin Brownlee, 235–61. Durham, NC: Duke University Press, 2001.

Medieval and Early Renaissance Medicine: An Introduction to Knowledge and Practice. Chicago: University of Chicago Press, 1990.

Skalli, Cedric Cohen. "The Humanist Rhetoric of Don Isaac Abravanel: Rhetoric, History and Tradition in His Introductions and Letters." PhD dissertation, Tel Aviv University, 2005.

Skinner, Quentin, Eckhard Kessler, and Jill Kraye, eds. *The Cambridge History of Renaissance Philosophy*. Cambridge: Cambridge University Press, 1988.

Smith, Pamela H. *The Body of the Artisan: Art and Experience in the Scientific Revolution*. Chicago: University of Chicago Press, 2004.

The Business of Alchemy: Science and Culture in the Holy Roman Empire. Princeton: Princeton University Press, 1994.

Smith, Pamela, and Benjamin Schmidt, eds. *Making Knowledge in Early Modern Europe: Practices, Objects, and Texts, 1400–1800*. Chicago: University of Chicago Press, 2007.

Spierling, Karen. *Infant Baptism in Reformation Geneva: The Shaping of a Community, 1536–1564*. Burlington, VT: Ashgate, 2005.

Spini, Giorgio. *Tra rinascimento e riforma*. Florence: La Nuova Italia, 1940.

Stannard, Jerry. "P. A. Mattioli: Sixteenth-Century Commentator on Dioscorides." *University of Kansas Library Bibliographic Contributions* 1 (1969): 59–81.

Starnes, DeWitt. *Renaissance Dictionaries: English-Latin and Latin-English*. Austin: University of Texas Press, 1954.

Steinke, H. "Medical Correspondence in Early Modern Europe. An Introduction." *Gesnerus* 61:3–4 (2004): 139–60.

Steinmetz, David, ed. *The Bible in the Sixteenth Century*. Durham, NC: Duke University Press, 1990.

Steinschneider, Moritz. "Lapidarien, ein kulturgeschichtliches Versuch." In *Semitic Studies (in Honor of Dr. A. Kohut)*, 1:42–72. Berlin: S. Calvary, 1897.

Stenhouse, William. *Reading Inscriptions and Writing Ancient History: Historical Scholarship in the Late Renaissance*. London: Institute of Classical Studies University of London School of Advanced Study, 2005.

Stinger, Charles. "Italian Renaissance Learning and the Church Fathers." In *The Reception of the Church Fathers in the West: From the Carolingians to the Maurists*, edited by Irena Backus, 473–510. Leiden: Brill, 2001.

Stolzenberg, Daniel. "Egyptian Oedipus: Antiquarianism, Oriental Studies and Occult Philosophy in the Work of Athanasius Kircher." PhD dissertation, Stanford University, 2003.

The Great Art of Knowing: The Baroque Encyclopedia of Athanasius Kircher. Stanford: Stanford University Libraries, 2001.

Stow, Kenneth. *Theater of Acculturation: the Roman Ghetto in the Sixteenth Century*. Seattle: University of Washington Press, 2001.

Sutcliffe, Edmund. "The Council of Trent on the Authentia of the Vulgate." *Journal of Theological Studies* 49 (1948): 35–42.

Swan, Claudia. "Making Sense of Medical Collections in Early Modern Holland: The Uses of Wonder." In *Making Knowledge in Early Modern Europe*, edited by Pamela Smith and Benjamin Schmidt, 199–213. Chicago: University of Chicago Press, 2007.

Sznol, Shifra. "Medieval and Jewish Greek Lexicography: The Arukh of Nathan Ben Jehiel." *Erytheia* 30 (2009): 107–28.

Ta-Shema, Israel. "The Italian Setting of Sefer HeArukh by Rabbi Nathan bar Yehiel of Rome." In Ta-Shema, *Studies in Medieval Rabbinic Literature,* vol. 3*: Italy and Byzantium*, 3–8. Jerusalem: Bialik, 2005.

"Sefer 'Ta'Alumot Ḥokhma' of Rabbi Elihu Galeno." In Ta-Shema, *Studies in Medieval Rabbinic Literature,* vol. 3*: Italy and Byzantium*, 331–35. Jerusalem: Bialik, 2005.

Toaff, Ariel. *Gli ebrei a Perugia*. Perugia: Deputazione di storia patria per l'Umbria, 1975.

The Jews in Umbria. Leiden: Brill, 1993.

Love, Work, and Death: Jewish Life in Medieval Umbria. London: Littman Library of Jewish Civilization, 1996.

Mostri giudei: l'immaginario ebraico dal medioevo alla prima età moderna. Bologna: Il Mulino, 1996.

Toellner, Richard. "Zum Begriff der Autorität in der Medizin der Renaissance." In *Humanismus und Medizin*, edited by Rudolf Schmitz and Gundolf Keil, 159–79. Weinheim: Acta Humaniora, 1984.

Touati, Charles. *La pensée philosophique et théologique de Gersonide*. Paris: Éditions de minuit, 1973.

Trevor-Roper, H. *The Plunder of the Arts in the Seventeenth Century*. London: Thames & Hudson, 1970.

Trinkaus, Charles. *In Our Image and Likeness: Humanity and Divinity in Italian Humanist Thought*. Chicago: University of Chicago Press, 1970.

Turner, John Douglas. *Sethian Gnosticism and the Platonic Tradition*. Louvain: Éditions Peeters, 2001.

Tuzi, Stefania. *Le colonne e il tempio di Salomone: la storia, la leggenda, la fortuna*. Rome: Gangemi, 2002.

Twersky, Isidore. *Rabbi Moses Naḥmanides: Explorations in His Religious and Literary Virtuosity*. Cambridge, MA: Harvard University Press, 1983.

Vajda, G. *La theologie ascétique de Bahya ibn Pakuda*. Paris: Imprimerie Nationale, 1947.

van der Eijk, Philip J. *Diocles of Carystus: A Collection of the Fragments with Translation and Commentary*. Boston: Brill, 2000.

Van Liere, Katherine Elliot. "Humanism and Scholasticism in the Sixteenth-Century Academy." *Renaissance Quarterly* 53:1 (2000): 57–84.

Vanzan Marchini, N. E. "Medici ebrei e assistenza cristiana nella Venezia del '500." *La Rassegna Mensile di Israel* 45:4–5 (1979): 132–61.

Veltri, Giuseppe. "Il lector prudens e la biblioteca della sapienza antica: Pietro Colonna Galatino, Amato Lusitano e Azaria de' Rossi." In *Hebraica hereditas: studi in onore di Cesare Colafemmina*, edited by Giancarlo Lacerenza, 369–86. Naples: L'Orientale, 2005.

"Jüdische Einstellung zu den Wissenschaften im 16. Und 17. Jahrhundert: das Prinzip der praktisch-empirischen Anwendbarkeit." In *Judentum zwischen Tradition und Moderne*, edited by Gerd Biegel and Michael Graetz, 149–59. Heidelberg: Universitätsverlag C. Winter, 2002.

Viallon-Schoneveld, Marie. *Le boire et le manger au XVIe siècle: actes du XIe colloque du Puy-En-Velay*. Saint-Etienne: Publications de l'Université de Saint-Étienne, 2004.

Visiani de, Roberto. *L'orto botanico di Padova*. Padua, 1842.

Vosté, J.-M. "La Volgata al Concilio di Trento." *Biblica* 27:4 (1946): 301–19.

Wallace, William A. "Traditional Natural Philosophy." In *The Cambridge History of Renaissance Philosophy*, edited by Charles B. Schmitt and Quentin Skinner, 201–35. Cambridge: Cambridge University Press, 1988.

Weil, Gérard. *Élie Lévita: humaniste et massorète (1469–1549)*. Leiden: Brill, 1963.

Weinberg, Joanna. "Azariah de' Rossi and Septuagint Traditions." *Italia* (1985): 7–35.

"The Beautiful Soul: Azariah de' Rossi's Quest for Truth." In *Cultural Intermediaries: Jewish Intellectuals in Early Modern Italy*, edited by David Ruderman and Giuseppe Veltri, 109–26. Philadelphia: University of Pennsylvania Press, 2004.

"The Quest for Historical Philo in Sixteenth-Century Jewish Historiography." In *Jewish History: Essays in Honour of Chimen Abramsky*, edited by A. R. Rapoport-Albert and S. Zipperstein, 163–87. London: P. Halban, 1988.

"A Sixteenth-Century Hebraic Approach to the New Testament." In *History of Scholarship*, edited by C. R. Ligot and J.-L. Quantin, 231–49. Oxford: Oxford University Press, 2006.

Weisz, Max. *Katalog der hebräischen Handschriften und Bücher in der Bibliothek des Professors Dr. David Kaufmann*. Frankfurt: Kauffmann, 1906.

Williams, Arnold. *The Common Expositor: An Account of the Commentaries on Genesis, 1527–1633*. Chapel Hill: University of North Carolina Press, 1948.

Wilson, N. G. *From Byzantium to Italy: Greek Studies in the Italian Renaissance.* Baltimore: Johns Hopkins University Press, 1992.

Würthwein, Ernst. *The Text of the Old Testament.* Translated by Erroll F. Rhodes. London: SCM Press, 1980.

Yaari, Abraham. "The Burning of the Talmud in Italy." In Yaari, *Meḥkarei sefer: perakim be-toldot ha-sefer ha-'ivri*, 198–234. Jerusalem: Mosad Ha-Rav Kuk, 1958.

Yerushalmi, Yosef. *From Spanish Court to Italian Ghetto: Isaac Cordoso. A Study in Seventeenth-Century Marranism and Jewish Apologetics.* New York: Columbia University Press, 1971.

Zanca, Attilio. *Notizie sulla vita e sulle opere di Marcello Donati da Mantova (1538–1602) medico, umanista, uomo di stato.* Pisa: Giardini, 1964.

Zinguer, Ilana. *L'Hébreu au temps de la Renaissance.* Leiden: Brill, 1992.

Zoller, I. "I medici ebrei laureati a Siena negli anni 1543–1694." *Rivista Israelitica* 10 (1913): 60–70, 100–10.

Index